Digestive Wellness

4ᵀᴴ EDITION

Strengthen the Immune System and
Prevent Disease Through Healthy Digestion

Elizabeth Lipski, Ph.D., CCN, CHN

Mc
Graw
Hill

New York Chicago San Francisco Lisbon London Madrid Mexico City
Milan New Delhi San Juan Seoul Singapore Sydney Toronto

7 8 9 10 11 12 13 14 15   QFR/QFR   1 9 8 7 6

ISBN   978-0-07-166899-6
MHID   0-07-166899-3

e-ISBN   978-0-07-170161-7
e-MHID   0-07-170161-3

Library of Congress Cataloging-in-Publication Data
Lipski, Elizabeth.
    Digestive wellness : strengthen the immune system and prevent disease through healthy digestion, 4th ed. / by Elizabeth Lipski.
        p. cm.
Includes index.
ISBN 978-0-07-166899-6   MHID 0-07-166899-3
    1. Indigestion—Popular works.   2. Digestion—Popular works.
RC827 .L57   2011
616.3'32

                                                           2011032638

Interior design by Sue Hartman

McGraw-Hill books are available at special quantity discounts to use as premiums and sales promotions or for use in corporate training programs. To contact a representative, please e-mail us at bulksales@mcgraw-hill.com.

This book is printed on acid-free paper.

This book is dedicated to Chris Dennen,
husband, friend, coworker, and playmate. Your unwavering love and support
allow me to spread my creative wings and fly. You are the banks of my river.

CONTENTS

Why Is Your Gut Making You Sick?

Doctors are trained to identify diseases by where they are located. If you have asthma, it's considered a lung problem; if you have rheumatoid arthritis, it must be a joint problem; if you have acne, doctors see it as a skin problem; if you are overweight, you must have a metabolism problem; if you have allergies, immune imbalance is blamed. Doctors who understand health this way are both right and wrong. Sometimes the causes of your symptoms do have some relationship to their location, but that's far from the whole story.

As we come to understand disease in the 21st century, our old ways of defining illness based on symptoms and location in the body are not very useful. Instead, by understanding the origins of disease and the way in which the body operates as one whole, integrated ecosystem we now know that symptoms appearing in one area of the body may be caused by imbalances in an entirely different system. Everything is connected. The center of that connection is the gut. Nowhere are those connections made clearer, and nowhere will you find a better owner's manual for your gut and how to keep it healthy, than in Dr. Lipski's updated edition of *Digestive Wellness*, which I have used successfully in my practice for more than a decade.

If your skin is bad or you have allergies, can't seem to lose weight, suffer from an autoimmune disease, struggle with fibromyalgia, or have recurring headaches, the real reason may be that your *gut is unhealthy*. This may be true even if you have *never* had any digestive complaints.

There are many other possible imbalances in your body's operating system that may drive illness as well. These include problems with hormones, immune function, detoxification, energy production, and more. But very often the gut may be at the root of your chronic symptoms.

SYMPTOMS THROUGHOUT THE BODY ARE RESOLVED BY TREATING THE GUT

Many today *do* have digestive problems, including reflux or heartburn, irritable bowel syndrome, bloating, constipation, diarrhea, and colitis. In fact, belly problems account for more than 100 million doctor's visits and billions in health-care costs annually. But gut problems cause disease far beyond the gut. In medical school I learned that patients with colitis could also have inflamed joints and eyes and that patients with liver failure could be cured of delirium by taking antibiotics that killed the toxin-producing bacteria in their gut. Could it be that when things are not quite right down below it affects the health of our entire body, including many diseases we haven't linked before to imbalances in the digestive system?

The answer is a resounding yes. Normalizing gut function is one of the most important things I do for patients, and it's so simple. The "side effects" of treating the gut are quite extraordinary. My patients find relief from allergies, acne, arthritis, headaches, autoimmune disease, depression, attention deficit, and more—often after years or decades of suffering. Here are a few examples of the results I have achieved by addressing imbalances in the function and flora of the gut:

- A 58-year-old woman with many years of worsening allergies, asthma, and sinusitis who was on frequent antibiotics and didn't respond to any of the usual therapies was cured by eliminating a worm she harbored in her gut called Strongyloides.
- A 52-year-old woman who had suffered with daily headaches and frequent migraines for years found relief by clearing out the overgrowth of bad bugs in her small intestine with a new nonabsorbed antibiotic called Xifaxan.
- A six-year-old girl with severe behavioral problems including violence, disruptive behavior in school, and depression was treated for bacterial yeast overgrowth, and in less than 10 days her behavioral issues and depression were resolved.
- A three-year-old boy with autism started talking after treating a parasite called giardia in his gut.

These are not miracle cures but common results that occur when you normalize gut function and flora through improved diet, increased fiber intake, daily probiotic supplementation, enzyme therapy, the use of nutrients that repair the gut lining, and the direct treatment of bad bugs in the gut with herbs or medication.

A number of recent studies have made all these seemingly strange reversals in symptoms understandable.

RESEARCH LINKING GUT FLORA AND INFLAMMATION TO CHRONIC ILLNESS

Scientists compared gut flora or bacteria from children in Florence, Italy, who ate a diet high in meat, fat, and sugar to children from a West African village in Burkina Faso who ate beans, whole grains, vegetables, and nuts. The bugs in the guts of the African children were healthier, more diverse, better at regulating inflammation and infection, and better at extracting energy from fiber. The bugs in the guts of the Italian children produced by-products that create inflammation; promote allergy, asthma, and autoimmunity; and lead to obesity.

Why is this important?

In the West our increased use of vaccinations and antibiotics, along with enhancements in hygiene, have led to health improvements for many. Yet these same factors have dramatically changed the ecosystem of bugs in our gut, and this has a broad impact on health that is still largely unrecognized. Our diet has changed significantly in the past 10,000 years, and even more in the past 100 years with the industrialization of our food supply. This highly processed, high-sugar, high-fat, low-fiber diet has dramatically altered the bacteria that historically grew in our digestive tracts, and the change has not been good. Many other modern inventions including antibiotics (both those prescribed to us and those in our food supply), acid blockers, anti-inflammatory medication, aspirin, steroids, and chronic stress all injure the gut, alter our gut flora, and lead to systemic inflammation and chronic disease. Is your gut contributing to your chronic disease or symptoms? It is very likely it is.

Think of your gut as one big ecosystem. It contains 500 to 1,000 species of bacteria that amount to three pounds of your total weight. There are more than 100 trillion microbial cells. There is 100 times more bacterial DNA than human DNA in your body. A whole new field of research has emerged on the human "microbiome" and how it interacts to create health or disease and even weight gain or weight loss. These bugs control digestion, metabolism, inflammation, and your risk of cancer. These bugs produce vitamins, beneficial nutrients, and molecules that sustain your body and your ecosystem through a symbiotic relationship with you. The gut microbiome, probiotics, and prebiotics are well covered here in *Digestive Wellness*.

When the balance of bacteria in your gut is optimal, this DNA works for you to great effect. For example, some good bacteria produce short-chain fatty acids. These healthy fats reduce inflammation and modulate your immune system. Bad bugs, on the other hand, produce fats that promote allergy and asthma, eczema, and inflammation throughout your body.

Another recent study found that the bacterial fingerprint of gut flora of autistic children differs dramatically from healthy children. Simply by looking at the by-products of their intestinal bacteria (which are excreted in the urine—a test I do regularly in my practice called organic acids testing), researchers could distinguish between autistic and normal children.

Think about this: Problems with gut flora are linked to autism. Can bacteria in the gut actually affect the brain? They can. Toxins, metabolic by-products, and inflammatory molecules produced by these unfriendly bacteria can all adversely impact the brain. I explore the links between gut function and brain function in much greater detail in my book, *The UltraMind Solution*, and you'll also find much about that here and in *Digestive Wellness for Children*.

Autoimmune diseases are also linked to changes in gut flora. A recent study showed that children who use antibiotics for acne may alter normal flora, and this, in turn, can trigger changes that lead to autoimmune disease such as inflammatory bowel disease or colitis.

The connections between gut flora and system-wide health don't stop there. A recent study in the *New England Journal of Medicine* found that you could cure or prevent delirium and brain fog in patients with liver failure by giving them an anti-biotic. Toxins from bacteria were scrambling their brains. Remove the bacteria that produce the toxins, and their symptoms clear up practically overnight.

Other similar studies have found that clearing out overgrowth of bad bugs with a nonabsorbed antibiotic can be an effective treatment for restless leg syndrome and fibromyalgia.

Even obesity has been linked to changes in our gut ecosystem that are the result of a high-fat, processed, inflammatory diet. This has been termed "microobesity." Bad bugs produce toxins called lipopolysaccharides (LPS) that trigger inflammation and insulin resistance or prediabetes and thus promote weight gain. You'll find a chapter in *Digestive Wellness* that discusses the role of obesity, insulin resistance, and diabetes in more detail.

It seems remarkable, but the little critters living inside of you have been linked to everything from autism to obesity, from allergies to autoimmunity, from fibro-myalgia to restless leg syndrome, from delirium to eczema to asthma. In fact, more links between chronic illness and gut bacteria are discovered every day.

These bacteria thrive on what you feed them. If you feed them whole, fresh, real foods, good bugs will grow. If you feed them junk, bad bugs will grow. And when the population of bugs changes, the bad bugs begin to produce nasty toxins. Instead of *symbiosis*—a mutually beneficial relationship between you and your bugs—you create *dysbiosis*—a harmful interaction between bugs and host.

The ecosystem in your gut must be healthy for you to be healthy. When unfriendly bacteria grow in there, the friendly bacteria are pushed out and a toxic environment develops. This toxic environment affects your body and your metabolism in surprising ways.

If you have a chronic illness, even if you don't have digestive symptoms, you might want to consider what is living inside your gut. *Digestive Wellness* is the user's manual for the most important organ in the body, which connects to every other system in the body. A healthy gut is the center of a healthy life. Tending to the garden within can be the answer to many seemingly unrelated health problems.

Mark Hyman, M.D.

References

Bass, N. M., Bass, K. D., Mullen, K. D., Sanyal, A., et al. (2010). "Rifaximin treatment in hepatic encephalopathy." *New England Journal of Medicine*, 362(12): 1071–81.

Cani, P. D., Amar, J., Iglesias, M. A., et al. (2007). "Metabolic endotoxemia initiates obesity and insulin resistance." *Diabetes*, 56(7): 1761–72.

De Filippo, C., De Filippo, D., Cavalieri, D., Di Paola, M., et al. (2010). "Impact of diet in shaping gut microbiota revealed by a comparative study in children from Europe and rural Africa." *Proceedings from the National Academy of Science USA*, 107 (33): 14691–96.

Margolis, D. J., Margolis, M., Fanelli, M., Hoffstad, O., and Lewis, J. D. (2010). "Potential association between the oral tetracycline class of antimicrobials used to treat acne and inflammatory bowel disease." *American Journal of Gastroenterology*, 105(12): 2610–16. Epub 2010 Aug 10.

Pimentel, M., Pimentel, D., Wallace, D., Hallegua, D., et al. (2004). "A link between irritable bowel syndrome and fibromyalgia may be related to findings on lactulose breath testing." *Annals of Rheumatic Disease*, 63(4): 450–52.

Sandin, A., Bråbäck, L., Norin, E., and Björkstén, B. (2009). "Faecal short chain fatty acid pattern and allergy in early childhood." *Acta Paediatrica*, 98(59): 823–27.

Weinstock, L. B., Fern, S. E., and Duntley, S. P. (2008). "Restless legs syndrome in patients with irritable bowel syndrome: Response to small intestinal bacterial overgrowth therapy." *Digestive Diseases and Science*, 53(5): 1252–56.

Yap, I. K., Yap, M., Angley, M., Veselkov, K. A., et al. (2010). "Urinary metabolic phenotyping differentiates children with autism from their unaffected siblings and age-matched controls." *Journal of Proteome Research*, 9(6): 2996–3004.

ACKNOWLEDGMENTS

Digestive Wellness takes a functional medicine approach to digestive and systemic health issues. It's foundation rests on the ideas of many people whose minds have helped inform my own—people like Jeffrey Bland, Ph.D., Sidney Baker, M.D., Leo Galland, M.D., Russel Jaffe, M.D., Ph.D., Daniel Hardt, N.D., Sally Fallon, M.S., Patrick Hanaway, M.D., Gerard Mullin, M.D., Paula Bartholomy, D.Sc., the faculty at the Institute for Functional Medicine, plus hundreds of colleagues and thousands of clients who have taught me so much.

I also would like to thank Mary Therese Church, Peter McCurdy, Nancy Hall, and the editors at McGraw-Hill for their careful handling of the manuscript and thoughtful edits.

I'd also like to thank my mom, Sylvia Lipski, who has been a consistent role model of strength, courage, and generosity, working for what she believes in, teaching me about the importance of family and relationships, and supporting her children's freedom even when she didn't really "get" what we were doing.

INTRODUCTION

Welcome to the fourth edition of *Digestive Wellness.* The original idea for this book grew from the emergence of an idea: what if imbalances in the digestive system caused not only digestive symptoms, complaints, and disease but also symptoms, imbalances, and disease throughout the body? And what if by balancing our digestion we could have more energy, think more clearly, experience less pain, and have a better quality of life?

It's estimated that scientific knowledge doubles every two to three years. That means, conservatively, that there is 32 times as much known now as when *Digestive Wellness* was first published in 1995. What we once thought of as a simple system becomes more complex with each advance of knowledge. In *Digestive Wellness* we'll explore each of these topics more fully.

Research on probiotics, genetics, metabolism, neurotransmitters, the immune system, hormones, and the impact our environment has on health has mushroomed. Whole new fields such as genomics, proteomics, and the study of the microbiome have been founded. Yet the basic principles of great health—whole natural food, rest, satisfying work, communicative relationships, and movement—haven't changed.

This book takes the science and melds it with the practical. I've spent the past 30 years working with clients, talking with colleagues and experts, and delving into the research to see how to interpret the research into something more basic: *How can we help people to actually feel better?*

WHAT'S NEW IN THIS EDITION

My understanding of how to assess digestive imbalances and disease has grown and continues to change nearly every day. One of the places where I have learned the most is by being on a team at the Institute for Functional Medicine. A group of us discussed what was known, what was believed, what seemed to work, and what we saw in our practices. From this consensus, Patrick Hanaway, M.D., Gerard E. Mullin, M.D., Tom Sult, M.D., Dan Lukaczer, ND, and I developed a 2½ day course that we have taught to more than 600 clinicians. For me, the main shift was in how we assess digestive imbalances and diseases. We call this the DIGIN model.

The DIGIN model allows us to look at the underlying mechanisms to assess and finally to come up with a plan for restoring health. These areas are:

- D: Digestion and absorption
- I: Intestinal permeabilty
- G: Gut microbiome
- I: Inflammation and immune
- N: Nervous system

A DIAGNOSIS IS NOT A CURE—IT'S A STARTING POINT

Two people can have the same diagnosis but different treatment. Two can have different diagnoses and have the same treatment. People with the same diagnosis may have different reasons for it. In the past several weeks, I've worked with four people who had been diagnosed with irritable bowel syndrome. We discovered that each of them had a different issue yet the same diagnosis. The first person had a low-grade infection, called small intestinal bacterial overgrowth. The second had food sensitivities to dairy and gluten-containing grains. The third had a parasitic infection. And the fourth realized that rest, stress management, and exercise were the key to her bowel issues.

On the other hand, it's also possible for people with different diagnoses to have the same underlying issues. As you'll read later on, people with irritable bowel syndrome, fibromyalgia, restless leg syndrome, and interstitial cystitis may all have small intestinal bacterial overgrowth as the underlying cause. When treated with antibiotic or antimicrobial herbs, they improve.

Now, let's discover more about the fascinating digestive system.

This edition of *Digestive Wellness* is built around this model. Most of the materials in these chapters are entirely new. The DIGIN model provides the big picture. Later, if more still needs to be done, we focus on details that are specific to each body part and type of imbalance or condition.

A lot of new topics are addressed in this book. There are chapters on the elimination diet and on restorative foods. For the first time, we discuss biofilms and biofilm protocols. As the research unfolds, so expand the chapters. There are now sections on fatty liver, gastroparesis, pancreatitis, and microscopic colitis. You'll also find chapters on the GI link to autoimmune diseases, interstitial cystitis, rosacea, cardiovascular disease, osteoporosis, obesity and metabolic syndrome, Sjögren's disease, and diabetes.

Plus, every page has been updated based on the latest research studies.

TWENTY-FIRST-CENTURY MEDICINE: FUNCTIONAL MEDICINE

In *Digestive Wellness*, you'll find a functional medicine approach seen through the lens of a nutrition professional. What is functional medicine (FM)? The original idea was developed by Jeffrey Bland, Ph.D., and David Jones, M.D., and continues to be refined and expanded by the thousands of health professionals who use it every day. FM, as evolved through the Institute for Functional Medicine in Gig Harbor, Washington, incorporates all of what is considered to be the best medical practices while also embracing a wide philosophy of health and healing. It offers clinicians a system for quickly assessing and evaluating underlying antecedents and triggers of disease. Functional medicine cuts across all disciplines and includes all types of clinicians—medical doctors, naturopathic physicians, chiropractic physicians, acupuncturists, nutritionists, nurses, physical therapists, psychologists, massage therapists, and more. It blends the best of science with the art and care of the person to find a personalized, patient-centered approach toward well-being.

In functional medicine, finding the underlying triggers of illness and listening to the person's story are key. For example, I recently had a client whose main complaints were stomach pain, diarrhea, fatigue, and a feeling that she was failing. She'd been to many doctors without respite. She'd tried many approaches. After a single conversation, it became apparent to me that she had detoxification issues. Her health issues all began about a year after she moved into a brand-new home that was off-gassing toxic chemicals. Treating her digestive systems would have been the norm, yet finding a way to gently detoxify her achieved the best results. On the other hand, I recently worked with a client whose main complaints were depression and fatigue. Although she didn't at first express issues with digestion, supporting her digestive system and an elimination diet were key to her improved health.

Functional medicine embraces person-centered therapies rather than setting protocols. It recognizes and honors the biochemical uniqueness of each person. Throughout this book, use your own story and initial triggers of disease to guide you. Recognize that one size does not fit all, and try what makes sense. Begin with the recommendations on diet and lifestyle. If you aren't eating well, sleeping, moving, or spending time to relax and renew, begin with small changes in lifestyle.

Here's what you'll find in the new *Digestive Wellness*:

Digestive Wellness is divided into four parts. In Part I, we walk through the digestive system. This grounds you in a basic understanding of the system, which makes the rest of the book easier to "digest."

Part II delves into what I consider to be the heart of the book, the DIGIN model. The DIGIN essentials work for many health conditions, and once these are balanced and corrected, health emerges. The features of DIGIN are as follows:

- **Digestion (Chapter 3):** We move through fundamentals, such as how you can know whether you are digesting and absorbing your food. If you aren't, how can you balance that?
- **Intestinal Permeability (Chapter 4):** Increased intestinal permeability, also called leaky gut, is explained along with what issues and symptoms it's related to and how to heal from it.
- **Gut Microbiome (Chapters 5–8):** Next, we move into the gut microbiome and look at healthy gut ecology, biofilms, prebiotics, and probiotics.
- **Immune/Inflammation (Chapter 9):** We then move into the role of the immune system and inflammation in the gut, specifically how to recognize it and heal it.
- **Enteric Nervous System (Chapter 10):** The gut has more nerve endings than the spine and more neurotransmitters than the brain. Here we look at the role of neurotransmitters, stress, and their role in digestive health.

Finally in this section, functional laboratory testing and self-tests are also discussed. If you read only one section, read Part II.

In Part III, you will find the specifics about bringing your body back into balance: food, the elimination diet, restorative foods, everything you'd like to know about food sensitivities, managing stress, acid-alkaline balance, and detoxification and cleansing programs.

Part IV offers specific healing methods for a wide number of digestive health conditions. We begin with the mouth and traverse the entire digestive tract, discussing each organ in turn. Here you'll get specific ideas about what to do about heartburn, irritable bowel syndrome, bad breath, and so much more. And finally in Part V, we explore systemic illnesses that have digestive components. Specific research is discussed along with specific healing modalities and functional lab tests.

Throughout the book are exercises and questionnaires designed to increase your self-awareness of mind and body; this awareness will help you shop more wisely, breathe more deeply, relax more fully, and live more freely. Even though we may not be aware of it, we all practice medical self-care. When we get a headache, we take an aspirin, lie down, or go for a walk. If we have indigestion, we take an antacid, eat an umeboshi plum, or drink ginger tea. We know when we're too sick to go to work. Most of the time, we make our own assessment and treatment plan, expecting that the problem will pass with time. When these plans fail, we seek professional help. This book will expose you to more plans, new ideas, and the tools to be your own health expert. Just as one tool won't work for every job, not all of these tools will work for you. But some will, and even the failures may give you useful information.

Digestive Wellness is about taking control of your lifestyle to increase your chances of getting healthier and more vibrant each year. It's informative and practical, and it puts you in the driver's seat. Since the first edition, many thousands of people have been helped from its pages. I hope that you and your loved ones will be among them.

DIGESTIVE AND LIFESTYLE QUESTIONNAIRE

Date: _____

PART 1

This questionnaire will help you assess your lifestyle and digestive status. It is not meant as a replacement for a physician's care. The answers will help you focus your attention on specific areas of need.

MEDICATIONS CURRENTLY USED

Circle any of the following medications you are taking. Add to this list any other medications that you take.

Antacids	Aspirin	Prednisone
Antibiotic	Cortisone	Stool softeners
Antifungals	Laxatives	Tylenol
Anti-inflammatories	Oral contraceptives	Ulcer medications
Other _____		

FOOD, NUTRITION, AND LIFESTYLE

Circle if you eat, drink, or use:

Alcohol	Coffee	Margarine
Candy	Fast foods	Soft drinks
Chewing tobacco	Fried foods	Sweets or pastries
Cigarettes	Luncheon meats	

Circle if you:

Diet often

Do not exercise regularly

Are under excessive stress

Are exposed to chemicals at work

Are exposed to cigarette smoke

How often do you cook meals from scratch? _____

How often do you eat meals at home? _____

How often do you eat meals out? _____

INTERPRETATION OF QUESTIONNAIRE PART 1

■ Medications

- ■ Medications are good indicators that your body is in some sort of imbalance.
- ■ Medications have drug/nutrient interactions. Some nutrient needs may be increased, some decreased; some nutrients may block absorption or usefulness of the drug. You may want to read a book, ask your pharmacist, or look online for drug-nutrient interactions to see if there are specific nutrients or herbs that you *should* or *should not* be taking with your medications.

■ Foods, Drinks, Tobacco

- ■ Candy, alcohol, sweets, and soft drinks: These "empty-calorie foods" contain few nutrients; however, nutrients are needed to metabolize them, and they replace healthy foods in our diets. These foods have a detrimental effect on most digestive problems; for instance, simple sugars feed yeasts, bacteria, and parasites.
- ■ Cigarettes and chewing tobacco: Make sure to take a good antioxidant supplement and lots of vitamin C to compensate for the stress the tobacco causes. Tobacco has a negative effect on the digestive system, it ages you, and it increases your risk of lung cancer.

- Luncheon meats, pastries, fast foods, and margarine: If you eat these foods you are probably getting too much of the wrong kinds of fat: restructured, nutrient-depleted fats. Margarine and most pastries also contain hydrogenated oils, which are absorbed into our cells but are detrimental to our health. They make the cell membranes stiff and stifle the intake of nutrients and outgo of wastes, promote free radical activity, and contribute to atherosclerosis and inflammatory diseases.

- The oils used in deep-frying are used over and over. This creates a breakdown of the oil and increases inflammation throughout your body. Eating fried foods on occasion won't hurt you, but as a part of your general diet, it's not recommended.

- Coffee, tea, energy drinks, and soft drinks that contain caffeine are a mixed bag. On one hand, coffee and tea provide polyphenols and antioxidant nutrients. If you like drinking coffee or tea, that's fine. If you need to drink coffee or tea to maintain your energy throughout the day, that's an issue. Try snacking on healthful foods every few hours to see if that works as effectively. Take naps if you are tired, rather than pushing on.

- As far as energy drinks and soft drinks, my opinion is that these are chemical soups, food-like substances that have no place in our diet. Live on the energy that you have. Paying attention to what your body needs rather than what your mind wants is one of the keys to enduring health.

■ Lifestyle

- Diet often: Weight problems can be caused by a hypoactive thyroid, food sensitivities, poor food choices, sedentary lifestyle, imbalance in the gut microbiome, and emotional and social overeating. Chronic dieting leads to further metabolic slowdown. A wellness-centered approach works best for the overweight person.

- Lack of routine exercise: Exercise is the great stress reducer and enhances the health of our whole body, including our digestive system. Regular exercise at least three times a week for 20 to 30 minutes can significantly reduce the risk of cardiovascular disease, help your bowels to move more regularly, and increase your total sense of well-being.

- High stress level: This indicates the need for a good exercise program, ways of nurturing oneself, and training to increase emotional heartiness. Food choices usually suffer during stressful periods, while nutrient needs are increased. Supplementation may be indicated.

- Exposure to chemicals: Prolonged exposure to chemicals can cause environmental illness, which can manifest as obvious illness or as nondiagnosable complaints of confusion, chronic fatigue, headaches, or just not feeling right. Metabolic clearing and low-temperature saunas are important.
- Exposure to cigarette smoke: Research indicates that secondhand smoke is detrimental to a healthy respiratory system. If you cannot get away from smokers, buy them "smokeless" ashtrays, open windows whenever possible, and take antioxidant supplements.
- Cooking meals from scratch: Cooking is self-love. Home-cooked meals are generally less expensive, and depending on what you cook, they can be more nutrient dense. A simple meal can be made from scratch in 20–30 minutes.
- Eating meals out: If you eat out for most of your meals, make healthful selections. Choose restaurants that serve salads, vegetables, and high-quality food whenever possible.

PART 2

This part of the questionnaire will help you discover where your digestive system is having problems. It is a screening tool and does not constitute an exact diagnosis of your problem. However, it can point you in the right direction in determining where the highest priorities lie in your healing process.

Circle the number that best describes the intensity of your symptoms. If you do not know the answer to a question, leave it blank. Add the totals for each section to assess which areas need your attention.

    0 = Symptom is not present/rarely present
    1 = Mild/sometimes
    2 = Moderate/often
    3 = Severe/almost always

SECTION A: HYPOACIDITY OF THE STOMACH

1. Burping	0	1	2	3
2. Fullness for extended time after meals	0	1	2	3
3. Bloating	0	1	2	3
4. Poor appetite	0	1	2	3
5. Stomach upsets easily	0	1	2	3
6. History of constipation	0	1	2	3
7. Known food allergies	0	1	2	3
8. Iron-deficiency anemia	0	1	2	3
9. Nausea after taking supplements	0	1	2	3

Total: _____

    Score 0–4: Low priority

    Score 5–9: Moderate priority

    Score 10 or above: High priority

SECTION B: HYPOFUNCTION OF SMALL INTESTINES AND/OR PANCREAS

1. Abdominal cramps	0	1	2	3
2. Indigestion one to three hours after eating	0	1	2	3
3. Fatigue after eating	0	1	2	3
4. Lower bowel gas	0	1	2	3
5. Alternating constipation and diarrhea	0	1	2	3
6. Diarrhea	0	1	2	3
7. Roughage and fiber cause constipation	0	1	2	3
8. Mucus in stools	0	1	2	3
9. Stool poorly formed	0	1	2	3
10. Shiny stool	0	1	2	3
11. Three or more large bowel movements daily	0	1	2	3
12. Dry, flaky skin and/or dry, brittle hair	0	1	2	3
13. Pain in left side under rib cage or chronic stomach pain	0	1	2	3
14. Acne	0	1	2	3
15. Food allergies	0	1	2	3
16. Difficulty gaining weight	0	1	2	3
17. Foul-smelling stool	0	1	2	3
18. Gallstones/history of gallbladder disease	0	1	2	3
19. Undigested food in stool	0	1	2	3
20. Nausea	0	1	2	3
21. Acid reflux/heartburn	0	1	2	3
22. Connective tissue disease: lupus, rheumatoid arthritis, Sjögren's	0	1	2	3
23. Alcoholism, diabetes, osteoporosis	0	1	2	3

Total: _____

    Score 0–6: Low priority

    Score 6–10: Moderate priority

    Score 10 or above: High priority

SECTION C: GASTRIC REFLUX

1. Sour taste in mouth 0   1   2   3
2. Regurgitate undigested food into mouth 0   1   2   3
3. Frequent nocturnal coughing 0   1   2   3
4. Burning sensation from citrus on way to stomach 0   1   2   3
5. Heartburn 0   1   2   3
6. Burping 0   1   2   3
7. Difficulty swallowing solids or liquids 0   1   2   3

Total: _____

    Score 0–3: Low priority

    Score 4–6: Moderate priority

    Score 7 or above: High priority

SECTION D: ULCERS OR TOO MUCH STOMACH ACID IN THE WRONG PLACE

1. Stomach pains 0   1   2   3
2. Stomach pains before or after meals 0   1   2   3
3. Dependency on antacids for heartburn/acid reflux 0   1   2   3
4. Chronic abdominal pain 0   1   2   3
5. Butterfly sensations in stomach 0   1   2   3
6. Burping or bloating 0   1   2   3
7. Stomach pain when emotionally upset 0   1   2   3
8. Sudden, acute indigestion 0   1   2   3
9. Relief of symptoms by carbonated drinks 0   1   2   3
10. Relief of stomach pain by drinking cream or milk 0   1   2   3
11. History or family history of ulcer or gastritis 0   1   2   3
12. Current ulcer 0   1   2   3
13. Black stool when not taking iron supplements 0   1   2   3
14. Use or previous use of pain medications: aspirin, ibuprofen, etc. ... 0   1   2   3

Total: _____

    Score 0–4: Low priority

    Score 5–8: Moderate Priority

    Score 9 or above: High priority

SECTION E: LIVER AND GALLBLADDER

1. Intolerance to greasy foods 0   1   2   3
2. Headaches after eating 0   1   2   3
3. Light-colored stool 0   1   2   3
4. Foul-smelling stool 0   1   2   3
5. Less than one bowel movement daily 0   1   2   3
6. Constipation 0   1   2   3
7. Hard stool 0   1   2   3
8. Sour taste in mouth 0   1   2   3
9. Gray-colored skin 0   1   2   3
10. Yellow in whites of eyes 0   1   2   3
11. Bad breath 0   1   2   3
12. Body odor 0   1   2   3
13. Fatigue and sleepiness after eating 0   1   2   3
14. Pain in right side under rib cage 0   1   2   3
15. Pain when passing stool 0   1   2   3
16. Water retention 0   1   2   3
17. Painful big toe 0   1   2   3
18. Pain radiates along outside of leg 0   1   2   3
19. Dry skin or hair 0   1   2   3
20. Red blood in stool
    No = 0   More than two years ago = 1   Current = 2   Chronic − 3
21. Have had jaundice or hepatitis
    No = 0   More than two years ago = 1   Current = 2   Chronic = 3
22. High blood cholesterol and low HDL cholesterol   No = 0   Unknown   Yes = 2
23. Cholesterol level above 200   No = 0   Unknown   Yes = 2
24. Triglyceride level above 115   No = 0   Unknown   Yes = 2-3

Total: _____

Score 0–2: Low priority
Score 3–5: Moderate priority
Score 6 or above: High priority

SECTION F: SMALL INTESTINAL BACTERIAL OVERGROWTH

1. Excessive gas/flatulence 0   1   2   3
2. Abdominal bloating and distension, especially with sugar, fiber, or carbohydrates 0   1   2   3
3. Diarrhea 0   1   2   3
4. Abdominal pain 0   1   2   3
5. Irritable bowel syndrome 0   1   2   3
6. Fibromyalgia 0   1   2   3
7. Restless leg syndrome 0   1   2   3
8. Intolerance to probiotic supplements 0   1   2   3
9. Scored 9 or more on Section A 0   1   2   3
10. Are taking antacids or proton pump inhibitors for heartburn/GERD 0   1   2   3

Total: _____

     Score 0–4: Low priority

     Score 5–9: Moderate priority

     Score 10 or above: High priority

SECTION G: INTESTINAL PERMEABILITY/LEAKY GUT SYNDROME DYSBIOSIS

1. Constipation and/or diarrhea 0   1   2   3
2. Abdominal pain or bloating 0   1   2   3
3. Mucus or blood in stool 0   1   2   3
4. Joint pain or swelling, or arthritis 0   1   2   3
5. Chronic or frequent fatigue or tiredness 0   1   2   3
6. Food allergy or food sensitivities or intolerance 0   1   2   3
7. Sinus or nasal congestion 0   1   2   3
8. Chronic or frequent inflammations 0   1   2   3
9. Eczema, skin rashes, or hives (urticaria) 0   1   2   3
10. Asthma, hay fever, or airborne allergies 0   1   2   3
11. Confusion, poor memory, or mood swings 0   1   2   3
12. Use of nonsteroidal anti-inflammatory drugs (aspirin, Tylenol, Motrin) 0   1   2   3
13. History of antibiotic use 0   1   2   3
14. Alcohol consumption, or alcohol makes you feel sick 0   1   2   3

15. Ulcerative colitis, Crohn's disease, or celiac disease 0   1   2   3

16. Headaches or migraine headaches 0   1   2   3

17. Chronic nasal congestion 0   1   2   3

Total: _____

    Score 1–5: Low priority

    Score 6–10: Mild priority

    Score 7–19: Moderate priority

    Score 20 or above: High priority

SECTION H: GLUTEN SENSITIVITY

Digestive

  1. Bloating and/or gas 0   1   2   3

  2. Constipation and/or diarrhea 0   1   2   3

  3. Nausea 0   1   2   3

  4. Weight trouble 0   1   2   3

  5. Iron-deficiency anemia 0   1   2   3

Hormonal

  6. Fatigue 0   1   2   3

  7. Sleep problems 0   1   2   3

  8. Depression, anxiety, and/or mood swings 0   1   2   3

  9. Menstrual problems 0   1   2   3

10. Infertility 0   1   2   3

11. Thyroid problems 0   1   2   3

12. Osteoporosis or osteopenia 0   1   2   3

Neurological

13. Headaches and/or migraines 0   1   2   3

14. Memory problems 0   1   2   3

15. Joint pains or aches 0   1   2   3

16. Fibromyalgia 0   1   2   3

17. Brain fog 0   1   2   3

Immune System

18. Get infections easily 0   1   2   3
19. History or family history of arthritis, any type 0   1   2   3
20. History or family history of cancer 0   1   2   3
21. History or family history of autoimmune disease 0   1   2   3
22. History or family history of celiac disease 0   1   2   3

Total: _____

    Score 0–6: Low priority

    Score 6–10: Moderate priority

    Score 10 or above: High priority

The section on gluten intolerance was adapted with permission from: Drs. Vikki and Richard Petersen, DC, CCN, *The Gluten Effect,* True Health Publishing, 2009; http://www.healthnowmedical.com. Sunnyvale, CA.

SECTION I: COLON/LARGE INTESTINE

1. Seasonal or recurring diarrhea 0   1   2   3
2. Frequent and recurrent infections (colds) 0   1   2   3
3. Bladder and kidney infections 0   1   2   3
4. Vaginal yeast infection 0   1   2   3
5. Abdominal cramps 0   1   2   3
6. Toe and fingernail fungus 0   1   2   3
7. Alternating diarrhea and constipation 0   1   2   3
8. Constipation 0   1   2   3
9. History of antibiotic use 0   1   2   3
10. Meat eater

        Never = 0   Rarely = 1   Often = 2   Daily = 3

11. Rapidly failing vision 0   1   2   3
12. Recurrent stomach pain 0   1   2   3
13. Blood or pus in stool 0   1   2   3
14. Family history of inflammatory bowel disease 0   1   2   3

Total: _____

    Score 0–5: Low priority

    Score 6–9: Moderate priority

    Score 10 or above: High priority

PART I

Fundamentals

In Part I, we begin to really look at the digestive system in its glory and wonder. We'll examine the role it plays in our overall health, metabolism, and immunity. Join me as we take a voyage through the digestive system. You'll learn more about the structure and function of the digestive organs and how they work in concert to keep us well.

CHAPTER 1

Changing the Way You Feel: When in Doubt, Begin in the Gut

"I am a cardiovascular surgeon infatuated with the challenge and promise of 'high-tech' medicine and surgery. Nonetheless, I have become convinced that the most overlooked tool in our medical arsenal is harnessing the body's own ability to heal through nutritional excellence."

—Mehmet Oz, M.D.

When working with clients, I always begin by looking at simple solutions. Recently, a woman in her mid-50s came to see me. Her neck, back, and wrists hurt. She was losing strength in her right arm and hand and was experiencing numbness in her hand. Her memory was "going down the tubes." Her anxiety and stress levels were high and she wasn't sleeping well. Her neurologist had diagnosed her with some sort of undifferentiated autoimmune disease. She was about 35 pounds overweight, which she wanted to lose to see if that made a difference in how she felt. Her lifestyle was terrific; she ate whole foods and a well-balanced diet. She taught pilates and did gentle yoga practices daily. Over the past few months she'd been getting a massage weekly.

So, you're asking, what does this have to do with digestive wellness? Sometimes systemic pain and autoimmune disease can be modulated with changes in diet and lifestyle. The word *diet* comes from the Greek word *diata*, which literally means "our manner of living." Our diet consists of everything we take in. So, I recommended several things. First, I recommended that she see a chiropractor or osteopath to determine whether the weakness and numbness on the right side of her body could be helped with manipulative therapy. Second, I recommended that she go on an elimination diet for two weeks. Third, I recommended that she rest when tired. These are simple solutions.

After three weeks her neck, arm, and hand pain were nearly gone, and her memory was improving. She lost four pounds, had better energy, and was sleeping better. It was hard to rest during the day, but she was doing it. We added some gut-supportive nutrients, and she continued with what she'd been doing.

When she walked into my office after three months she had lost 22 pounds "without trying." Her energy level was high, and she was experiencing *no* pain at all anywhere in her body. She was sleeping well and felt entirely healthy. Even though she still had stress in her life, she felt terrific. When I asked about her autoimmune symptoms, she looked at me, threw her arms up, and said, "What autoimmune disease?"

Certainly not everyone gets such benefit from simple solutions, but people often do. This book gives you a step-by-step outline as to what you can do.

WHY DIGESTION?

There is currently an epidemic of digestive illness in our country, one that is directly related to the foods we eat and the way we live. Between 30 and 40 percent of us complain about digestive issues, accounting for 104.7 million doctor visits a year. According to the Digestive Disease Clearinghouse and Information Center in 2004, about 69 percent of all doctor visits were for digestive issues. Year after year, medications for digestive illness top the pharmaceutical bestseller list. In 2007, 4 of the top 20 drugs were for GI issues. In 2008, Nexium and Prilosec, both used for heartburn, were the third and fourth bestselling drugs in the United States. Of the top 10 medications prescribed for digestive complaints, a little more than half were for gastroesophageal reflux disease (GERD), also known as heartburn.

Healthy Digestion Is the Seat of Total Health

The digestive system is like a river that runs through us. Each day we put pounds of foreign substances (food, drinks, medications, and supplements) into our mouths hoping that our bodies will be able to sort out friend from foe. And generally our bodies do a terrific job, even though much of what we put in our mouths was foreign to the environment even 100 years ago. Because of this interface, the digestive system is the seat of our immune system, runs our metabolism, makes vitamins, and communicates with *every* other cell in our bodies. The purpose of the digestive system, also lovingly called "the gut," is to bring nutrients to each cell of your body. When this doesn't occur, we feel tired and sluggish, can't think clearly, and begin to develop symptoms of illness. If left untended, these symptoms can develop into full-blown health problems.

Surprising Information About Your Digestive System
Research into the functioning of the digestive system has yielded surprising results, turning the arena of digestive health on its head.

- If spread flat, your digestive system would cover a tennis court.
- Roughly 70 percent of your immune system is located in the digestive system.
- You have 10 times as many microbes in your body as cells in your body. These microbes live in communities that live in symbiosis with you. The health of these communities determines your overall health. Collectively these communities are called the microbiome.
- You have 100 times more DNA in your microbiome than in the cells of your body. The DNA in your cells and in your microbiome talk to each other.
- You have three and a half to four and a half pounds of bacteria in your digestive system that help to make vitamins, protect you against infection, and run your metabolism. Collectively this is called the microbiome.
- The digestive system is often called the "second brain" because if the vagus nerve, which connects the brain and the digestive system, is cut, the digestive system functions fine on its own. This system is called the enteric nervous system (ENS).
- Your gut manufactures significantly more neurotransmitters, such as serotonin, than the brain. In fact, 80 to 90 percent of your serotonin is made in the gut, and every class of brain neurotransmitter has been found in the gut.
- You eat food to ultimately nourish all of your cells. If you make poor food choices *or* if your body cannot digest, absorb, and utilize the food due to poor digestive function, you probably will eventually develop signs, symptoms, and finally a diagnosable illness. Digestive insufficiencies contribute to a wide range of health issues, including migraine headaches, depression, arthritis, foggy thinking, autoimmune illness, autism, fibromyalgia, chronic fatigue, multiple sclerosis, and more.
- And finally, foods that are terrific for others may or may not be healthful for you.

WHAT CAUSES DIGESTIVE ILLNESS

We are each given a set of genes called our "genotype." As we know from the many research studies that have been done on identical twins, our genetics are only part of the picture. The things that we do, say, are exposed to, feel, eat, and hang out with make up our environment. In Buddhist terms you might say that our "dharma," or the way we live our life, affects the way our genes react. (See Figure 1.1.) If you are an optimist, then your genes get happy messages. If you are depressed, your genes get unhappy messages. Candice Pert, in her groundbreaking book *Molecules of Emotion*, explains that when we are happy, dopamine sits on our receptor sites and blocks cold viruses from those sites. Therefore, happy people get fewer colds. In fact, subsequent research finds that happy people get 65 percent fewer colds than unhappy people do. This can be simplified into the following equation:

$$\text{Genes} + \text{Environment} = \text{Health Status}$$

In fact, the only factor we can't control is our genetic makeup, and even that is more malleable than we previously believed. To illustrate this point, here are two recent studies on the effect of lifestyle and diet on how our genes behave. The Functional Genomics and Nutrition Study (FUNGENUT) looked to see whether different carbohydrate sources would change the way genes worked. Participants ate 25 percent of their calories either as rye bread and dark pasta or as oat-wheat bread and potatoes. Those who ate the rye and dark pasta diet had 62 genes that were up-regulated (turned on). The genes that were affected were related to better handling

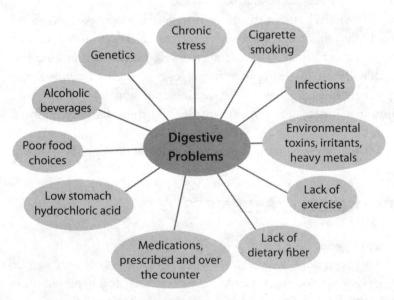

Figure 1.1   **Causes of digestive imbalance.**

of stress and reductions in inflammatory markers. Dean Ornish, M.D., performed genetic testing on 30 men who had low-risk prostate cancer. Eighteen of these men's cancer-protective genes were down-regulated (turned off) and 388 of their cancer-promoting genes were up-regulated. For three months, they changed their life-styles to include a low-fat, whole-foods, plant-based diet; daily stress-management techniques; moderate exercise; and participation in a support group. At the end of the study, the cancer-protective genes were significantly turned on and the cancer-promoting genes had been significantly turned off. While so far no genetic studies of this type have been done on digestive issues, we can anticipate many of them in the future. The few studies that we do have illustrate that small changes in lifestyle can have dramatic impacts on how genes express themselves.

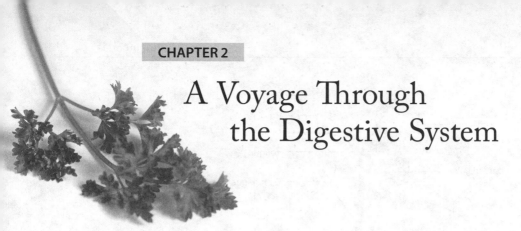

CHAPTER 2

A Voyage Through the Digestive System

"The surface area of the digestive mucosae, measuring up and down and around all the folds, rugae, villi, and microvilli, is about the size of a tennis court."

—Sydney Baker, M.D.

The digestive system is self-running and self-healing. Because this beautiful, intricate system works automatically, the average person knows very little about it. Let's take a trip through the digestive system to see what miraculous events occur inside us every moment of our lives.

The digestive system (also called the alimentary system, the gut, and the gastrointestinal system) comprises the mouth, pharynx, esophagus, stomach, small intestine, and large intestine (colon) (Figure 2.1). There are also accessory digestive organs that are outside of the digestive tract and these include our teeth, tongue, salivary glands, gall bladder, pancreas, and liver. Think of the digestive tract as a 16- to 23-foot tubular set of muscles that runs from the mouth to the anus. At its most basic, its function is to turn food into molecules that our cells can use for energy, maintenance, growth, and repair and waste products. On a deeper level it helps run our metabolism and protects us from infections and foreign substances that may come in on our food.

The digestive system is like an irrigation system. A large source of water gets narrower and narrower, finally getting water to each tiny portion of a field. If the water becomes blocked upstream, the plants wither and die. In the body, the unblocked flow of nutrients is critical for optimal health and function. Along the way, the body breaks down food protein into amino acids, starches into glucose, and fats into fatty acids and glycerol. Enzymes, vitamins, and minerals are also absorbed. The cells use these raw materials for energy, growth, and repair. If digestive wellness is compromised, our cells lose their capacity to function fully. Unlike a field, the body is inno-

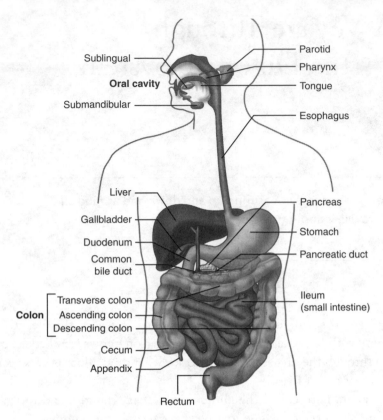

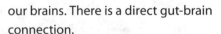

Figure 2.1   **The digestive system.**

THE DIGESTIVE SYSTEM IS WEBLIKE

The digestive system is complex. While we think of it as just something that digests food, here are some of its other less obvious functions.

- **Muscular:** The digestive structure is muscles.
- **Immune:** Most of the immune system lies in the digestive system.
- **Neurological:** The enteric nervous system has more nerve endings than our spines and more neurotransmitters than our brains. There is a direct gut-brain connection.
- **Endocrine:** There are more than 16 known digestive hormones, such as gastrin, ghrelin, and secretin.
- **Cardiovascular:** Probiotic bacteria help normalize cholesterol and triglyceride levels.
- **Metabolic:** The commensal bacteria in the digestive system drive the body's metabolism.

vative and will try to find ways to make things work. Eventually, however, its ability to seek new pathways fails, and we feel unwell. This is especially apparent in the lining of the digestive tract, which repairs and replaces itself every three to five days.

YOU AREN'T ONLY WHAT YOU EAT

Eating healthful foods is the right place to start, and that's where we focus much of our attention, but many people eat all the "right" foods and still have digestive and other health problems. Typically we digest and absorb 90 to 97 percent of the food that we eat. The rest is typically plant fibers that serve to create bulk and to create short-chain fatty acids in our colon. Yet, the best diet in the world won't help if you aren't digesting properly. You must be able to digest foods; break them down into tiny particles; absorb the food mash; take that through the intestinal lining and into the bloodstream; assimilate nutrients and calories into the cells where they can be used; and eliminate waste products through the kidneys, bowels, lymph system, and skin. Health can and does break down at any of these phases. For example, people with lots of intestinal gas are often fermenting their food rather than digesting it. Difficulty with absorption can cause people to have food sensitivities, fatigue, skin rashes, and migraine headaches. In people with celiac disease, the gut may be so inflamed that they have malabsorption issues. Diabetics have a problem with assimilation of glucose into the cells. Constipation and diarrhea are problems of elimination.

A GUIDED TOUR THROUGH THE DIGESTIVE SYSTEM

To gain a thorough understanding of how the digestive system works, let's take a guided tour starting at the brain and ending at the colon.

Brain
Before you even put food into your mouth, any sound, sight, odor, taste, or texture associated with food can trigger the body to prepare for the food that will arrive. If you imagine eating a piece of pizza, you can taste the tangy sauce and creamy cheese and feel the texture of the crust. Digestive juices, saliva, enzymes, and digestive hormones begin to flow in anticipation of the food to come. As a result your body "revs up" to prepare for the work of digestion, and your heart rate and blood flow can change. (See Chapter 10, "The Enteric Nervous System," for more information.)

THE DIGESTIVE PROCESS

Eating (also called ingestion or the cephalic phase) is voluntary and begins when materials are put in the mouth. This is our portal for all nutrients to enter the body and involves the mouth, teeth, tongue, and parotid and salivary glands. Food choices are related to lifestyle, personal values, and cultural customs.

Digestion occurs in the mouth, stomach, and small intestine and requires cooperation from the liver and pancreas. Mechanically, foods are chewed in the mouth and churned in the small and large intestine to break the foods into small pieces so that they can be fully digested. Proper levels of hydrochloric acid, bile, enzymes, and intestinal bacteria are critical for full digestive capacity.

Secretion is ongoing. Every day the walls of the digestive tract secrete about seven quarts of water, acid, buffers, and enzymes into the lumen (inside) of the digestive tract. Secretion occurs throughout the entire digestive tract. These secretions help maintain pH levels, send water into the gut to lubricate it and keep things moving, and trigger enzymes to digest foods and facilitate the digestive process. Hydration is essential for this phase of digestion to work properly.

Mixing and propulsion are muscular functions. Whatever we eat is squeezed through the digestive system by a rhythmic muscular contraction called peristalsis. Sets of smooth muscles throughout the digestive tract contract and relax, alternately, pushing food through the esophagus to the stomach and through the intestines. (Think of a snake swallowing a mouse.) When the food has been swallowed it is acidified, liquefied, neutralized, and homogenized until it's broken down into usable particles. From the time you swallow, this process is involuntary and can occur even if you stand on your head. (When my son, Arthur, was seven years old, he demonstrated this by eating upside-down. Yes, the food went down—or rather, up—as usual!)

Absorption occurs when digested food molecules are taken through the epithelial cell lining of the small intestine into the bloodstream and through the portal vein to the liver, where they are filtered. From the bloodstream they pass to the cells. Until food is absorbed, it is essentially outside the body—in a tube going through it. If the gut is inflamed, as with gluten intolerance or celiac disease, there can be malabsorption, which is typified by an inability to gain weight, lack of growth in children, anemia, and diarrhea.

Assimilation is the process by which fuel and nutrients enter the cells. Technically this isn't part of the digestive system, but it is the ultimate goal of the digestive process.

Elimination is the last step. In digestion we excrete wastes by having bowel movements (defecation). These wastes are comprised of indigestible food components, waste products, bacteria, cells from the mucosal lining that are being sloughed off, and food that has not been absorbed.

Mouth

The main function of the mouth is chewing and liquefying food. The salivary glands, located under the tongue, produce saliva, which softens food, begins dissolving soluble components, and helps keep the mouth and teeth clean. Saliva contains amylase, an enzyme for splitting carbohydrates, and lipase, a fat-digesting enzyme. Only a small percentage of starches are digested by the amylase in your mouth, but they continue to work for about another hour until the stomach acid inactivates the enzymes. On the other hand, the lipases become activated once reaching the stomach, beginning the process of fat digestion. Saliva also has clotting factors, helps to buffer acids, allows us to swallow, and protects our teeth, oral mucosa, and esophagus. Saliva also reabsorbs nitrates from our foods, primarily green leafy vegetables and beets. These nitrates are converted into nitrites by bacteria on our tongues, concentrating this a thousand times higher than those found in plasma. When this nitrite-rich saliva gets swallowed into acidic gastric juics, it converts into nitric oxide (NO), reducing inflammation throughout the body.

Chewing also stimulates the parotid glands, behind the ears in the jaw, to release hormones that stimulate the thymus to produce T cells, which are the core of the protective immune system.

Healthy teeth and gums are critical for proper digestion. Many people eat so fast, they barely chew their food at all and then wash it down with liquids. That means the stomach receives chunks of food instead of mush. This undermines the function of the teeth, which is to increase the surface area of the food. These people often complain of indigestion or gas. In *May All Be Fed*, John Robbins describes three men who survived in a concentration camp during World War II by chewing their food very well, while their compatriots perished. Simply by chewing food thoroughly we can enhance digestion and eliminate some problems of indigestion.

The most common problems that occur in the mouth are sores on the lips or tongue—usually canker or cold sores (herpes)—and tooth and gum problems.

Esophagus

The esophagus is the tube that passes from the mouth to the stomach. Here peristalsis begins to push the food along the digestive tract. Well-chewed food passes through the esophagus in about six seconds, but dry food can get stuck and take minutes to pass. At the bottom of the esophagus is a little door called the cardiac or esophageal sphincter. It separates the esophagus from the stomach, keeping stomach acid and food from coming back up. It remains closed most of the time, opening when a peristaltic wave, triggered by swallowing, relaxes the sphincter. The most common esophageal problems are heartburn (also called gastroesophageal reflux disease, or GERD), hiatal hernia, Barrett's esophagus, and eosinophilic esophagitis (EE).

Stomach: The Body's Blender

The stomach is the body's blender. It chops, dices, and liquefies as it changes food into a soupy liquid called chyme, which is the beginning of the process of protein digestion. The stomach is located under the rib cage, just under the heart.

After reaching your stomach, your food may stay in the top part of your stomach for up to an hour. Here the salivary amylase continues to break down starches. Most food stays in the stomach two to four hours—less with a low-fat meal, more with a high-fat or high-fiber meal. When the stomach has finished its job, chyme (the mixture of food mash and gastric juices) has the consistency of split-pea soup. Over several hours it passes in small amounts through the pyloric valve into the duodenum, the first 12 inches of the small intestine. Chronic stress lengthens the amount of time that food stays in the stomach, while short-term stress usually shortens the emptying time. Most of us have experienced a nervous stomach, or a feeling in the pit of the stomach, or a stomach that feels like it's filled with rocks.

Once food enters your stomach, gentle mixing waves begin chopping up your food and increasing surface area. The hormone gastrin is also produced in the stomach and stimulates the production of gastric juices. Gastric juices are comprised of enzymes, hydrochloric acid, hormones, and intrinsic factor. For example, protein molecules are composed of chains of amino acids—up to 200 amino acids strung together. The stomach produces a hormone called pepsinogen. When pepsinogen is exposed to hydrochloric acid, it turns into pepsin, which begins protein digestion, breaking the protein you eat into short chains called peptides.

Hydrochloric acid (HCl), produced by millions of parietal cells in the stomach lining, begins to break apart these protein chains. The parietal cells use huge amounts of ATP energy to concentrate acids to the low pH of about 1 that is required by the stomach. HCl also kills microbes that come in with food, protecting us against food poisoning, parasites, and bacterial infections. The hydrochloric acid in your stomach is so strong that it would burn your skin and clothing if spilled on you. Yet, the stomach is protected by a thick coating of mucus (mucopolysaccharides), which keeps the acid from burning through the stomach lining. When the mucous layer of the stomach breaks down, HCl burns a hole in the stomach lining, causing a gastric ulcer. Hydrochloric acid production is stimulated by the presence of gastrin, acetylcholine (a neurotransmitter), or histamine. The stomach also produces small amounts of lipase, enzymes that digest fat. Most foods are digested and absorbed farther down the gastrointestinal tract, but alcohol, water, and certain salts are absorbed directly from the stomach into the bloodstream. That's why we feel the effects of alcohol so quickly.

Intrinsic factor is made in the stomach in the parietal cells, and it binds vitamin B_{12} so that it can be readily absorbed in the intestines. Without adequate amounts of intrinsic factor, we do not utilize vitamin B_{12} from our food, and pernicious anemia may occur. The main symptoms are dementia, depression, nervous system problems, muscle weakness, and fatigue. This is why many people benefit from vitamin B_{12} injections, under a physician's care, or use of sublingual B_{12} or even B_{12} in a nasal spray. I remember one elderly woman who had normal serum B_{12} levels, but she felt enormously different when B_{12} shots were added to her regimen. This simple, inexpensive therapy can dramatically affect quality of life for those who need it. By the time serum B_{12} levels are low, your tissues are depleted of vitamin B_{12}. A newer test to detect early B_{12} deficiencies is called the methylmalonic acid test (MMA). Levels of methylmalonic acid rise when our bodies cannot transform vitamin B_{12} to create energy. High levels of MMA indicate early B_{12} insufficiency. Recently, researchers have remarked that probably the best test for B_{12} is just taking sublingual B_{12} supplements or a trial of B_{12} shots to see if you feel better. I have seen this to be true; when people need B_{12} and take it, their energy and sense of well-being soar. People who try B_{12} and have sufficiency already don't notice a thing.

Hydrochloric acid is also produced by the parietal cells. As the parietal cells become less efficient, the production of both hydrochloric acid and intrinsic factor falls.

The most common problems associated with the stomach are upset stomach, gastric ulcers, and underproduction of hydrochloric acid.

The GI Mucosa

The GI mucosa, depicted in Figure 2.2, is the inner lining of the digestive tract. It consists of the lumen, which is the space inside the digestive tube; the epithelial layer; the lamina propria; and the muscularis mucosae, or smooth muscles. The entire mucosa is a large mucous membrane, not unlike the tissues inside of your nose. It is here that our food makes contact with us and is eventually absorbed in the intestines. It is home to trillions of bacteria and fungi and is the center of our body's immune system. It is your body's first line of defense against infections and other invaders.

The primary layers of the gut mucosa (also called gut-associated lymphoid tissue, or GALT) include the epithelium, the lamina propria, and the muscularis mucosae. The epithelium is comprised of a single layer of cells that come into direct contact with your food. This layer of cells is held together in tight junctions (desmosomes)

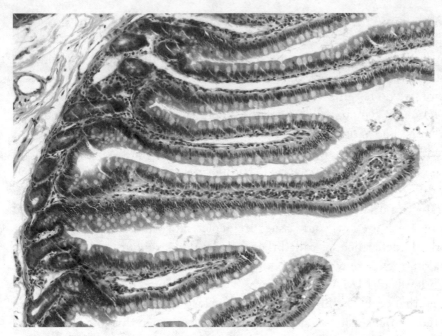

Figure 2.2   **The GI mucosa.** *(The McGraw-Hill Companies, Inc./Al Telser photographer)*

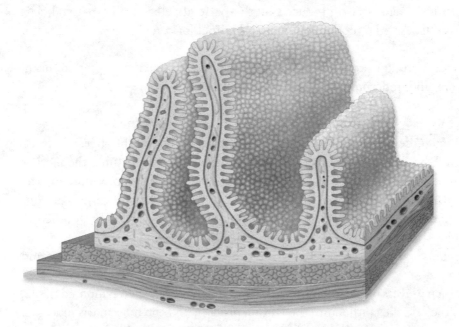

Figure 2.3   **Lamina propria and epithelial tissue.** *(The McGraw-Hill Companies, Inc.)*

that prevent leakage of molecules between the cells. (See Chapter 4.) This epithelial layer replaces itself every five to seven days and uses glutamine as its primary energy source. There are exocrine cells among the epithelial cells that secrete mucus and fluid as well as endocrine cells that release hormones.

The lamina propria connects the digestive system to the lymphatic system for digestion of fats and to the blood for absorption of nutrients (Figure 2.3). The lamina propria is where lymphatic nodules, lymphocytes, plasma cells, and macrophages form the first line of defense against infections. These are lymphatic nodes (like the ones that swell in your throat when you have a bad cold) that run throughout the digestive system but are most prominent in the tonsils, small intestine, appendix, and large intestine. The lymphatic system circulates fluids throughout your body, drains excess fluids from the fluid between cells (interstitial fluid), initiates immune response against infection and allergy, transports the fat-soluble vitamins A, D, E, and K, and brings digested fats into the bloodstream, among other things.

The lamina propria is also where cytokines, such as IL-6, IL-10, TNF-alfa, and others, are produced. Some cytokines are inflammatory, while others are healing.

The final layer of the GALT is the muscularis mucosae, which is a thin layer of smooth muscle that runs from the stomach through the small intestine. (See Chapter 9.)

Small Intestine

The small intestine is hardly small. If this coiled-up garden hose were stretched out, it would average 15 to 20 feet long. If spread flat, it would cover a surface the size of a tennis court. Here food is completely digested and absorbed. Nutrients are absorbed through hundreds of small, fingerlike folds called villi in the epithelium, which are covered, in turn, by millions of microvilli. (Think of them as small loops on a towel that then have smaller threads projecting from them.) The villi and microvilli are only one cell layer thick, but they perform multiple functions of producing digestive enzymes, absorbing nutrients, and blocking absorption of substances that aren't useful to the body.

The intestinal wall has a paradoxical function: it allows nutrients to pass into the bloodstream while blocking the absorption of foreign substances found in chemicals, bacterial products, and other large molecules found in food. Some foods we eat and medications we use irritate the intestinal wall, and it can lose the ability to discern between nutrients and foreign substances. When this occurs, there is a problem of increased intestinal permeability, commonly known as "leaky gut syndrome." This syndrome contributes to skin problems, food sensitivities, osteoarthritis, migraine headaches, and chronic fatigue syndrome. (See Chapter 4.)

The small intestine has three parts: the duodenum, the jejunum, and the ileum. The duodenum is the first 12 inches of the small intestine, the jejunum composes about 40 percent of the digestive system (about 11 feet), and the ileum composes the last segment (about 8 feet). The jejunum and ileum are connected by the ileocecal valve. Each nutrient is absorbed at specific parts of the small intestine. The duodenum has an acidic environment that facilitates absorption of some minerals, including chlorine, sulfur, calcium, copper, iron, thiamin, manganese, and zinc. We also begin the process of absorbing fat-soluble vitamins (A, D, E), fats, and some water-soluble vitamins (B_1, B_2, B_6, C, and folic acid). People with low hydrochloric acid levels may become deficient in one or more of these nutrients because they need acid for absorption. In the jejunum, we continue absorption of nutrients plus sugars, proteins, and amino acids. In the ileum, we finish the job of digesting many nutrients and add absorption of cholesterol, B_{12}, and bile salts. And finally, in the colon, we absorb potassium, water, salt, vitamin K, and short-chain fatty acids. If you look at the nutrient absorption chart in Figure 2.4 you can see specifically where each nutrient is absorbed along the digestive tract.

Pancreas

The pancreas has two main roles: to aid in the digestion of food and to produce insulin and glucagon, which regulate blood sugar levels, thereby maintaining both digestive and global function.

When food passes from the stomach to the duodenum, cholecystokinin is secreted and enhanced by secretin. This stimulates the pancreas to secrete bicarbonate-rich alkaline fluid, essentially baking soda, which neutralizes the acidity of the chyme. The hydrochloric acid has already finished its work and a more neutral pH is where the rest of the digestive system functions best. The pancreas also manufactures and secretes specific digestive enzymes. Pancreatic amylase digests starches and sugars. The protein-splitting enzymes are called trypsin, chymotrypsin, carboxypeptidase, and elastase (also called pancreatic elastase). Pancreatic lipase and colipase break fats into fatty acids and glycerol. Ribonuclease and deoxyribonuclease digest old RNA and DNA. Once our food has been fully digested, nutrients can be absorbed into the bloodstream and used by the cells. Low secretion of pancreatic enzymes can lead to nutritional deficiencies. For example, vitamin B_{12} requires protein-splitting enzymes to separate it from its carrier molecule, so poor pancreatic function can lead directly to vitamin B_{12} deficiencies.

The second role of the pancreas is the production of hormones, including insulin, glucagon, somatostatin, and pancreatic polypeptide in the pancreatic islets (also called islets of Langerhans). Insulin is secreted when blood sugar levels rise; gluca-

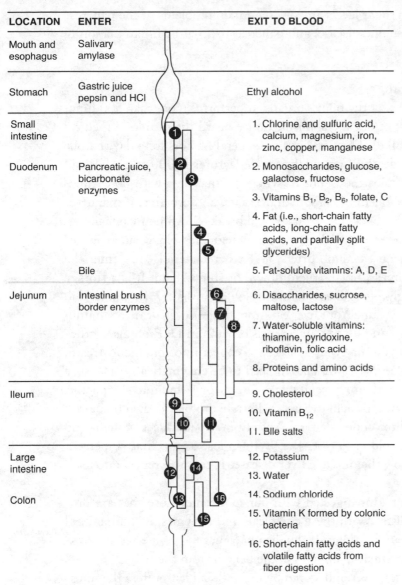

LOCATION	ENTER		EXIT TO BLOOD
Mouth and esophagus	Salivary amylase		
Stomach	Gastric juice pepsin and HCl		Ethyl alcohol
Small intestine			1. Chlorine and sulfuric acid, calcium, magnesium, iron, zinc, copper, manganese
Duodenum	Pancreatic juice, bicarbonate enzymes		2. Monosaccharides, glucose, galactose, fructose
			3. Vitamins B_1, B_2, B_6, folate, C
			4. Fat (i.e., short-chain fatty acids, long-chain fatty acids, and partially split glycerides)
	Bile		5. Fat-soluble vitamins: A, D, E
Jejunum	Intestinal brush border enzymes		6. Disaccharides, sucrose, maltose, lactose
			7. Water-soluble vitamins: thiamine, pyridoxine, riboflavin, folic acid
			8. Proteins and amino acids
Ileum			9. Cholesterol
			10. Vitamin B_{12}
			11. Bile salts
Large intestine			12. Potassium
			13. Water
Colon			14. Sodium chloride
			15. Vitamin K formed by colonic bacteria
			16. Short-chain fatty acids and volatile fatty acids from fiber digestion

Figure 2.4 **Nutrient absorption chart.**

gon is secreted when blood sugar levels are low. Common problems in the pancreas are diabetes, which is a systemic disease, and pancreatitis, that is, inflammation of the pancreas.

Liver: The Body's Fuel Filter

The liver is the most complex of the body's organs. It performs more than 500 functions and is critical to most of our metabolism. I once heard the dean of a medical school say, "I'd rather run all of the operations of General Motors for a day than be my own liver." Your four-and-a-half-pound liver manufactures 13,000 chemicals and has 2,000 enzyme systems, plus thousands of synergists that help with body functions. It regulates the metabolism of carbohydrates, fats, and proteins; it manufactures bile to emulsify fats for digestion; it makes and breaks down many hormones, including cholesterol, testosterone, and estrogens; it regulates blood sugar levels; it processes all food, nutrients, alcohol, drugs, and other materials that enter the bloodstream and lets them pass, breaks them down, or stores them. It is a storage house for many nutrients: glycogen, fats, vitamin B_{12}, vitamins A, D, E, and K, and zinc, iron, copper, and magnesium. Your liver can store five to seven years of vitamin B_{12}, four years of vitamin A, and up to four months of vitamin D. Proteins synthesized in your liver transport vitamin A, iron, zinc, and copper into your bloodstream. Practically all vitamins and minerals we take in need to be enzymatically processed by the liver before we can use them. Several vitamins are converted into their active forms: carotene to vitamin A, folic acid to 5-methyltetrahydrofolic acid, and vitamin D to its active form 25-hydroxycholecalciferol. Your liver also produces proteins and lipoproteins that allow your blood to clot. The liver can lose as much as 70 percent of its capability and not show diagnosable liver disease. It can also regenerate itself after being injured.

The liver breaks down toxins ingested with our foods and those that are produced by bacterial metabolism. With these chemicals and enzymes, it "humanizes" nutrients so that the cells can use them. If the liver becomes too congested to enzymatically process these nutrients, we do not get the benefit from them.

Bile, manufactured by the liver and stored by the gallbladder, buffers the intestinal contents due to its high concentration of bicarbonates. It also emulsifies fats. Bile is a soaplike substance made of bile salts, cholesterol, and lecithin. It makes fats more water-soluble, increasing their surface area so that the enzymes can split them for the cells to use. It's essential for absorption of fats, the fat-soluble vitamins A, D, E, and K, and some minerals. Bile also secretes immunoglobulins that protect our intestinal mucosa. Drugs and other toxins are eliminated from the liver through bile. The brown color of stool comes from the yellow color of bilirubin in bile.

The liver is also part of our immune system. The Kupffer cells filter bacteria and debris from the blood. The liver also stores environmental toxins like radioactive substances, pesticides, herbicides, food preservatives, and dyes. The liver will detoxify what it can, but if it can't break down a particular substance, it stores it there and in tissues throughout the body.

Gallbladder: A Holding Tank for Bile

The gallbladder is a pear-shaped organ that lies just below the liver. The gallbladder's function is to store and concentrate bile, which is produced by the liver. When you eat a food that contains fat, cholecystokinin is released from the duodenum, which stimulates the gallbladder and liver to release bile into the common duct that connects the liver, gallbladder, and pancreas to the duodenum. Bile emulsifies the fats, cholesterol, and fat-soluble vitamins you've eaten by breaking them into tiny globules. These create a greater surface area for the fat-splitting enzymes (lipase) to act on during digestion.

The most common problem of the gallbladder is gallstones. When bile becomes too concentrated, stones may form, which can cause pain, nausea, and discomfort. Another common issue is bile reflux, where bile backs up into the stomach. Gallbladder disease is directly related to diet.

Appendix

The appendix is a small, fingerlike sac that extends off the beginning of the colon. Until recently, the function of the appendix was a mystery. Now we know it contains a great deal of lymphatic tissue and is important for fetal and early childhood development. Hormones produced in the appendix beginning about the 11th week of pregnancy help regulate fetal metabolism. The appendix contains a lot of lymphatic tissue and is especially important in immune health in the first decades of life. In the developmental years, the appendix produces secretory IgA and helps with the maturation of B-lymphocytes (a type of white blood cell). These functions help to support local immune function.

Large Intestine or Colon

When all nutrients have been absorbed, water, bacteria, and fiber pass through the ileocecal valve to the large intestine and colon. The ileocecal valve is located by your right hip bone and separates the contents of the small and large intestines.

The colon is short, only three to five feet long. Its job is to absorb water and remaining nutrients from the chyme and form stool. Two and a half gallons of water pass through the colon each day, two-thirds of which come from body fluids. The efficient colon pulls 80 percent of the water out of the chyme, which is absorbed into the bloodstream.

The large intestine has three main parts: the ascending colon (up the right side of the body), the transverse colon (straight across the belly under the ribs), and the descending colon (down the left side of the body) to the rectum, where feces exit the body. Stool begins to form in the transverse colon. If the chyme passes through the colon too quickly, water is not absorbed, causing diarrhea. Stool that sits too long in the colon becomes dry and hard to pass, leading to constipation. About two-thirds of stool is composed of water and undigested fiber and food products. The other third is composed of living and dead bacteria.

The large intestine contains the majority of commensal and probiotic bacteria by far. In the colon, bifidobacteria ferment fibers that become short-chain fatty acids: butyric, propionic, acetic, and valerate. Butyric acid is the main fuel of the colonic cells. Low butyric acid levels or an inability of the colon bacteria to properly metabolize butyric acid has been associated with ulcerative colitis, colon cancer, active colitis, and inflammatory bowel disease.

When the stool is finally well formed, it gets pushed down into the descending colon and then into the rectum. It is held there until there is sufficient volume to have a bowel movement. Two sphincters—rings of muscle—control bowel movements. When enough feces have collected, the internal sphincter relaxes and your mind gets the signal that it's time to relieve yourself. The external sphincter opens when you command it. Because this is voluntary, you can have the urge to defecate but wait until it's convenient. If you ignore the urge, water keeps being absorbed back into the body and the stool gets dry and hard. Some people are chronically constipated because they don't want to take the time to have a bowel movement or don't like to have bowel movements at work. This book is about listening to your body signals. Take the time when your body calls you, not when it's convenient or ideal.

Many health problems arise in the colon: appendicitis, constipation, diarrhea, diverticular disease, Crohn's disease, ulcerative colitis, rectal polyps, colon cancer, irritable bowel syndrome, parasites, and hemorrhoids.

WHAT GOES IN, MUST COME OUT!

We can learn a lot about ourselves from stool. Dennis Burkitt, M.D., father of the fiber theory, found that on average people on Western diets excreted only 5 ounces of stool daily, whereas Africans eating traditional diets passed 16 ounces. Well-formed stool tells us when it wants to come out; we don't need to coax it. It looks like a brown banana with a point at one end, is well hydrated, and just slips out easily. Stool that looks like little balls all wadded together has been in the colon too long. The longer waste materials sit in the colon, the more concentrated the bile acids become; concentrated bile acids irritate the lining of the colon. Hormones that have been broken down by the body are also excreted via our feces. If the stools sit in the colon for too long, these hormones are reabsorbed into the bloodstream, increasing the risk for estrogen-dependent cancers. Betaglucuronidase, an enzyme that may activate formation of cancer-causing substances in the colon, can be measured in stool as a marker of hormone reabsorption.

Frequency of bowel movements is a good health indicator. How often do you have a bowel movement? People on good diets generally have one to three bowel movements each day. If you are not having a daily bowel movement, there can be many causes.

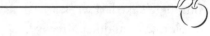

TESTING BOWEL TRANSIT TIME

Transit time is how long it takes from the time you eat a food until it comes out the other end. Buy charcoal tablets at a drug or health-food store, and take about 1,000 mg. Depending on the particular product, this can be two to four capsules. Note exactly when you took the charcoal. When you see darkened stool (charcoal will turn the stool black), calculate how many hours since you took the charcoal tablets. That is your transit time. You can also do the test with beets. Eating three or four whole beets will turn stool a deep garnet red.

The Results

- Less than 12 hours: This usually indicates that you are not absorbing all the nutrients you should from your food. You may have malabsorption problems.

- Twelve to 24 hours is optimal.
- More than 24 hours: This indicates that wastes are sitting inside your colon too long. Poor transit time greatly increases the risk of colon disease. Substances that were supposed to be eliminated get absorbed back into the bloodstream, and they can interfere with and irritate your system. Take action now! Increase your fiber intake by eating more fruit, vegetables, whole grains, and legumes. Drink lots of water every day. Get 30 minutes of exercise at least three times a week.

First, take a close look at your diet. You probably aren't eating enough fiber. If that's the case, increase your intake of fruits, vegetables, whole grains, and legumes. These foods are generally high in magnesium, which helps normalize peristalsis. Make sure that you are drinking enough fluids. Coffee and soft drinks don't count! And get regular exercise!

Another good indicator of your colon's health is your bowel transit time—how long it takes food to move from the first swallow until it exits the body. When your system is working well, the average amount of time is 12 to 24 hours. On average, Americans have a transit time that is way too long—48 to 96 hours—because we don't eat enough high-fiber foods, take in enough magnesium, or drink enough water. You can do a simple home test to determine your transit time, which gives you important information about the way your body works.

EXERCISE: CLEAN UP YOUR DIET!

Let's take a look at what foods you are eating and begin the process of cleaning up your diet. Take last week's food diary. Get out some crayons or markers. You're going to color! (If you don't already keep a food diary, you will find instructions on how to do so in Chapter 12.)

- **Circle the following foods red:** Sugar, caffeine, alcohol, junk foods, fried foods, high-fat foods, pastries, donuts, chips, microwave popcorn, highly processed foods, soft drinks, diet soft drinks, diet foods
- **Circle the following foods blue:** Dairy products: milk, cheese, yogurt, ice cream, frozen yogurt, ice milk
- **Circle the following foods green:** Fruits and vegetables
- **Circle the following foods yellow:** Protein foods: fish, poultry, beef, pork, lamb, veal, legumes, soy products
- **Circle the following foods purple:** Nuts and seeds, oils, butter, margarine
- **Circle the following foods black:** Grains: wheat, bread, cereal, corn, rice, millet, buckwheat, bulgur, quinoa, amaranth, barley, oats, rye

Look at those circles. Is there one food group that dominates your diary? If you eliminated one of these categories from your diet, which would be the easiest to give up and which would be the most difficult? Sometimes the ones that are the hardest to give up are the ones that are causing us the most trouble. They temporarily make us feel better, even though they are really making us sicker. Why? Our bodies may react negatively to cigarettes, dairy products, caffeine, sugar, wheat, pork, beef, citrus fruits, or any other foods, yet we crave them.

This week, focus on the foods you circled in red and eliminate all of them. Sugars ferment and can contribute to your digestive problems. Get rid of soft drinks, cookies, pastries, donuts, and sugar added to coffee or tea. We're not talking about perfection here. Let's just make some progress. Why? These foods make it harder for your body to be healthy. High-sugar foods deplete our nutrient stores. We need most of the B-complex vitamins, chromium, manganese, and potassium to metabolize these foods properly, but sweets don't have any of these nutrients. So we take nutrients out of storage, and eventually our tissues become depleted.

After a couple of weeks, fruit begins to taste really sweet, which is just how it ought to taste. Once, I realized that it had been months since I had had any chocolate. I began to feel deprived, so I bought a big chocolate bar for my family and friends. I ate a few squares and was totally satisfied. I hope that eventually you can be satisfied with just a little bit, too. But if you can't, you're really better off without any. Once I was sick and was craving sweets like crazy. My doctor told me it was the bacteria—both good and bad—that wanted the energy. So starve those bad guys out. The helpful bacteria can adapt with real food.

PART II

The DIGIN Model and the 5 Rs

In conventional medicine, a clinician makes a diagnosis and there are standard therapies for each diagnosis. In functional medicine, there is no cookie-cutter approach. Finding the underlying mechanisms of disease rather than focusing on symptom relief is the goal. Two people with the same diagnosis may need completely different therapies. At the same time, two people with completely dissimilar diagnoses may benefit from the same therapy. For example, irritable bowel syndrome, migraine headaches, attention deficit disorder, and fibromyalgia may seem like different diagnoses, but they may all have the underlying cause of leaky gut syndrome or food intolerances. On the other hand, three people with irritable bowel syndrome could have completely different underlying causes, including small intestinal bacterial infection, a deficiency of protective bacteria, too little fiber, food sensitivities, lactose intolerance, celiac disease, imbalances in neurotransmitters, or stress-induced IBS, to name a few.

So how do we begin looking for underlying mechanisms? I call it the DIGIN approach. In the following chapters we'll explore each aspect of this model (see Figure II.1). I consider this section to be the heart of the book. No matter what the diagnosis, there is probably some aspect of this model that will help bring you back into better balance.

THE DIGIN MODEL FOR ASSESSMENT OF DIGESTIVE ISSUES

DIGIN is an acronym for the five primary categories of digestive imbalances:

- **D**igestion/absorption
- **I**ntestinal permeability
- **G**astrointestinal microbiota

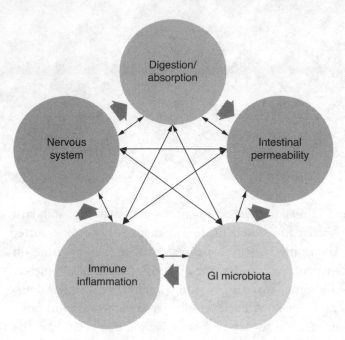

Figure II.1   **The DIGIN model.**

- **I**mmune function and inflammation
- Enteric **n**ervous system

By assessing each of these areas, you can discover how to best get your body back into balance.

THE 5 RS

The principles of repair in functional medicine are fairly simple. As one of the pioneers in the field, Sidney Baker, M.D., said: Get rid of what you don't need, and get what you do need. The 4 Rs were originally put together by Jeffrey Bland, Ph.D., and Metagenics. Recently at the Institute for Functional Medicine, we've updated this to the 5 R Program, which includes:

- **Remove:** Nutrient-depleted food, processed foods, poor-quality fats and oils, parasites, metals, infections, foods that don't agree with us. This is the critical first step.
- **Replace:** Processed foods with whole foods, nutrients, digestive enzymes, hydrochloric acid, bile salts.

- **Reinoculate (Repopulate):** Beneficial probiotics and prebiotics from food and supplements.
- **Repair:** Using foods and supplements such as glutamine, gamma-oryzanol, duodenum glandular, N-acetyl glucosamine, fiber, boswellia, geranium, licorice, quercetin, goldenseal, wormwood, aloe, celandine, cranesbill, marshmallow root, rice protein powders, essential fatty acids, okra, cabbage, fasting.
- **Rebalance:** Stress management, improved sleep habits, exercise and movement, changes of attitude and belief systems. Come to a new sense of who you are. Accept that and regroup your lifestyle to promote a healthier way of living and being.

The 5 Rs are sprinkled throughout this section of the book and continue in Part III, "Coming Back into Balance."

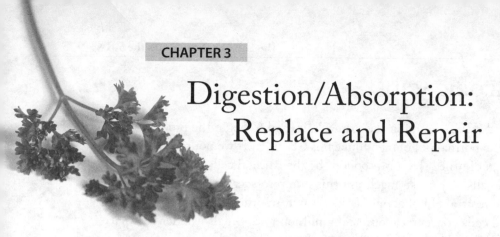

CHAPTER 3

Digestion/Absorption: Replace and Repair

"Things which matter most must never be at the mercy of things which matter least."

—Goethe

If you cannot digest and absorb your food, your cells won't get the nourishment that they need to function properly. Many health issues begin because people aren't fully digesting and/or absorbing their food. This can occur from five main reasons:

- Poor chewing and rushed eating
- Hydrochloric acid insufficiency
- Bile salt insufficiency
- Enzyme insufficiency
- Lack of dietary fiber

In today's rushed culture, we often don't chew our food well or even really pay much attention to what we are eating. I'm as guilty as anyone, reading while I eat or eating while driving in the car. Yet, the simple act of using our teeth for the purpose for which they were designed can dramatically improve our health.

Eating mindfully or consciously can help you digest food more efficiently and minimize digestive issues. It is an old custom to chew each bite 30 times. When drinking liquids, we also need to slow down and pay attention to pacing.

HYDROCHLORIC ACID

Hydrochloric acid (HCl), found in the stomach, is used to begin the process of protein digestion. The normal pH of our stomach is 0.8 to 1.5. If we poured this acid on our hands, we'd get burned. HCl is produced by the parietal cells in your stomach.

The parietal cells of your stomach use this pump to secrete gastric juice. Most of our body has a neutral pH of about 7.0, like water. In order to create hydrochloric acid, our parietal cells concentrate our acid a million fold. Small wonder that parietal cells are stuffed with mitochondria, our cellular energy factories, and use huge amounts of energy as they carry out this enormous concentration of protons.

The mucous layer in the stomach protects it from this acid. HCl triggers pepsin secretion. Pepsin cleaves large protein molecules so that they can be more easily broken down by digestive enzymes in the small intestine. In the duodenum, the high acid environment allows for absorption of minerals such as iron, calcium, magnesium, zinc, and copper. Stomach acid also provides our first defense against food poisoning, H. pylori, parasites, fungi, and other infections. Without adequate acid, we leave ourselves open to decreased immune resistance. A couple of tip-offs that people may have low stomach acid levels is that they often belch and burp, develop food poisoning, or have been diagnosed with small intestinal bacterial overgrowth (SIBO).

In the current medical system, it is believed that excess stomach acid causes much disease. According to a Gallup poll, 44 percent of us experience heartburn at least once a month and 7 percent of us have it once a week or more. We are quick to blame this discomfort on excess acid. In fact, drugs to block stomach acid production have blockbuster sales. In 2007, Nexium, Protonix/Pantozol, and AcipHex were all in the top 25 drugs, making up about 10 percent of *all* top drug sales. This doesn't include over-the-counter sales for Zantac, Prilosec, Tums, and other antacids.

Chronic use of antacids and acid-blocking drugs contribute to long-term problems. They increase the incidence of SIBO; decrease mineral, folic acid, and B_{12} absorption; open us up to more food-borne infections; and cause dependence because when we stop using them we feel even worse than before we began. Jonathan Wright, in *Why Stomach Acid Is Good for You*, has found that many people with diseases such as type 1 diabetes, osteoporosis, childhood asthma, chronic fatigue, depression, and other illnesses have atypically low levels of HCl in their stomachs. When they are supported with HCl plus pepsin, digestive enzymes, nutrients, stress management, and other supportive treatment, their health issues improve or resolve.

Acid blockers and antacids *do* help us feel better. But is the cause too much acid or too much acid in the wrong place?

Between the esophagus and the stomach is a circular muscle called the lower esophageal sphincter (LES). It opens to allow food to pass from the esophagus into the stomach. In some people, the LES opens inappropriately for brief moments. This allows stomach acid to back up, or "reflux," into the esophagus. Even small amounts of this cause tissue damage and burning.

The problem, however, is typically due not to an overall excess of stomach acid, but to acid where it doesn't belong. As we age, stomach acid levels decline while heartburn increases. In addition, the LES works less effectively in many of us as

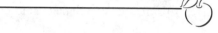

CLINICAL CLUES OF LOW STOMACH ACID

- Bloating, belching, burning, and flatulence immediately after meals
- A sense of fullness after eating just a few bites of food
- Feeling as though food sits in stomach undigested for hours
- Indigestion, diarrhea, or constipation
- Multiple food allergies
- Nausea after taking supplements
- Itching around the rectum
- Weak, peeling, and cracked fingernails
- Dilated blood vessels in the cheeks and nose (in nonalcoholics)
- Acne
- Iron deficiency
- Chronic intestinal parasites or abnormal flora
- Undigested food in stool
- Chronic candida infections
- Upper digestive tract gassiness

The following are diseases associated with low gastric acidity:

- Addison's disease
- Asthma
- Celiac disease
- Chronic autoimmune disorders
- Chronic hives
- Dermatitis herpetiformis (herpes)
- Diabetes
- Eczema
- Gallbladder disease
- Graves disease
- Hepatitis
- Hyper- and hypothyroidism
- Lupus erythematosis
- Myasthenia gravis
- Osteoporosis
- Pernicious anemia
- Psoriasis
- Rheumatoid arthritis
- Rosacea
- Sjögren's syndrome
- Thyrotoxicosis
- Vitiligo

Used with permission from Michael Murray, N.D., "Indigestion, Antacids, Achlorhydria and H. pylori," *American Journal of Natural Medicine* (January–February 1997): 11–16.

we get older. Nicotine, caffeine, high-fat meals, orange juice, tomatoes and tomato-based products like spaghetti sauce, spicy foods, and alcohol can weaken the LES. Carminitive herbs, such as peppermint and spearmint, also relax the LES and can increase acid reflux.

The symptoms of too little stomach acid and too much are similar. Typically I hear about belching, burping, and food that feels as if it sits in the stomach undigested for hours. Some of the clues that might alert you that you have low stomach acid appear on page 33.

What causes too little stomach acid? Food sensitivities and stress play a role. Additionally, chlorine and fluoride in drinking water can block its production, and a stressful lifestyle can deplete acid output.

Testing for Low Hydrochloric Acid Levels

You can do a home test to determine whether your HCl levels are optimal. For definitive results, find a physician who can measure your HCl levels with a Heidelberg capsule test or the SmartPill test. (See Chapter 11, "Functional Medicine/Functional Testing.")

Options for Increasing HCl Naturally

If you have determined through testing that your HCl levels are low, you can try the following.

- Take betaine HCl with pepsin with meals that contain protein. Dosage: 300 to 750 mg per capsule.
- Consider stress management to naturally allow your stomach to come into balance again.
- Chiropractic adjustments can improve blood flow to the stomach and help normalize HCl production.
- You can also stimulate HCl production by using bitters. Bitters have long been used to promote better digestion. They typically have gentian plus other herbs. They probably work by increasing saliva, HCl, pepsin, bile, and digestive enzymes. Sweetish (Swedish) bitters can be found in health-food stores and some drugstores. Compari bitters are also effective and are found where alcoholic beverages are sold.
- Some people find relief by using diluted vinegar. Apple cider vinegar seems to work best. Begin with 1 teaspoon in 8 teaspoons of water. Gradually increase the amount of vinegar until you get the desired effect.

- Umeboshi plums are found in the Asian section of grocery and health-food stores. Umeboshi plums are salted, pickled plums that can relieve most indigestion and alkalize the body. They can be eaten whole or used as the base for tea, to replace salt and vinegar in salad dressings, or as umeboshi vinegar.
- Use protein-splitting enzymes to aid digestion of protein foods. The most common ones include bromelain (from pineapple stems), papain (from papaya), and mixed protease enzymes (also called proteolytic enzymes). (See the section later in this chapter on enzymes for more information.)

BILE SALTS

Bile is a soaplike substance secreted by the liver. Bile salts emulsify the fats from our food. By increasing the surface area of the molecules, our lipase (fat-splitting) enzymes can digest fats and absorb fat-soluble vitamins (A, D, E, and K) more efficiently. Bile is made from cholesterol; it sequesters cholesterol and is a main way in which we eliminate cholesterol from our bodies. When our bile acid levels are high, our body stops making more cholesterol; conversely, when our bile acid levels are low, our bodies can make up to 15 times more cholesterol. Bile also helps make calcium and iron more absorbable. See Figure 3.1.

People who have had their gallbladders removed don't concentrate bile acids. People with liver and gallbladder issues and people who have had their ileum removed often benefit from taking extra bile salts. While I haven't seen any studies on the supplemental use of bile to lower high serum cholesterol levels, it's something to consider.

Typical tests for bile acid insufficiency include endoscopy, testing for fats in stool, and comprehensive stool testing that tests for various fats.

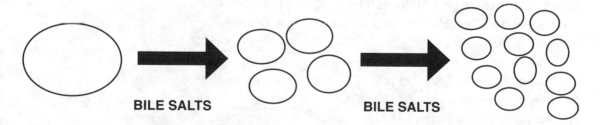

BILE SALTS   BILE SALTS

Figure 3.1 **This is how bile salts emulsify the fat we eat.**

If you have had your gallbladder removed, have liver disease, or experience a failure to absorb fats, consider using bile salts. A typical dosage would be between 200 to 1,000 mg with food. Taurine at dosages of 500 to 2,000 mg daily also enhances your body's ability to make bile salts.

Foods and herbs that help stimulate bile are called cholagogues. Cholagogic foods include radishes, dandelion, chicory, mustard greens, turnip greens, and artichokes. You can often find cholagogue herbs in combination that will typically have dandelion and one or more of the following herbs: wormwood, greater celandine, boldo, blue flag, and fringe tree.

ENZYMES

An enzyme is a protein that catalyzes (triggers a change without being changed itself) a reaction to speed up, slow down, or change a small number of chemical reactions. Since each enzyme can make only a "small" change, we need many of them. Some enzymes also have a nonprotein part—a metal molecule, a vitamin, or another molecule attached to them. These are called coenzymes. Most of the B-complex vitamins are coenzymes. Enzymes work in our bodies to conserve energy. Without them, much more heat and calories would be needed to perform the same jobs.

Metabolic Enzymes

We have 2,700 known enzymes in our bodies. All enzymes are very specific for their jobs. Each one binds to a specific type of substance and does one specific type of job. They are needed for *every* chemical reaction that occurs in the human body. We

CLINICAL CLUES OF BILE INSUFFICIENCY

- Have had your gallbladder removed or have gallbladder issues
- Liver disease
- Thyroid issues (hypothyroid or hyperthyroid)
- Ileostomy (removal of part of your ileum)
- Incomplete digestion/absorption of fats
- Steatorrhea (stools that have a lot of fat in them; they typically are frothy, smell bad, and are tan or light in color)
- Diarrhea
- Abdominal discomfort
- Gas and bloating
- Decreased absorption of nutrients
- Water retention
- Low serum albumin levels
- Bleeding tendency (vitamin K deficiency)
- Weight loss
- Growth failure in children

use them to make energy, think, and control blood sugar levels. We cannot utilize a vitamin, a mineral, or a fat; make or break down cells; or remove wastes without enzymes. Our immune system and nervous system cannot work without enzymes. We use them to build cartilage and bone, give our skin elasticity, keep our blood from clotting, build and break down hormones, and everything else. And if we don't have enough enzymes, we don't feel as well as we could. We make enzymes from the proteins we eat and by recycling them. In order for enzymes to work properly, they need to be synthesized correctly and be in a correct pH and temperature.

Digestive Enzymes

Our digestive system uses enzymes to break down the food we eat. (HCl and bile also help in the process of digestion.) We make most of our digestive enzymes in the pancreas, but enzymes are produced throughout the digestive system, beginning with amylase in our saliva. We have separate enzymes for digesting fats, carbohydrates, proteins, pectins, and phytic acid. The fat-splitting enzymes are called lipases, the carbohydrate-splitting enzymes are called amylases, and the protein-splitting enzymes are called proteases. Pectins are found in fruits, such as apples and pears. Pectinase enzymes help break them down. Phytic acid is found primarily in grains and beans. Phytic acid binds minerals, and we cannot use them if they are bound. Phytase enzymes help break them down, releasing minerals as a result.

Digestive Enzyme Insufficiencies. Many people have enzyme deficiencies, making them unable to adequately digest specific foods or food groups. Lactose intolerance, fructose intolerance, and lack of gluten-splitting enzymes are the most common of these.

- **Lactose intolerance:** It's estimated that about 25 percent of Americans and 75 percent of the world's population is lactose intolerant. It's most prevalent in people of Asian, African, or Mediterranean descent. In the United States, virtually all people of Asian ancestry and 80 percent of African Americans are lactose intolerant. Interestingly enough, most people can tolerate small amounts of dairy products. Even more can tolerate lactose-free milk or eat dairy products when they take lactase enzyme supplements.
- **Gluten intolerance/Celiac disease:** Celiac disease affects 1 in 133 people, 3 million Americans. About 40 percent of us have the correct genes to develop celiac disease, and it is estimated that up to 15 percent of us are gluten intolerant. People with celiac disease cannot fully digest gliaden, a protein found in wheat, barley, rye, spelt, and kamut. (See section on celiac disease and gluten intolerance in Chapter 24.)

- **Fructose intolerance:** This disorder affects 1 in 20,000 people who have fructose 1-phosphate aldolase deficiency. This is typically found in infancy or early childhood with children who refuse to eat sweet foods or who get ill from them. Typical symptoms include vomiting, failure to thrive, liver changes, jaundice, acidosis, blood clotting disorders, hypoglycemia, and possibly seizures.
- **Disaccharide intolerance:** Some people lack the ability to break apart two-molecule sugars, such as lactose, maltose, and sucrose. These deficiencies are quite rare, yet many people with dysbiosis find that they benefit from a specific carbohydrate diet until their gut has healed.

Enzymes in Our Foods

Foods can be a good source of enzymes if we are eating fresh, locally grown foods or if we are eating fermented or cultured foods. Enzymes are what ripen tomatoes or bananas sitting on our counter. Enzymes are also what continue to "compost" those tomatoes and bananas if we don't eat them fast enough.

Foods have the highest enzyme activity level when they are fresh or when they are fermenting. So, growing your own or buying local gives you the most enzyme activity. Raw fish, such as sushi or sashimi, is rich in active enzymes. Raw milk is high in enzymes. Fresh pineapple has bromelain enzymes, but canning or cooking deactivates the bromelain. Soy sauce is rich in enzymes to help digest the protein in the meal.

Cooked, packaged, or processed foods are enzyme depleted. Cooking at temperatures as low as 118 degrees Fahrenheit destroys enzymes. Since these kinds of foods are what we eat, most of us will benefit from enzyme supplementation.

Supplemental Enzymes and Their Clinical Use

Studies reveal that about 10 percent of 10-year-olds have enzyme deficiencies, 20 percent of 20-year-olds have enzyme deficiencies, 50 percent of 50-year-olds have enzyme deficiencies, and so on. This can occur from stress or low-grade inflammation in the stomach, called gastritis, and infections, such as H. pylori.

Enzyme deficiencies are obvious in children with cystic fibrosis, but less obvious as a pivotal factor in type 2 diabetes and obesity in our children. Enzyme supplementation has been helpful in the treatment of these health problems.

Supplemental enzymes have also been used successfully to treat several types of arthritis in adults, working more effectively than drug treatment. Moreover, they have been used successfully to treat children and adults with food allergies, eosinophilic gastroenteritis, asthma, and other illnesses. Along with probiotics, they are the first thing I think of when working with children and adults who are failing to thrive. Other diseases that enzymes have been used clinically for include Crohn's disease, ulcerative colitis, hay fever, pulmonary fibrosis, sinusitis, multiple sclerosis, bladder infections, and in breaking up and preventing blood clots. The effect on blood clots also protects us from heart disease.

Protein-splitting enzymes are used to reduce swelling and pain throughout the body and can be used to treat injuries. In one study, soccer players were given enzymes or placebos after they were injured. Injuries healed more quickly when enzymes were given, sometimes up to twice as fast. They can be used to reduce the time that bruises take to heal by about 50 percent.

Enzymes have also been used for decades in cancer treatment, especially in Europe. I recently heard oncologist Dr. Mahesh Kanojia speak at a medical conference. He said that use of Aspergillus-derived protein splitting, also called proteolytic enzymes, enzyme supplements lessens the side effects of chemotherapy, including hair loss, and enhances the results of the treatments. Nicholas Gonzales, M.D., in New York, uses pancreatic enzyme supplements as a critical part of his individualized programs for people with all types of cancers. The National Institutes of Health (NIH) was so impressed, they funded a study to reproduce his work. This study did not show effectiveness of Dr. Gonzales's treatments, but he has contested the way in which the evaluation was performed.

According to Dr. Brad Rachman, proteolytic enzymes improve protein digestion and decrease the quantity of antigens that leak into the bloodstream. This can reduce issues with food allergies and food sensitivities.

Categories of Enzyme Supplements

There are three major types of supplemental enzyme products: pancreatic enzymes, enzymes grown on a fungal base, and plant-based enzymes.

Pancreatic enzymes have been used and are part of common medical practice for illnesses such as cystic fibrosis. They are actually derived from animal pancreatic tissue. They work well to assist with digestion and to help stabilize blood glucose levels in people with diabetes and hypoglycemia. When I was in my 20s I suffered from hypoglycemia; I took pancreatic enzymes several times a day for about a year and found my hypoglycemia to be nearly 100 percent gone. The difficulty with pancreatic enzymes is that they work in a limited pH range, at 8 or above. This pH is too alkaline to function in the stomach, where a large part of digestion takes place. In cystic fibrosis a small percentage of children become allergic to pancreatic enzymes.

More recently, enzymes have been grown on a fungal base of Aspergillus niger and Aspergillus oryzae. New to the United States, these enzymes have been used in food production for centuries and clinically for more than 50 years in Japan. There are hundreds of species of Aspergillus, but these two have been found to be completely free of mycotoxins (substances produced from fungi that are toxic). These enzymes are blended like wine to ensure that they work in the high acid environment of the stomach and through the small and large intestines, which have a more neutral pH. They also are not derived from an animal protein and have been found to cause fewer allergic issues in people.

Plant-based enzymes, such as bromelain and papain, are protein-splitting enzymes. Bromelain is derived from the green stems of pineapple plants, and papain comes from green papayas. They are useful for reducing inflammation and pain and for digestion of protein.

Enzymes are rated by their activity level rather than by counting milligrams or micrograms of them. When you purchase enzyme supplement products, you will see units such as DU, HUT, FCCLU, CU, IAU, and many others to express the level of enzyme activity. If you look at an enzyme label and it measures the enzymes only in milligrams or micrograms, you cannot know if there are any active enzymes in the product at all. Enzyme supplements are very stable and will last for at least three years, so many labels do not have expiration dates.

DIETARY FIBER

Insufficient dietary fiber intake is yet another reason people may not be absorbing or digesting their foods appropriately. In fact, most of us eat half as much fiber as our ancestors did. Soluble fiber (found in fruit, beans, barley, rice, flaxseed, and psyllium) helps bind bile acids, regulates cholesterol and blood sugar levels, and keeps our intestinal pH in balance. Insoluble fiber (found in bran, vegetables, whole grains, and carrots) helps keep us regular and normalizes peristalsis. Insoluble fiber is fermented in our large intestines by beneficial bifidobacteria to produce butyrate and other short-chain fats that provide fuel and cell maintenance in our large intestines. Soluble fiber helps to regulate both constipation-type and diarrhea-type irritable bowel syndrome. Improvement in bowel function may help prevent diverticulosis, appendicitis, colon polyps, colon cancer, hemorrhoids, and varicose veins. Diets high in soluble fiber are helpful to people with irritable bowel syndrome, Crohn's disease, hiatal hernia, and peptic ulcer. Dietary fiber also helps prevent obesity by slowing down digestion and the release of glucose and insulin. Fiber has been shown to normalize serum cholesterol levels. High-fiber diets reduce the risk of heart disease, high blood pressure, and certain types of cancer. See Chapter 12 for more information on increasing high-fiber foods in your diet.

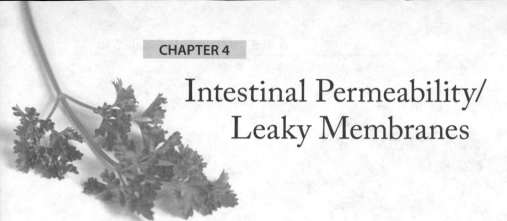

CHAPTER 4

Intestinal Permeability/ Leaky Membranes

The foot bone connected to the leg bone,
The leg bone connected to the knee bone,
The knee bone connected to the thigh bone,
The thigh bone connected to the back bone,
The back bone connected to the neck bone,
The neck bone connected to the head bone

—African American spiritual/children's song

Leaky gut syndrome is really a nickname for the more formal term *increased intestinal permeability*, which underlies an enormous variety of illnesses and symptoms. It's not a disease or an illness itself. It's a symptom of inflammation and imbalance that has many causes. The list of health conditions associated with increased intestinal permeability grows each year as we increase our knowledge of the synergy between digestion and the immune system. Currently there are more than 8,000 research articles on intestinal permeability.

The small intestines have a paradoxical function. It allows only properly digested fats, proteins, and starches to pass through so they can be assimilated, while providing a barrier to keep out bacterial products, foreign substances, and large undigested molecules. This is called the barrier function of the gastrointestinal mucosal lining. This surface is often called the brush border because under a microscope its villi and microvilli look like bristles on a brush.

In between cells are junctions called desmosomes. Normally, desmosomes form tight junctions and do not permit large molecules to pass through. When the area is irritated and inflamed, however, these junctions loosen up, allowing larger molecules to pass through. The substances that pass through the intracellular junctions are seen by our immune system as foreign, stimulating an antibody reaction. When

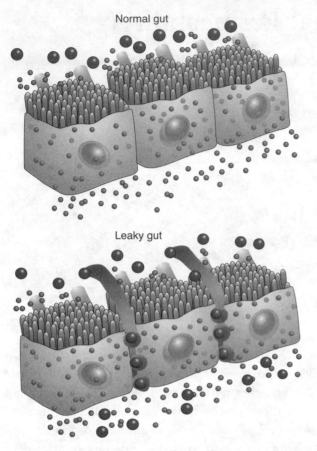

Figure 4.1 **Leaky gut syndrome.** (Used with permission from Genova Diagnostic Laboratory.)

the intestinal lining is damaged, larger substances of particle size are allowed to pass directly, again triggering an antibody reaction. (See Figure 4.1.)

When the intestinal lining is damaged even more, substances larger than particle size—disease-causing bacteria, fungi, potentially toxic molecules, and undigested food particles—are allowed to pass directly through the weakened cell membranes. They go directly into the bloodstream, activating antibodies and alarm substances called cytokines. The cytokines alert our lymphocytes (white blood cells) to battle the particles. Oxidants are produced in the battle, causing irritation and inflammation far from the digestive system. Inflammation on this brush border can prevent small nutrients and food molecules from passing into the gut lumen. This is the primary cause of malabsorption.

Intestinal mucus normally blocks bacteria from moving to other parts of the body. But when the cells are leaking, bacteria can pass into the bloodstream and travel throughout the body. When intestinal bacteria colonize in other parts of the body, we call it bacterial translocation, and it is often found in people with leaky gut syndrome. For example, Blastocystis hominis, a bacteria that causes GI problems, has been found in the synovial fluid in the knee of an arthritis patient. Surgery or tube feeding in hospitals can also cause bacterial translocation.

Here's how leaky gut syndrome works. Imagine that your cells need a kernel of corn. They are screaming out, "Hey, send me a kernel of corn." The bloodstream replies, "I have a can of corn, but I don't have a can opener." So the can goes around and around while the cells starve for corn. Finally, our immune system reacts by making antibodies against the can of corn, treating the corn as if it were a foreign invader. Your immune system has mobilized to finish the job of incomplete digestion, but this puts unneeded stress on it. The next time you eat corn, your body already has antibodies to react against it, which triggers the immune system, and so on. As time goes on, people with leaky gut syndrome tend to become more and more sensitive to a wider variety of foods and environmental contaminants.

Depending on our own susceptibilities, we may develop a wide variety of signs, symptoms, and health problems. Leaky gut syndrome is associated with the following medical problems: allergies, celiac disease, Crohn's disease, HIV, and malabsorption syndromes. It is also linked to autoimmune diseases such as AIDS, ankylosing spondylitis, asthma, atopy, bronchitis, eczema, food and environmental sensitivities, other allergic disorders, psoriasis, Reiter's syndrome, rheumatoid arthritis, Sjögren's syndrome, and skin irritations.

The listed conditions can arise from a variety of causes, but leaky gut syndrome may underlie more classic diagnoses. If you have any of the common symptoms or disorders associated with leaky gut syndrome, ask your physician to order an intestinal permeability test to see if it is causing your problem. In addition to clinical conditions, people with leaky gut syndrome display a wide variety of symptoms.

Leaky gut syndrome puts an extra burden on the liver. All foods pass directly from the bloodstream through the liver for filtration. The liver "humanizes" the food and either lets it pass or changes it, breaking down or storing all toxic or foreign substances. Water-soluble toxins are easily excreted, but the breakdown of fat-soluble toxins is a two-stage process that requires more energy. When the liver is bombarded by inflammatory irritants from incomplete digestion, it has less energy to neutralize chemical substances. When overwhelmed, it stores these toxins in fat cells, much the same way that we put boxes in the garage or basement to deal with at a later date. If the liver has time later, it can deal with the stored toxins, but most commonly it is busy dealing with what is newly coming in and never catches up. These toxins provide a continued source of inflammation to the body. Increased intestinal permeability has been found to be a factor in liver diseases, such as cirrhosis.

CLINICAL CLUES ASSOCIATED WITH LEAKY GUT SYNDROME

- Abdominal pain
- Aggressive behavior
- Anxiety
- Asthma
- Bed wetting
- Bloating
- Chronic joint pain
- Chronic muscle pain
- Confusion
- Constipation
- Diarrhea
- Fatigue and malaise
- Fevers of unknown origin
- Fuzzy thinking
- Gas
- Indigestion
- Mood swings
- Nervousness
- Poor exercise tolerance
- Poor immunity
- Poor memory
- Recurrent bladder infections
- Recurrent vaginal infections
- Shortness of breath
- Toxic feelings

The following are common clinical conditions associated with intestinal permeability:

- Acne
- Alcoholism

- Ankylosing spondylitis
- Arthritis
- Autism
- Behcet's syndrome
- Burns (severe)
- Celiac disease
- Chemotherapy for cancer treatment
- Childhood hyperactivity
- Chronic fatigue syndrome
- Cirrhosis
- Crohn's disease
- Cystic fibrosis
- Eczema
- Endotoxemia
- Environmental illness
- Food allergy and food sensitivity
- Giardia
- Hives
- HIV-positive status
- Intestinal infections
- Irritable bowel syndrome
- Liver dysfunction
- Malnutrition
- Multiple chemical sensitivities
- NSAIDs enteropathy
- Pancreatic insufficiency
- Psoriasis
- Schizophrenia
- Trauma
- Ulcerative colitis

TESTING FOR LEAKY GUT (INTESTINAL PERMEABILITY)

Typically, I don't recommend lactolose, mannitol testing for leaky gut. Rather, I use the clinical observations to determine the likelihood. Leaky gut is a symptom not a cause, so I look deeper. Does the client have food allergies or intolerances? Does he or she have parasites, yeast infections, or bacterial infections? Could high stress levels or medications be the cause of the leaky gut? Typically I will recommend a comprehensive stool analysis and/or look for food sensitivities. But for those of you who want something on paper proving that you have leaky gut, the lactulose-mannitol test is the gold standard. (See Chapter 11, "Functional Medicine/Functional Testing.")

WHAT CAUSES LEAKY GUT SYNDROME?

Leaky gut syndrome has no single cause, but some of the most common are chronic stress, dysbiosis, environmental contaminants, gastrointestinal disease, immune overload, overuse of alcoholic beverages, poor food choices, presence of pathogenic bacteria, parasites and yeasts, and prolonged use of NSAIDs. Let's discuss some of these one at a time.

Chronic Stress
Prolonged stress changes the immune system's ability to respond quickly and affects our ability to heal. It's like the story of the boy who cried wolf. If we keep hollering that there's a wolf every time we're late for an appointment or we need to finish a project by a deadline, our bodies can't tell the difference between this type of stress and real stress—like meeting a vicious dog in the woods or a death in the family. Our body reacts to these stressors by producing less secretory IgA (sIgA) (one of the first lines of immune defense) and less DHEA (an antiaging, antistress adrenal hormone) and by slowing down digestion and peristalsis, reducing blood flow to digestive organs, and producing toxic metabolites. Meditation, guided imagery, relaxation, and a good sense of humor can help us deal with daily stresses. We can learn to let small problems and traumas wash over us, not taking them too seriously.

Dysbiosis
The presence of dysbiosis contributes to leaky gut syndrome. Candida push their way into the lining of the intestinal wall and break down the brush borders. Candida

must be evaluated when leaky gut syndrome is suspected. Blastocystis hominis, giardia, helicobacter, salmonella, shigella, Yersinia enterocolitica, amoebas, and other parasites also irritate the intestinal lining and cause gastrointestinal symptoms. People who have or have had digestive illness or liver problems have an increased tendency to leaky gut syndrome. Which came first: the chicken or the egg?

Environmental Contaminants

Daily exposure to hundreds of household and environmental chemicals puts stress on our immune defenses and the body's ability to repair itself. This leads to chronic delay of necessary routine repairs. Our immune systems can pay attention to only so many places at one time, and parts of the body far away from the digestive system are affected. Connective tissue begins to break down, and we lose trace minerals like calcium, potassium, and magnesium. Environmental chemicals deplete our reserves of buffering minerals, causing acidosis in the cells and tissue and cell swelling. This is known as leaky cells—like having major internal plumbing problems!

Overconsumption of Alcoholic Beverages

Alcoholic drinks contain few nutrients but take many nutrients to metabolize. The most noteworthy of these are the B-complex vitamins. In fact, alcoholic beverages contain substances that are toxic to our cells. When alcohol is metabolized in the liver, the toxins are either broken down or stored by the body. Alcohol abuse puts a strain on the liver, which affects digestive competency, and also damages the intestinal tract.

Poor Food Choices

Low-fiber diets cause an increase in transit time, allowing toxic by-products of digestion to concentrate and irritate the gut mucosa. In addition, diets of highly processed foods injure our intestinal lining. Processed foods invariably are low in nutrients and fiber, with high levels of food additives, restructured fats, and sugar. These foods promote inflammation of the GI tract.

It's also important to note that even foods we normally think of as healthful, such as milk, wheat, and eggs, can be irritating to the gut lining.

Use of Medication

Nonsteroidal drugs such as Advil, aspirin, and Motrin, damage brush borders, allowing microbes, partially digested food particles, and toxins to enter the bloodstream. Birth control pills and steroid drugs also create conditions that help feed fungi, which damage the lining. Chemotherapy drugs and radiation therapy can also significantly disrupt GI balance.

Food and Environmental Sensitivities

Food and environmental sensitivities are usually the result of leaky gut syndrome. The prevalence of these sensitivities is more widely recognized today than in the past; 24 percent of American adults claim they have food and environmental sensitivities. These sensitivities, also called delayed hypersensitivity reactions, differ from true food allergies, also called type I or immediate hypersensitivity reactions.

Lectins

Lectins are found primarily in legumes and induce mast cells to produce histamine. They also bind to the intestinal mucosa, making it more porous and leaky.

RESTORING GUT INTEGRITY

If you believe you suffer from leaky gut, it's best to work with a health professional who can help you determine the underlying factors. Fortunately, you can find many ways to heal your gut. Some involve changing your habits, like chewing your food more completely; others involve taking specific supplements that will help your body repair itself. If you have food allergies or sensitivities, deal with them. Find out if you have an infection of some sort and get appropriate treatment. Replenish your bacterial flora with probiotics and prebiotics such as fructooligosaccharides (FOS). You may need to support your digestive function with enzymes, bitters, or hydrochloric acid tablets.

The following are steps you can take to help repair your gut. Supportive foods and supplemental nutrients can help repair the mucosal lining directly. Cabbage juice, cabbage family foods, bone broths, vegetable broths, fresh vegetable juices, aloe vera juice, okra, and slippery elm tea and lozenges all have a healing effect on the small intestine.

- Unlike the brain, which uses glucose for energy, the cells of the small intestine depend on glutamine as their main fuel and for maintenance and repair. Glutamine is the first nutrient I think of to repair a leaky gut. Glutamine is alkalizing to the body. It decreases the incidence of infection and stimulates the production of sIgA. Glutamine has also been shown to decrease the risk of bacterial translocation. Dosages can range from 1 to 30 grams daily, depending on your needs. Begin with 1 to 3 grams daily. Too much glutamine will probably constipate you, so that's a good gauge of how much you need. Many people find that they feel stronger and have more endurance when they take glutamine.

- Zinc may be an essential nutrient for gut repair. The type of zinc that shows the most promise for digestive healing is zinc carnosine. A typical dose is 75 mg of zinc carnosine twice daily.

- Take probiotics. L. plantarum is specifically soothing to the small intestine. (See Chapter 6 for more on probiotics.)

- Quercetin helps to heal leaky gut and also helps to modulate allergies by preventing histamine release. Be sure to get a high-quality quercetin product. I use Perque Pain Guard and Repair Guard, which couples quercetin with grape seed extract. The Repair Guard also contains pomegranate extract for antioxidant support. I wouldn't mention a brand, except in this case, it simply works better than other products. Take between 500 and 3,000 mg daily.

- Take proteolytic enzymes (protease, or protein-splitting enzymes) between meals. Protease helps to support immune function and also breaks down immune complexes. Dosage varies with product.

- Taking digestive enzymes with meals may ensure that all foods are completely digested. Take one to two digestive enzymes with meals.

Additional Supplements

- **Gamma oryzanol:** A compound found in rice bran oil, gamma oryzanol is a useful therapeutic tool in treating gastritis, irritable bowel syndrome, and ulcers. It has a healing effect throughout the digestive tract and can help normalize cholesterol and serum triglycerides, menopausal symptoms, and depression. Take 100 mg three times daily for three weeks or longer.

- **Seacure:** Seacure is a supplement made from deep-ocean white fish that has been broken down into peptides and amino acids. I don't know why, but the product is soothing and healing to the gut. This product is stinky; keeping it frozen can help with that. Take six capsules daily in divided doses.

- **Vitamin A:** Vitamin A is an essential nutrient for mucous membranes. Vitamin A is a two-edged sword, so monitor serum retinol levels and/or get your vitamin A from carotenoids, which can be converted into vitamin A in most, but not all, people. Plant foods that are rich sources of carotenoids are all green, yellow, and orange vegetables. Take 5,000 IU daily of preformed vitamin A and up to 25,000 IU carotenoids daily.

■ **Vitamin C:** With its strong antioxidant properties, vitamin C binds viruses and toxins to chelate them out of the body. Take 500 to 10,000 mg or more daily.

■ **Deglycyrrhized licorice:** Licorice root has many health-enhancing properties. It's soothing to the mucous membranes of the digestive tract, and chewable licorice can help reduce inflammation and pain. It promotes healing of mucous membranes by stimulating production of prostaglandins that promote healing and cell proliferation. It also has antibiotic and antioxidant properties. Use only deglycerrhized licorice; whole licorice root can raise blood pressure levels and lower potassium levels. Take two tablets between meals as needed up to four times daily.

■ **Antioxidant support:** Once the intestinal tract has been damaged, free radicals are often produced in quantities too large for the body to process. This causes inflammation and irritation, which exacerbate a leaky gut. So try eating antioxidant-rich foods like beans, fruits, vegetables, nuts, and seeds. Increasing use of antioxidant nutrients such as vitamin E, selenium, N-acetyl cysteine, superoxide dismutase (SOD), zinc (especially carnosine), manganese, copper, coenzyme Q10, lipoic acid, and vitamin C can help quench the free-radical fire.

■ **Phosphatidylcholine:** Research indicates that phosphatidylcholine helps to reduce intestinal permeability. Phosphatidylcholine is found in the mucous gel of the intestinal lumen and protects the GI tract. Take 2,000 to 4,000 mg daily.

As you can see, increased intestinal permeability (leaky gut) can underlie many different health conditions and contribute to ill health. Taking the steps mentioned here can help renew your health, yet this is an often overlooked factor in medicine today.

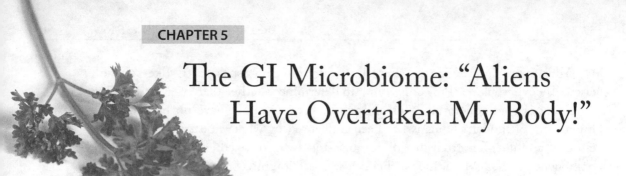

CHAPTER 5

The GI Microbiome: "Aliens Have Overtaken My Body!"

"Within these regions battles rage; populations rise and fall; affected just as we are by local environmental conditions, industry thrives and constant defense is exercised against interlopers and dangerous aliens who may enter unannounced; colonists roam and settle—some permanently, some only briefly, in general we have in miniature many of terrestrial life's vicissitudes, problems and solutions."

—Natasha Trenev and Leo Chaitow, *Probiotics*

We live in a great symbiotic harmony with bacteria. Our soils are filled with them. They thrive in our waters, in the hottest places on earth, below the seas, and in the air. On a personal level, bacteria comprise 10 percent of our dry body weight. Their story is one of wonder and the creation of life. They terraformed our planet and created oxygen in the air we breathe. They were the very first "world wide web" and were the first self-propelled beings on this planet. They are the initial substance of life, and without them plants and animals could not survive.

You have 10 times more bacteria in your gut than you have cells in your body. And those bacteria comprise 99 percent of the DNA in your body. If only 1 percent of our DNA is human, and 99 percent is alien, you have to ask the question, who hosts whom? These bacteria are called your microbiota and live in your digestive tract, skin, eyes, airways, blood, mouth, and vagina. You have billions of microbes in your mouth, many billions in your small intestine, and hundreds of trillions in your large intestine (half of the colon's volume). Each day, you produce several ounces of these microbes and eliminate several ounces in stool.

The microbiota function much like an organ, and they act as a major part of the immune system. They protect us from microbial and parasitic diseases, influence the effects of drugs, affect whether we are fat or thin, affect our nutritional status and overall health, and contribute to our rate of aging.

Your microbiota is like a fingerprint; yours probably isn't exactly like anyone else's. The Microbiome Project is trying to determine whether there is a "core" balance that is common to all of us and what effects it might have on health. The microbiota of modern humans has been influenced by what we eat as well as our climate, and it differs from that of our ancestors, who traveled less and ate a more homogeneous diet. Medications, chemicals, C-section births, breast-feeding versus bottle-feeding, stress, diet, and lifestyle all affect the balance if these gut bacteria. Bacterial infections, antibiotics use, high stress levels, excessive alcohol intake, poor diet, and a number of other factors can disrupt the delicate balance of beneficial bacteria in our gut. Often, disease-producing bacteria and fungi will proliferate, causing symptoms such as diarrhea, bloating, and gas. If left unchecked, they can contribute to long-term conditions such as irritable bowel syndrome.

After the Human Genome Project discovered that we have fewer genes than fruit flies or carrots, the Human Microbiome Project (www.nihroadmap.nih.gov/hmp/) was funded by the National Institutes of Health (NIH) to study what types of microbes inhabit our digestive system and what's normal. Bacteria "talk" to each other, and when there are enough of them, they turn on to become harmful. This is called "quorum sensing." It's like waiting until you amass enough troops to actually be effective before you try to scale the castle wall. It's believed that the cross talk between our genes and our bacteria runs our metabolism and modulates our immune system. Researchers for the Human Microbiome Project are exploring how microbes affect our metabolism, immune system, nutritional intake, and development and how they communicate with our genes and each other. All very cool!

THE GOOD, THE BAD, AND THE UGLY

You have somewhere between 500 and 1,000 types of bacteria in your digestive system, each type having hundreds of different strains. Although genetic research has discovered 40,000 different bacteria in the GI of different people so far, 80 to 90 percent of these are from two bacterial families or phyla. Bacteriodetes includes Bacteroides and Prevotella; the Firmicutes family includes Clostridium, Enterococcus, Lactobacillus, and Raminococcus. The next most common phylum is Actinobacteria, which includes Bifidobacteria, followed by Proteobacteria such as H. pylori and Escherichia (E. coli is an example of Escherichia). They have coevolved with humans; they come in in cultured and fermented food, from putting our fingers in our mouths, through being born, and other events. They weigh several pounds and have the same metabolic capacity as your liver. Some are permanent residents; others are just passing through.

Collectively these bacteria are called commensals, which means they are the normal bacteria in your gut. There is much yet to be learned about the benefits of commensal microbes that live within us. We are really at the edge of a frontier. In addition to commensal bacteria you have probiotic bacteria, or probiotics, which are beneficial to you, as well as pathogenic or disease-causing bacteria. You also have fungi and possibly some parasites in your microbiota.

Microbes that make us sick are called pathogens. These can cause acute or chronic illness. Some bacteria are extremely virulent and cause sudden and violent illness. Our body reacts to virulent bacteria, such as salmonella, with diarrhea, fever, loss of appetite, and vomiting. The body screams, "Get this stuff out of me!" and attempts to rapidly flush or starve it out. Most disease-causing microbes thrive at human body temperature, while fever kills them by overheating them. Some produce toxins that are more inflammatory than the bacteria.

Bacteria that cause chronic illness are generally weak organisms of low virulence. They are often found in small quantities in all of us and have been assumed to be harmless. But when given the opportunity to thrive, they can and do cause illness.

WHERE DO THEY COME FROM?

Until birth, we receive predigested food from our mothers, and our digestive tract is sterile. The trip down the birth canal then initiates us into the world of microbes that thrive everywhere. Babies are subsequently exposed to bacteria in breast milk and formula and when sucking on nipples, fingers, and toes. With every breath and touch, bacteria flock to an infant's skin and mucous membranes. In no time, every conceivable space in the colon is occupied by microbes. Within the first few days of life, colonization of E. coli and streptococcus occurs. Within a week of birth, bifido bacteria, bacteroides, and clostridium are established in bottle-fed babies. Breast-fed infants have increased numbers of lactobacillus and bifidobacteria species. As babies begin eating solid foods, they begin developing a balance of microbes that are more like adults.

The first two years of life are critical for our long-term immune responses. It's when we set up our lifelong microbiota fingerprint. Bacterial colonization patterns set up in infancy continue to prevail throughout our lifetime—and the foods and drugs to which we expose our children dramatically affect this delicate balance. The balance of these microbes change dynamically depending on the mother's microbes, place of delivery, whether there was a vaginal or C-section birth, whether the baby came to full term or was premature, hygiene (which when excessive can disrupt normal balance), use of antibiotics, having siblings or not, whether a baby is breast-fed or bottle-fed, and the foods that are eaten. This process normally happens in a predictable way, and, once established, the colonies flourish.

Babies who are unable to properly colonize friendly flora, however, can become irritable and colicky and have gas pains, diaper rash, or eczema. Babies who *don't* develop the right balance of beneficial bacteria are also more susceptible as they age to diarrhea, constipation, irritable bowel syndrome, allergy, asthma, and eczema. They are more prone to acne and severe gingivitis.

In a study of growth rate and probiotic supplementation, babies given bifido-bacteria showed better growth during their first six months of life; in another study, supplemental Lactobacillus acidophilus and L. casei decreased the severity and inci-dence of bronchitis and pneumonia in babies aged six months to two years. Adding probiotics to infant formula can reduce the need for antibiotics and can help prevent

---

PROBIOTIC BACTERIA HELP US IN MANY WAYS

Digestive

- Digest lactose
- Digest proteins to free amino acids
- Balance intestinal pH
- Improve or prevent irritable bowel syndrome
- Stop diarrhea
- Regulate peristalsis and improve diarrhea, constipation, IBS
- Reduce intestinal inflammation
- Protect gums and teeth

Nutritional

- Manufacture vitamins B_1, B_2, B_3, B_5, B_6, B_{12}, and K
- Increase absorption of minerals
- Minimize or eliminate lactose intolerance
- Aid in protein digestion
- Manufacture essential fatty acids and short-chain fatty acids
- Convert flavonoids to usable forms

Immune

- Prevent and treat diarrhea from antibiotics
- Prevent infection by producing antibiotic and antifungal substances
- Prevent and alleviate eczema, asthma, and allergies
- Prevent food poisoning
- Decrease severity and duration of respira-tory and other infections
- Break down bacterial toxins
- Protect against toxic substances
- Have antitumor and anticancer effects
- Prevent and control thrush, vaginal yeast infection, and bladder infection
- Break down and prevent synthesis of bacterial toxins
- Activate mucosal-associated lymphoid tissue (MALT)
- Protect and modulate autoimmune diseases

infections in preterm infants by giving their immune systems a boost. I've seen colicky babies become calm in less than 24 hours when given Bifidobacteria infantis—what a blessing!

THE MANY BENEFITS OF PROBIOTIC BACTERIA

Intestinal microbes play an important role in our ability to fight infectious disease, providing a front line in our immune defense. Friendly microbes also manufacture many nutrients, including vitamin K and several of the B-complex vitamins: biotin, B_1, B_2, B_3, B_5, B_6, B_{12}, and folic acid. Certain acid-secreting species increase our absorption of minerals including calcium, copper, iron, magnesium, and manganese. Probiotics improve peristalsis, help normalize bowel transit time, and are also

Heart
- Normalize serum cholesterol and triglycerides
- Support healthy blood pressure levels

Metabolic
- Break down and rebuild hormones
- Promote optimal growth
- Promote healthy metabolism and weight
- Break down bile acids
- Manufacture 5 to 10 percent of all short-chain fatty acids
- Reduce blood ammonia levels in people with cirrhosis and liver disease

Probiotic supplements may be beneficial for the following health conditions:
- Alcohol-induced liver disease
- Allergy, including food allergies
- Asthma
- Bacterial and fungal infections
- Bladder infections (recurrent)
- Cancer
- Complications from antibiotic therapy
- Constipation
- Dental health
- Diarrhea (all causes) in adults and children
- Eczema
- Elevated blood cholesterol
- Flatulence
- Hypertension
- Immune system stimulation
- Infectious diarrhea
- Inflammatory bowel diseases and pouchitis
- Irritable bowel syndrome
- Kidney stones
- Lactose intolerance
- Lupus erythematosus
- Necrotising enterocolitis
- Rheumatoid arthritis
- Small intestinal bacterial overgrowth
- Traveler's diarrhea and/or colitis
- Vaginal infections

important in preventing traveler's diarrhea. If you travel outside the United States, take a probiotic supplement daily, as studies show it significantly increases your ability to withstand the new microbes to which you will be exposed.

Native and supplemental probiotics help us in many additional ways. Some have antitumor and anticancer effects, and others help to keep our normal internal fungus population from proliferating out of control. Probiotics help us metabolize foreign substances like mercury and pesticides, protect us from damaging radiation and harmful pollutants, and break down and rebuild "used" hormones like estrogen. Although the mechanism is not yet understood, bacterial balance is also essential for healthy metabolism; many superthin people have been able to gain weight through the use of probiotic supplements.

BENEFITS OF SPECIFIC PROBIOTIC BACTERIA AND YEASTS

A probiotic is a specific type of bacteria or yeast that has been identified as a specific genus, species, and strain. Each type of probiotic has specific effects on the human body and is able to compete with disease-causing bacteria and reproduce in our intestinal tract for a week or two. Here are the criteria for probiotics:

Our two most important groups of intestinal flora are the lactobacilli, found mainly in the small intestine, and bifidobacteria, found primarily in the colon. Neither species is native to our digestive tract, but we can consume them in cultured dairy products or in supplements, and they "vacation" in us for up to 12 days in a mutually beneficial relationship. While on vacation they shore up the local economy, like all good tourists.

Lactobacilli and bifidobacteria secrete large amounts of acetic, formic, and lactic acid, which makes the intestinal environment inhospitable to invading microbes and helps prevent, or lessen the severity of, food poisoning. Some food-borne infections lead to chronic illness, causing heart and valve problems, immune system disorders, joint disease, and possibly even cancer. Use of supplemental acidophilus and bifidus can help prevent food poisoning by making the intestinal tract inhospitable to the invading microbes.

Lactobacilli manufacture antibiotics, such as acidophilin, produced by acidophilus, which are effective against many types of bacteria, including streptococcus and staph. Lactobacillus acidophilus and Lactobacillus bulgaricus have been shown to be effective in laboratory testing against the following pathogens: Bacillus subtilis,

CRITERIA FOR THE USE OF PROBIOTICS IN HUMANS

1. Identified at the genus, species, and strain level
   - The gold standard for species identification is DNA–DNA hybridization; 16S rRNA sequence determination is a suitable substitute, particularly if phenotypic tests are used for confirmation.
   - Strain typing should be performed by pulsed-field gel electrophoresis.
   - Strain should be deposited in an international culture collection.
2. Safe for food and clinical use
   - Nonpathogenic
   - Not degrading the intestinal mucosa
   - Not carrying transferable antibiotic resistance genes
   - Not conjugating bile acids
   - Susceptible to antibiotics
3. Able to survive intestinal transit; acid and bile tolerant
4. Able to adhere to mucosal surfaces
5. Able to colonize the human intestine or vagina (at least temporarily)
6. Producing antimicrobial substances
7. Able to antagonize pathogenic bacteria
8. Possessing clinically documented and validated health effects; at least one phase 2 study, preferably independent confirmation of results by another center
9. Stable during processing and storage

Used with permission from A. T. Borchers et al., "Probiotics and Immunity," *Journal of Gastroenterology* 44 (2009): 26–46. DOI 10.1007/s00535-008-2296-0.

Clostridium botulinum, Clostridium perfringens, Escherichia coli, Proteus mirabilis, Salmonella enteridis, Salmonella typhimurium, Shigella dysenteriae, Shigella paradysenteriae, Staphylococcus aureus, and Staphylococcus faecalis.

Candida albicans, a fungus that causes infections in nails and eyes, thrush, and yeast infections, is controlled by acidophilus. This works in at least two ways. First, acidophilus bacteria ferment glycogen into lactic acid, which changes the pH of the intestinal tract. Since candida and many other disease-causing microbes thrive in alkaline environments, this action discourages many disease-producing microbes. Second, specific strains of lactobacillus produce hydrogen peroxide, which kills candida directly. Studies show that supplementation with a hydrogen peroxide–producing strain of acidophilus, DDS-1, reduced the incidence of antibiotic-induced vaginal yeast infections threefold. Other probiotics have antitumor and anticancer effects. Probiotics also help us metabolize foreign substances, such as mercury and pesticides, and protect us from damaging radiation and harmful pollutants.

Saccharomyces boulardii, another probiotic, is a friendly yeast that enhances levels of sIgA. In France, it's called "yeast against yeast." It has been well studied

BENEFITS OF A FEW SPECIFIC PROBIOTIC BACTERIA

It is impossible in a book of this scope to describe all of our probiotic species, but the following lists highlight several of the most significant.

Benefits of Lactobacillus Acidophilus

- Prevents infections including candida, E. coli, H. pylori, and salmonella
- Prevents and treats antibiotic-associated diarrhea and traveler's diarrhea
- Aids digestion of lactose and dairy products
- Improves nutrient absorption
- Maintains integrity of intestinal tract
- Helps prevent vaginal and urinary tract infections

Benefits of Lactobacillus Reuteri

- Inhibits growth of disease-causing microbes including gram-negative and gram-positive bacteria, yeast, fungi, and protozoa
- Appears to inhibit adherence of pathogens in the gut
- Shortens duration of children's rotaviral infections, which cause diarrhea
- Has protective and therapeutic effect on vaginal infections

Benefits of Bifidobacteria Infantis

- Helps treat colic, cradle cap, and eczema in infants and babies
- May protect against bacteria that promote inflammatory bowel disease
- Helpful to alleviate the symptoms of irritable bowel syndrome
- With L. acidophilus, reduces illness and deaths from necrotizing enterocolitis (NEC) in infants
- Has antitumor properties in test research

and used clinically for more than 50 years. It is safe for people of all ages, including infants. It is resistant to antibiotics, except antifungal medications, so it can be used while taking antibiotics. It helps protect and restore normal flora, and it stimulates the production of sIgA and IgG, antibodies that are the first line of defense against pathogens. It also stimulates enzymatic production, helping to repair and maintain normal gut mucosa, and stimulates the activity of short-chain fatty acids and disaccharide enzymes, such as lactase, maltase, and sucrase, which can help prevent diarrhea.

When used therapeutically, S. boulardii is useful for stopping diarrhea caused by traveling, antibiotics, AIDS, and severe burns. It has also been used effectively in people with Crohn's disease, significantly reducing the number of bowel movements and diarrhea, and it has been used to help people with diarrhea-type irritable bowel syndrome.

S. boulardii helps protect against bacteria and bacterial toxins by preventing them from attaching to the intestinal mucosa or specific receptor sites. Studies have shown its effectiveness against disease-causing strains of E. coli, Clostridium difficile, cholera, and Entamoeba histolytica. Studies indicate that it may also be effective against salmonella, the main cause of food poisoning.

E. coli strain Nissle has also been used effectively in digestive diseases. It's best been studied for its role in protection from inflammatory bowel diseases and irritable bowel syndrome.

The GI Microbiome: Probiotics Naturally from Food and Supplements

Beneficial bacteria do not permanently stay in the gut, so we need to regularly get them from foods, such as yogurt or kefir, or use a supplement.

In healthy people, the composition of the intestinal population usually remains fairly constant, but it can become unbalanced by aging, diet, disease, drugs, poor health, or stress. Health problems resulting from unbalanced flora have now become widespread. Eating cultured dairy products and other foods can maintain colonies of friendly flora in people who are already healthy, but once disease-producing microbes get established, probiotic supplements may be necessary to rebalance the internal community. Until recently, it was believed that taking these supplements would cause the desired organisms to colonize in the gut; newer research indicates, however, that they probably don't. Instead it is believed that these are transient residents in our digestive system. They "vacation" in our bodies for up to 12 days. Just like tourists who boost local economies, these visitors have a beneficial effect on our intestinal ecosystem. This makes a great argument for eating cultured and fermented foods and/or taking probiotics on a regular basis.

Bacteria manufacture nutrients for their own benefit, but we can reap the rewards. Pretty much any food that is cultured or fermented contains probiotics and increased nutrients. By having cottage cheese and yogurt rather than milk (see Table 6.1), sauerkraut rather than cabbage, tofu and tempeh rather than soybeans, and wine rather than grapes, we obtain higher dietary levels of such nutrients as vitamins A, B-complex, and K.

Table 6.1   **Nutritionally Enhanced Dairy Foods**

Original Food	Fermented/Cultured Food	Increased Nutrition
Milk	Cheddar cheese	Vitamin B_1, 3x
Milk	Cottage cheese	Vitamin B_{12}, 5x
Milk	Yogurt	Vitamin B_{12}, 5–30x
Milk	Yogurt	Vitamin B_3, 50x
Skim milk	Low-fat yogurt	Vitamin A, 7–14x

With or without knowledge of the scientific principles involved, people around the world have long recognized the health benefits of fermented foods. They have been used for thousands of years. Fermentation is a low-cost, efficient, and easy-to-use process that preserves foods without the need for refrigeration or other high-tech processes. Traditional sauerkraut has historically been eaten by Europeans to combat ulcers and digestive problems. Asian cultures serve pickled daikon radish and kimchi as condiments and drink a sweet rice beverage called *amasake*. Lactose-intolerant people worldwide have relied for centuries on cultured dairy products such as cottage cheese, kefir, and yogurt; in India, the fermented dairy drink lassi is a household staple, and in Israel, yogurtlike *leban* is served daily. Each year, Japan produces more than a billion liters of soy sauce to use nationally. In many African cultures, fermented cassava products, such as gari and fufu, comprise about 50 percent of the calories eaten each day.

Many foods are fermented or cultured with the use of lactic-acid-producing bacteria, such as Lactobacillus, Leuconostoc, Pediococcus, and Streptococcus. During the fermentation process, carbohydrates are converted into lactic acid and organic acids that are used in our bodies for energy production. The lactic-acid-producing bacteria also inhibit the growth of disease-causing microbes. L. plantarum, one of the most soothing of all probiotics, creates the acid that's present in "sour" vegetables, such as sauerkraut. Leuconostoc mesenteroides is the main bacteria associated with sauerkraut and pickles. The Propionibacteriaceae family of bacteria provide the flavor and holes in Swiss cheese. The acetic-acid-producing bacteria, Acetobacter, change foods, such as apples and grapes, into vinegar.

Yogurt traditionally contains types of probiotic bacteria: Lactobacillus bulgaricus and Streptoccus thermophiles. Eli Mechnikoff won the Nobel Prize in 1908 for demonstrating that the bacteria in yogurt prevented and reversed bacterial infection.

He named L. bulgaricus after the long-lived, yogurt-loving peasants of Bulgaria. These "tourists" have a beneficial effect on our intestinal ecosystem by enhancing the production of bifidobacteria and having antitumor effects. L. bulgaricus also has antibiotic and antiherpes effects.

The traditional Japanese diet takes advantage of several fermented soy foods that have antibiotic properties. Miso paste, for example, contains 161 strains of aerobic bacteria, almost all of which compete successfully with the main food-poisoning agents E. coli and Staphylococcus aureus, and contains many lactic-acid-producing bacteria as well. Several microbes, including yeast and L. acidophilus, are used to brew health-giving soy sauce, also called shoyu or tamari. (In the United States, however, most soy sauce is manufactured with inorganic acids that break down the soybeans, rather than by fermentation with living microbes, so it doesn't have the same benefits.)

Probiotic-Rich Foods

Amasake	Kefir	Raw whey
Beer (microbrew)	Kimchi	Root and ginger
Black tea, oolong tea	Kombucha	beers
Buttermilk	Lassi	Sauerkraut
Cheese	Leban	Sourdough breads
Chocolate	Miso	(traditionally
Coconut kefir	Natto	made)
Coffee	Olives	Tempeh
Cottage cheese	Pickles (brine cured,	Wheat grass juice
Fermented sausages	not vinegar)	Wine
and meats	Pulke	Yogurt
Fermented vegetables	Raw vinegars	

Certain herbs also promote the growth of friendly flora. Polyphenols provide the colors in fruits, vegetables, beans, seeds, nuts, and grain. Polyphenols like those in green tea, red wine, apples, onions, and chocolate have been shown to increase the number of beneficial intestinal bacteria such as lactobacilli and bifidobacteria while decreasing the number of disease-causing bacteria. A significant increase in beneficial flora was also found when an extract of the herb Panax ginseng was tested in vitro on 107 types of human-dwelling bacteria. While more research needs to be done, it appears that here is just one more reason to eat our veggies!

PROBIOTIC SUPPLEMENTS

In addition to getting probiotics naturally from our food each day, they can be obtained by taking probiotic supplements. I am frequently asked about which probiotics to take, when to take them, and what type of dosage is required.

Buying Probiotic Supplements

The many probiotic supplements on the market look similar but can be extremely different in their effectiveness. Consumer Lab tested 25 probiotic products. Eight of them contained less than 1 percent of the number of probiotic bacteria listed on the label. It is important to use well-researched probiotics that have been found useful in clinical settings. So how can you know which products are best? Always look for a batch number and expiration date. Purchase your products from a health professional or store where someone has done the research for you.

Typically I look for mixed probiotic supplements that contain Lactobacillus acidophilus plus Bifidobacteria strains. However, there are times when you may choose to use a specific strain or specific probiotic. For example, for chronic diarrhea, you may choose to use Saccharomyces boulardii by itself. If you are lactose intolerant, you may choose to buy a dairy-free probiotic. However, some people find that by using dairy-based probiotics they become more lactose tolerant. The best test is to try them out and see what your body likes best.

What Types of Microbes Am I Looking For? Look for the normal gut flora such as lactobacilli and bifidobacteria. Supplements may also contain the species Lactobacillus casei, L. reuteri, Bifidobacteria longum, B. breve, L. lactis, L. rhamnosus, and others (see Table 6.2). Bifidobacteria infantis is the most appropriate choice for a newborn and is also useful for children and adults who have IBS.

More is being learned about specific strains of probiotics. Just as a poodle is not the same as an English setter, two strains of acidophilus or bifidobacteria can be very different. According to Natasha Trenev, an expert on probiotics, various strains of acidophilus can differ genetically by as much as 20 percent. This is a huge difference when you consider that the genetic difference between mice and man is about 2 percent.

Some supplements contain soil-based probiotics such as Bacillus laterosporus, B. subtilis, and L. sporonges (also known as B. coagulous), but research in peer-reviewed journals has yet to substantiate the many anecdotal stories of great success with these soil-based organisms. In fact, all of the literature seems to be about the disease potential of these bacteria. Therefore, I cannot recommend them at this point in time.

Viability and Potency. Most probiotics supply between 1 billion and 25 billion organisms per dose, and a few supply substantially more, up to 450 billion. The number, however, isn't the important thing, as some studies have shown supplements to be effective even when they contain only millions of organisms. What matters is whether the product contains living, viable organisms that adhere to the gut lining, are not destroyed by bile, and have benefit once in your body. Yet there is still much to be learned. Research indicates that even dead probiotics can have profound effects on the immune system.

Probiotics come in two main types: those that need refrigeration and those that don't. I generally prefer the refrigerated varieties. These delicate bacteria must be

Table 6.2   **Bacteria and Yeast Used as Probiotics in Supplements and Food**

Bifidobacteria	Lactobacilli	Streptococcus	Other Species
B. bifidum	L. acidophilus	S. thermophilus	Enterococcus faecium
B. breve	L. bulgaricus	S. jacium	Saccharomyces boulardii
B. longum	L. rhamnosus	S. jaecali	Lactococcus cremoris
B. adolescentis	L. casei	S. lactis	E. coli Nissle (not available in USA)
B. pseudocatenulatum	L. gasseri	S. salivarius	E. faccalis
B. catenulatum	L. brevis	S. cremoris	Aspergillus sp.
B. animalis lactis	L. debreuckii	S. diacetylactis	
B. thermophilum	L. lactis	S. intermedius	
B. angulatum	L. kefir	S. cerevisaie	
	L. yoghuni		
	L. plantarum		
	L. salavarius		
	L. reuteri		
	L. cellebiosus		
	L. fermentum		
	L. curvatus		

refrigerated in shipping, at the store, and in your home to ensure their life span and greatest potency. Probiotics will maintain potency at room temperature for short periods of time; for instance, if you are on vacation for a week or two you'll probably lose a few percentages of potency. If you left them out for several months, they'd be dead. I personally put a week's worth of probiotics in my supplement container so that I don't forget to take them.

Bacteria multiply very quickly, but they need enough food and protection to survive the trip through the stomach and into the intestinal tract, so many probiotic supplements also contain prebiotics such as fructooligosaccharide (FOS) and inulin, which provide nourishment for the bacteria (see the section "Prebiotics" later in this chapter).

What to Look for in a Probiotic Supplement

- Look for Lactobacillus acidophilus and Bifidobacteria bifidum.
- Choose an age-appropriate product. For a baby or toddler, B. infantis is appropriate; for children and adults, the most-studied strain of L. acidophilus is DDS-1.
- Choose a product that is condition appropriate when it's available. There are now supplements that are specific for lactose intolerance, sugar malabsorption, irritable bowel syndrome, and diarrhea. There may soon be other specific products for psoriasis, vaginal infections, inflammatory bowel disease, and other health conditions.
- Most of the best products come refrigerated. There are some viable products on the market that are stored at room temperature.
- Bacteria multiply very quickly, but they need enough food once they reach the intestines. Some products contain inulin, FOS, or other prebiotics that help the flora grow. This can vastly improve the viability of the product. Just note that some people bloat from FOS.
- Combination supplements with several types of flora are helpful. Bacteria compete for the same food supply, so look for freeze-dried products. Freeze-drying puts the flora into suspended animation, keeping them dormant until placed in water or in your body.

Finding the Appropriate Dosage

For daily prevention take 1 billion to 25 billion organisms daily.

Therapeutic dosages vary depending on the severity of the condition. You may find 1 billion or 2 billion organisms daily keep you well and rebalance you. Other people may need 25 billion to 100 billion organisms, or more. After antibiotics, I typically recommend doses between 30 billion and 100 billion organisms daily.

Studies on people with ulcerative colitis have found benefit in dosages of more than 2 trillion microorganisms daily.

Begin taking the probiotics at a low level and increase the dose slowly. If you experience bloating, diarrhea, gas, or worsening of symptoms, stop taking your probiotics. As the disease-producing bacteria and fungus are killed, they release chemicals that aggravate symptoms. Begin again with tiny amounts and build up your dosage slowly to avoid the die-off reaction. Symptoms like this usually tip you off that what you are doing is correct; however, if that's true, they begin to subside after a few days. Of course, if the symptoms continue, do go see a doctor.

PREBIOTICS

Prebiotics are saccharide (sugar) molecules that play an important role in health maintenance. Prebiotics also nourish and stimulate the growth of "good" bacteria while promoting a reduction in disease-causing bacteria such as clostridia, klebsiella, and enterobacter. Prebiotics work synergistically with probiotics and can be taken together for best results (together, they are called synbiotics). You will often find them in your probiotic supplements. Like probiotics, they acidify the intestinal environment, enhancing the absorption of essential minerals.

Benefits of Prebiotics
- Promote the growth of bifidobacteria and lactobacilli
- Lower colon pH
- Discourage growth of clostridia
- Prevent constipation and diarrhea
- Help keep blood sugar levels even
- Useful for people with liver disease to lower ammonia levels

The most common prebiotics are FOS and inulin. They typically come from Jerusalem artichoke and chicory. FOS has been shown to lower serum triglyceride levels and insulin levels. FOS and inulin also protect against colon cancer and help normalize insulin levels. These fibers have been shown to increase levels of acidophilus and bifidobacteria. Dosages as low as 2.75 grams daily in adults will dramatically increase bifidobacteria. They have also been shown to be antagonistic to at least eight bacteria, including salmonella, listeria, campylobacter, shigella, and vibrio.

Because of their health-building qualities, inulin and FOS are being investigated worldwide as possible functional food additives, but they are naturally found in our food already. On average, we consume about 2.5 grams per day of FOS alone. Honey is a good prebiotic food; in a recent test-tube study of prebiotics' effect on bifidobacteria, honey worked as well as FOS, galactooligosaccharide (GOS), and inulin in promoting the bacteria's production of lactic and acetic acid. Other foods with prebiotics include the following:

- Asparagus
- Bananas
- Burdock root
- Bran
- Chicory
- Chinese chives
- Cottage cheese
- Dandelion greens
- Eggplant
- Endive
- Fruit
- Garlic
- Green tea
- Honey
- Jerusalem artichokes
- Jicama
- Kefir
- Leeks
- Legumes
- Onions
- Peas
- Radicchio
- Rye
- Soybeans
- Sugar maple
- Wheat
- Yogurt

Many people experience gas and bloating when they start taking prebiotics, but these symptoms usually dissipate after a week or so; if they do occur, you can either continue your current dosage or lower the dosage and then increase it gradually. Human studies of prebiotic use show the greatest growth of helpful bacteria in the people who need it most, with benefits most evident at doses up to 10 grams daily. After you stop taking prebiotics, your internal bacteria will return to previous levels in about two to three weeks.

The GI Microbiome: Dysbiosis, a Good Neighborhood Gone Bad

Dysbiosis is not so much about the microbe as it is about the effect of that bacteria, yeast, or parasite on a susceptible person. It's about the relationship between the microbe and the host. Dysbiosis can occur in the digestive system as well as on your skin, vagina, lungs, nose, sinuses, ears, nails, or eyes. Typically dysbiosis doesn't appear as a classic type of infection. These imbalances generally simmer along. After all, if the microbes were too virulent, you'd die. It's in their best interests to learn to coexist with you and not make you too uncomfortable so that you also just learn to live with it! Dysbiosis may express itself as irritable bowel syndrome in one person, migraines in another, eczema, psoriasis, autoimmune illness, depression, and other illnesses.

The term *dysbiosis* was coined by Dr. Eli Metchnikoff early in the 20th century. It comes from *dys-*, which means "not," and *symbiosis*, which means "living together in mutual harmony." Dr. Metchnikoff was the first scientist to discover the useful properties of probiotics. He won the Nobel Prize in 1908 for his work on lactobacilli and their role in immunity and was a colleague of Louis Pasteur, succeeding him as the director of the Pasteur Institute in Paris.

Dr. Metchnikoff found that the bacteria in yogurt prevented and reversed bacterial infection. His research proved that lactobacilli could displace many disease-producing organisms and reduce the toxins they generated. He believed these endotoxins (toxins produced from substances inside the body) shortened life span. He advocated use of lactobacillus in the 1940s for ptomaine poisoning, a widely used therapy in Europe. He was also the first to note that these benefits were greatest in babies and in the eldery.

In more recent decades, Metchnikoff's work has taken a backseat to modern therapies, such as antibiotics and immunization programs, which scientists hoped would conquer infectious diseases. Microbes are extremely adaptable. In our efforts to eradicate them we have pushed them to evolve. Long before chemists created antibiotics, yeasts, fungi, and rival bacteria were producing antibiotics to ward each other off and establish neighborhoods. They became adept at evading each other's strategies and adapting for survival. Because people have used antibiotics indiscriminately in humans and animals, the bacteria have had a chance to learn from it, undergoing rapid mutations. They talk to each other and borrow plasmids, which are incorporated into their genetic structure. As they shuffle their components, learning new evolutionary dance steps, superstrains of bacteria have been created that no longer respond to any antibiotic treatment. For instance, our immune systems normally detect bacteria by information coded on the cell walls. Now, in response to antibiotics, some bacteria have survived by removing their cell walls, so they're able to enter the bloodstream and tissues unopposed, causing damage in organs and tissues. Given people's rapid movement between countries, these new microbes have spread quickly throughout the world, increasing the risk of even more mutation and enhancement of the microbial defense system.

Dysbiosis weakens our ability to protect ourselves from disease-causing microbes, which are generally composed of low-virulence organisms. Unlike salmonella, which causes immediate food-poisoning reactions, low-virulence microbes are insidious. They cause chronic problems that go undiagnosed in the great majority of cases. If left unrecognized and untreated, they become deep-seated and may cause chronic health problems, including joint pain, diarrhea, chronic fatigue syndrome, or colon disease.

Because most doctors in our culture do not yet recognize dysbiosis, often people do not get well. Published research has listed dysbiosis as the cause of arthritis, diarrhea, autoimmune illness, B_{12} deficiency, chronic fatigue syndrome, cystic acne, cystitis, the early stages of colon and breast cancer, eczema, fibromyalgia, food allergy or sensitivity, inflammatory bowel disease, irritable bowel syndrome, psoriasis, restless leg syndrome, and steatorrhea. These problems were previously unrecognized as being microbial in origin. Common dysbiotic bacteria are aeromonas, citrobacter, helicobacter, klebsiella, salmonella, shigella, Staphylococcus aureus, vibrio, and yersinia. Helicobacter, for example, is commonly found in people with ulcers. Citrobacter is implicated in diarrheal diseases. A common dysbiosis culprit, the candida fungus causes a wide variety of symptoms that range from gas and bloating to depression, mood swings, and premenstrual syndrome (PMS).

Common Symptoms and Diseases Associated with Dysbiosis

Arthritis	Foul-smelling stools
Asthma	Frequent indigestion
Autoimmune diseases	Gas
Bad breath	Gastritis
Belching	Inflammatory bowel disease
Bloating	Interstitial cystitis
Bowel urgency	Irritable bowel syndrome
Celiac disease	Itching in vagina, anus, or other
Constipation, chronic	mucous membranes
Cramping	Mucus or blood in stool
Cystic acne	Nausea after taking supplements
Depression or anxiety	Rectal itching
Diarrhea, chronic	Restless leg syndrome
Digestive infections that recur	Sinus congestion, chronic
Fatigue	Skin conditions
Fibromyalgia	Undigested food in stool
Food allergies, intolerances,	Weight loss due to malabsorption
sensitivities	

COMMON PATTERNS OF DYSBIOSIS

The lines between these types of dysbiosis often blur, and people often have more than one of these patterns.

- **Insufficiency dysbiosis:** This is when you don't have enough "good" probiotic in your digestive system. This is common in people who took antibiotics as young children and in people who are currently taking or have taken many antibiotics. Low-fiber diets are another cause. Insufficiency dysbiosis is often seen in people with irritable bowel syndrome and food sensitivities and is often coupled with putrefaction dysbiosis. To restore balance, eat probiotic- and prebiotic-rich food and/or take supplemental probiotics, and eat 25 to 40 grams of fiber each day.

- **Putrefaction dysbiosis:** This occurs when you don't have enough digestive enzymes, hydrochloric acid, and probiotic bacteria to enable you to fully digest your proteins. High-fat, high-animal-protein, low-fiber diets predispose people to putrefaction due to an increase of bacteroides bacteria, a decrease in beneficial bifidobacteria, and an increase in bile production. Bacteroides cause vitamin B_{12} deficiency by uncoupling the B_{12} from the intrinsic factor necessary for its use. Research has implicated putrefaction dysbiosis with hormone-related cancers such as breast, prostate, and colon cancer. Bacterial enzymes change bile acids into 33 substances formed in the colon that are tumor promoters. Bacterial enzymes, such as betaglucuronidase, re-create estrogens that were already broken down and put into the colon for excretion. These estrogens are reabsorbed into the bloodstream, increasing estrogen levels. Putrefaction dysbiosis can be corrected by eating more high-fiber foods, fruits, vegetables, and grains, and fewer meats and fats.

- **Fermentation dysbiosis:** We don't form gas; the bacteria in our gut do. They eat our carbohydrates, and the by-products of fermentation create gas. Eating sugar, fruit, beer, wine, starchy vegetables, and grains makes this worse. Typically a low-carbohydrate diet helps bring this back into balance. Think about implementing a low-carbohydrate type of diet such as Atkins, Anti-Fungal Diet, Specific Carbohydrate Diet (SCD), or Gut and Psychology Syndrome (GAPS) diet. (You can read more about these diets in Chapter 13.) Fermentation dysbiosis is typically coupled with bacterial and fungal dysbiosis.

- **Bacterial overgrowth dysbiosis:** Bacteria may move (translocate) from the colon into the small intestine, or they may grow in the small intestine due to low levels of hydrochloric acid. People experience this often as gas and bloating, diarrhea, discomfort, and sometimes constipation. Bacterial overgrowth is often coupled with fermentation dysbiosis. Common types include Clostridium difficile, H. pylori, infectious E. coli, and Clostridium perfringens. Think about implementing an Atkins, Specific Carbohydrate, or GAPS diet. (See "Small Intestinal Bacterial Overgrowth" and "Helicobacter Pylori" in Chapter 8.)

- **Fungal dysbiosis:** We normally have a fair number of Candida species, a diploid fungus in the yeast family, in our natural microbiome. Antibiotics, stress, sugar, steroids, and other medications can give them the opportunity to quickly grow, causing a myriad of ill effects. True to dysbiosis, these yeasts can colonize on skin (athlete's food, eczema, psoriasis), in the vagina, in the small intestine, in the nose (some chronic sinusitis), on the scalp (seborrhea, cradle cap), and elsewhere in the body. They are always coupled with fermentation dysbiosis. In fact, in rare people Candida manufacture enough alcohol to make people drunk. (See "Candida: The Masquerader" in Chapter 8.)

- **Parasitic dysbiosis:** Many people have amoebas, fluke, cysts, other protozoa, and other parasites. (See "Parasites" in Chapter 8.)

- **Immune-inflammatory dysbiosis:** Microbes produce toxins that affect the immune system by suppressing it. For example, gliotoxin is produced by Candida albicans. This leads to inflammation in the mucosal tissues of the small intestinal lumen. This inflammation can lead to leaky gut and malabsorption.

It can also set the stage for hypersensitivity-allergic dysbiosis in people who are susceptible.

■ **Hypersensitivity-allergic dysbiosis:** Some people have an exaggerated immune response to otherwise "normal" yeast and bacteria due to their genetic predisposition. Our body initially reacts to a microbe of some sort, but the antibodies formed to fight it are what set off autoimmune reactions. This is called gene mimicry. Ankylosing spondylitis, rheumatoid arthritis, reactive arthritis, Reiter's syndrome, and psoriatic arthritis also fall into this category. Other people may experience acne, IBS, eczema, or psoriasis. These people often have food intolerances, leaky gut, and environmental sensitivities as well. Replacing probiotic bacteria, avoiding foods that you are sensitive to, and repairing the intestinal mucosa are essential.

WHAT CAUSES DYSBIOSIS?

While there are many causes of dysbiosis, we generally bring it on ourselves. Constant high levels of stress, use of antacids and proton-pump inhibitors, exposure to manufactured chemicals, poor food choices, gluten sensitivity, chronic constipation, oral contraceptives, gastric surgery including gastric bypass surgery, and use of antibiotics and painkillers all change the healthy balance of the digestive tract.

Antibiotics

The most common cause of dysbiosis is the use of antibiotics, which change the balance of intestinal microbes. Not terribly specific, antibiotics simultaneously kill both harmful and helpful bacteria throughout our digestive system, mouth, vagina, and skin, leaving the territory to bacteria, parasites, viruses, and yeasts that are resistant to the antibiotic that was used. In a healthy gut, parasites may be present in small numbers and not cause symptoms, but if allowed to flourish they can cause diarrhea, illness, and weight loss. Most people can recover fairly easily from a single round of antibiotics, but even those with strong constitutions may have trouble regaining balance from repeated use of antibiotic drugs. I've worked with many clients whose doctors bounce them between antibiotic, antifungal, and antiparasitic drugs. Many feel better after a regimen like this, but some feel worse than before they began.

Antacids and Proton-Pump Inhibitors

These medications are designed to block hydrochloric acid production in the stomach. This acid acts as a first line of defense against microbes that come in as guests with our food. When blocked, our defense is gone.

Endotoxins

These microbes produce toxins that cause symptoms. The bacteria form chemicals that are poisonous to the cells around them and to the person they live in. A wide variety of substances are produced, including amines, ammonia, hydrogen sulfide, indoles, phenols, and secondary bile acids. These substances may hurt the intestinal lining directly by damaging the brush border and become absorbed into the bloodstream, causing system-wide effects. Initially, our body rushes white blood cells to the injured tissue to eat up the bacteria and carry away the debris via the lymphatic system. Cytokines and other inflammation markers rush to the scene. If all is in balance, the infection will soon go away. But if our immune system is overwhelmed, the dysbiosis will continue and we will eventually experience pain, discomfort, and leaky membranes.

Diet

Poor diet also contributes to dysbiosis. High-fat, high-protein diets and low-fiber diets can contribute to dysbiosis because these diets slow down bowel motility. A diet high in fat, sugar, and processed foods may not have enough nutrients to optimally nourish the body or repair and maintain the digestive organs. The nutrients most likely to be lacking are the antioxidants (vitamins C and E, beta-carotene, coenzyme Q10, glutathione, selenium, the sulfur amino acids, and zinc), the B-complex vitamins, calcium, essential fatty acids, and magnesium.

Ileocecal Valve Gets Stuck

Poor ileocecal valve function can contribute to dysbiosis. The valve's job is to keep waste matter in the colon from mixing with the useful material that is still being digested and absorbed in the small intestine. When this valve is stuck, either open or closed, dysbiotic problems can occur. Chiropractors can adjust the ileocecal valve to alleviate this problem.

TESTING FOR DYSBIOSIS OF ALL TYPES

This list offers the most common tests that are used to assess whether you have dysbiosis. You can find more detailed information on functional testing in Chapter 11.

- Crook's yeast questionnaire (for candida and fungal infection)
- Comprehensive stool testing
- Organic acid testing; this is the best test for candida and also can sometimes disclose small intestinal bacterial overgrowth (SIBO)
- Hydrogen or methane breath testing for SIBO

- Antigen tests for H. pylori, C. difficile, and others
- Working empirically and seeing how you respond

THERAPEUTIC DIETS FOR DYSBIOSIS

Many, many therapeutic programs are available for people to follow to rid themselves of candida, SIBO, and other bacterial infections. Remember that yeasts and bacteria eat sugars and carbohydrates, so all of these diets limit sugars and carbohydrates. I find that the diet is hugely successful when used along with probiotics. Sometimes medications, herbs, or homeopathic medicines are also needed to irradicate the infection itself.

TREATING DYSBIOSIS

You probably will use only some of these treatments. Choose one type of prebiotic fiber. Choose one type of herbal therapy *or* use a product that contains a combination of herbs.

Probiotics: Dose Depends on Severity of the Situation

Dosages of probiotic supplements vary depending on whether you are taking antibiotics and what stage of the pattern you are in. Dosages as high as 3.6 trillion microorganisms of VSL-3 have been used instead of steroids to stop ulcerative colitis flare-ups. Caution: Using dosages this high should be supervised by a physician.

- Lactobacillus: 10 billion to 100 billion live organisms daily or higher.
- Saccharomyces boulardii: 250 to 3,000 mg daily. Use specifically if you are taking antibiotics or experiencing diarrhea.
- Bifidobacterium (various species): 10 billion to 100 billion live organisms daily or higher.
- Combination products work well that contain Lactobacilli, Bifidobacterium, and other probiotic species.

Prebiotics

- Fructooligosaccharides (FOS) or inulin or larch arabinogalactins: 500 to 5,000 mg daily
- Modified citrus pectin: 3,000 to 5,000 mg daily
- High-soluble fiber

COMMON DIETS FOR DYSBIOSIS
- Elimination diet
- Body Ecology Diet
- Yeast diet
- Specific Carbohydrate Diet (SCD)
- Gut and Psychology Syndrome (GAPS) Diet

Herbal Therapy
- Garlic: Either several cloves of garlic eaten daily or standardized to 5,000 mcg allicin potential three times daily
- Goldenseal or berberine: Standardized to contain 200 to 400 mg of berberine; 200 to 400 mg three times daily
- Wormwood or Chinese wormwood: 1,000 to 3,000 mg three times daily
- Grapefruit seed extract: 250 to 500 mg three times daily
- Oregano (Origanum vulgare) oil: 200 mg three times daily
- Thyme (Thymus vulgaris): Standardized to contain thymol, 100 to 200 mg three times daily

Aromatic oils such as caraway, bitter orange, sweet fennel, star anise, lavender, peppermint, and Ajowan oils have been shown to inhibit disease-causing microbes while preserving healthy GI balance.

Pharmaceuticals
- Rifaxamin (brand name: Xifaxan): 1,200 mg daily seven days (for SIBO)
- Ciprofloxacin (brand names: Cipro, Proquin): 250 to 750 mg every 12 hours
- Norfloxacin (brand name: Noroxin): 250 to 750 mg every 12 hours
- Co-trimoxazole (brand names: Septra, Bacrim): 500 to 875 mg every 12 hours

As you can see from these recommendations, dosages can be complicated. When treating dysbiosis, I would advise you to work with someone experienced in this area. I've seen too many of my own clients who have been put on medication after medication. While sometimes medication is necessary, first try to heal the environment with diet and lifestyle change. Dietary change can have the most profound effect of all yet alone is typically not enough to permanently correct the dysbiosis. Use a combination of lifestyle change, diet, pre- and probiotics, and either herbal or pharmaceutical substances to get the best effect.

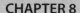

CHAPTER 8

The GI Microbiome: Specific and Common Dysbiosis Infections

In Chapter 7, we discussed dysbiosis in general terms. In this chapter we are breaking it down into some of the common, specific types. Here you will learn about H. pylori, chronic fungal infections, small intestinal bacterial overgrowth, and parasites.

HELICOBACTER PYLORI

In 1982, Australian physician Barry Marshall discovered the presence of Helicobacter pylori (H. pylori) between the stomach lining and the mucous membrane. Until their discovery, ulcers were believed to be caused by stress and lifestyle alone. In 2005 Marshall and J. Robin Warren won the Nobel Prize for their work. Because of their work, it's known that 90 percent of people with duodenal and stomach ulcers actually have an H. pylori infection that is easily treatable. H. pylori is also associated with gastric reflux (GERD), gastritis, stomach cancer, and stomach lymphoma.

H. pylori induces an immune response that brings inflammation and leaky gut. Because of this, it can wreak havoc throughout the body. It has been found to play a role in atherosclerosis, heart disease, idiopathic thrombocytopenia purpura, iron-deficiency anemia, inflammation in the iris of the eye (idiopathic anterior uveitis), Parkinson's disease, autoimmune thyroid diseases, GI lymphomas, ear infections, glaucoma, Sjögren's syndrome, food allergy, migraine headaches, lichen planus, purigo, Henoch-Schonlein purpurea, psoriasis, and rosacea.

It's present in about 50 percent of the world's population, yet only a small percentage get sick from it. This poses a curious question. Why do some people have helicobacter infection yet no GI upset? In fact, some scientists hypothesize that H. pylori actually protects us from allergies, eczema, and asthma. A recent study explored the protective effect of H. pylori in people from developing inflammatory bowel disease. They have found inverse relationships between the presence of H. pylori and the absence of these allergic conditions. It's probably due to a difference in genetics. If you have "lucky" genes in this case, you remain unaffected or even protected by the H. pylori.

Because many people have H. pylori and have no symptoms, conventionally it is treated only when someone has H. pylori and an ulcer, stomach cancer or precancerous lesions, mucosa-associated lymphoid tissue, or iron-deficiency anemia that doesn't respond to treatment. Many physicians also treat people with gastritis.

Conventional treatment is with triple therapy. This consists of two antibiotics (amoxicillin or metronidazole plus clarithromycin) and a proton-pump inhibitor for 14 days. Other doctors might use quadruple therapy: a proton-pump inhibitor, bismuth subsalicylate, tetracycline, and metronidazole (Flagyl) for 10 to 14 days. These treatments can have side effects: upset stomach, diarrhea, headache, a metallic taste in the mouth, a darkened tongue or stools, flushing when drinking alcohol, and sensitivity to the sun. Once treated, ulcers typically don't recur. After four weeks people are retested to see if the ulcer has healed and if the H. pylori has been eradicated. Despite treatment, 10 to 20 percent have a relapse of their ulcer within six months without aggravation from NSAID medications. Although this treatment has minor side effects, the overall outcome shows improved quality of living and less psychological stress after therapy.

There are many natural remedies for H. pylori that are being used by integrative clinicians. Many of these have excellent research. First of all, eating probiotic-rich foods can help heal and irradicate H. pylori infections. Broccoli sprouts or Brussels sprouts cooked (about 3 ounces daily), cabbage juice, sauerkraut juice, cranberry juice (about 2 cups daily), green tea as you'd like, yogurt, apples, moderate amounts of red wine or red grape juice, onions, and capers all have antibacterial effects on H. pylori. If you want to use a natural treatment, here are some suggestions:

- Deglycyrrhizinated licorice (DGL): 760 mg three times daily
- Mastic gum: 1 gram daily
- Zinc carnosine: 75 mg three or four times daily
- Sanogastril: One to three tablets daily
- Unripe plaintain powder: 5 to 10 grams daily

- Aloe vera juice: Use as directed three times daily after meals
- Fermented soy (Sano-Gastril): Two tablets three times daily chewed or sucked between meals
- Oil of oregano: 200 mg three times daily

Other natural substances that have been found to be useful include cat's claw, Dangshen, Dragon's blood (Dracaena cochinchinesis), ginger, Optiberry (combination of berries), parsley, evening primrose oil, probiotics, propolis, quercetin, reishi mushrooms, seabuckthorn, swallowroot (Decalepis hamiltonii), turmeric, curcumin, water hyssop (Baucopa monniera), and traditional Chinese medicine formulas.

CANDIDA: THE MASQUERADER

A prevalent and obvious form of dysbiosis is candidiasis, a fungal infection. Candida is a type of fungi that belongs to the yeast family, so it is commonly called a yeast infection. Although this section refers to candidiasis, the material applies to people with other types of fungal infections, such as Rhodotorula, Cryptococcus, and Rhodotorula species. These infections can appear in as oral thrush, eye fungi, vaginitis, skin rashes, or athlete's foot and can also contribute to systemic symptoms such as brain fog.

Candida is found in nearly everyone, and in small amounts it is compatible with good health. Candida is usually controlled by friendly flora, our immune defense system, and intestinal pH. After we've taken antibiotics, eaten too many sweets, drunk too much alcohol, or taken birth control pills or steroids, candida can overgrow, causing a variety of symptoms. In my experience, candida is an opportunistic infection. When we are susceptible and weakened, it can thrive. As our digestive system heals, it has difficulty thriving.

In the early 1980s, Orion Truss, M.D., noticed that many of his patients' other problems resolved when he treated them with Nystatin for fungal problems. Indeed, one patient had a complete reversal of multiple sclerosis. After hearing Dr. Truss lecture on his findings, Abram Hoffer, M.D., a doctor in the field of orthomolecular psychiatry, tried his first yeast protocol on a psychiatric patient who had suffered from depression for many years. One month after initiating Truss's program, she was mentally and emotionally sound or stable. They met with other doctors, including Sidney Baker, who also began seeing enormous changes in their patients. Soon the word began to spread among integrative clinicians of all sorts. Dr. Abram Hoffer stated that one-third of the world's population is affected by candidiasis. Typically if someone's problem is due to candida, when the person is treated you see remarkable effects; often the person is 80 percent better in just two weeks.

Candida can also colonize in the digestive tract, causing havoc everywhere in the body. Candida colonies produce powerful toxins, such as gliotoxin, aldehydes, and, rarely, alcohol, that are absorbed into the bloodstream and affect our immune system, hormone balance, and thought processes. Candida also lowers immunity by splitting secretory IgA molecules.

The most common symptoms are abdominal bloating, anxiety, constipation or diarrhea (or both), depression, environmental sensitivities, fatigue, feeling worse on damp or muggy days or in moldy places, food sensitivities, fuzzy thinking, insomnia, low blood sugar, mood swings, premenstrual syndrome, recurring vaginal or bladder infections, ringing in the ears, and sensitivities to perfume, cigarettes, or fabric odors. Although these symptoms are the most prevalent, candida has many faces, and many types of symptoms can occur.

Candida infections are usually triggered by use of antibiotics, birth control pills, steroid medications, and consumption of sugar. These drugs change the balance of the intestinal tract, killing the bacteria that keep candida in check, and the fungus quickly takes hold. Candida are like bullies that push their way into the intestinal lining, destroying cells and brush borders. Greater numbers of candida produce greater amounts of toxins, which further irritate and break down the intestinal lining, causing leaky gut. This damage allows macromolecules of partially digested food to pass through. The macromolecules are the perfect size for antibodies to respond to. Your immune system then goes on alert for these specific foods so the next time you eat them, your antibodies will be waiting. The net result is increased sensitivity to foods, other food substances, and the environment. (See Chapter 4, "Intestinal Permeability/Leaky Membranes.")

Healing Candida

First begin with a candida diet or the Body Ecology Diet. (Both are described in Chapter 13.) Herbs and medications don't work to permanently rebalance your system unless you change your diet.

Many substances are helpful in killing off candida. Garlic is my personal favorite—eat lots of it raw; women can use it as a vaginal suppository (make sure not to nick the garlic or it can sting!) or take in capsule form. Capryllic acid from coconuts, oleic acid from olive oil, oil of oregano, thyme oil, pau d'arco, olive leaf extract, and grapefruit seed extract are all valuable agents for killing candida. Mathake, a South American herb, has also been found to be extremely effective. While it isn't necessary to use all these health enhancers, you can buy many of them in combination products in health-food stores or from health professionals. Remember to take a good probiotic supplement or to eat lots of probiotic-rich foods while you are taking these products.

Typically when I am working with someone, I recommend probiotics and either a single or combination herbal product. If candida is the underlying problem, people feel dramatically better within two weeks. If so, I continue the herbs for 6 to 12 weeks or until no further improvement is noticed. After that I typically recommend a different herb or combination to kill the fungi that didn't respond to the first one. Many people also choose to use pharmaceutical drugs like Nystatin or Diflucan to treat candidiasis.

When the candida die, protein fragments and endotoxins are released, triggering an antibody response. This can initially produce a worsening of the person's symptoms and is commonly known as a die-off reaction, or a Herxheimer reaction. To avoid this, it is important to begin therapeutics gently, with small doses, and gradually increase. If your symptoms are still initially aggravated, cut back and increase supplements more gradually. Most people begin to feel dramatically better within two weeks. If you don't, you're probably not dealing with a candida problem. Ask your clinician to make therapeutic recommendations.

I recently advised a client to take probiotic supplements for peeling skin and a burning sensation on her feet. Although she scored low on the candida questionnaire (see Chapter 11), her symptoms fit those of candida. I advised her to take probiotics slowly, beginning with 5 billion organisms daily and working up gradually to 50 billion to 100 billion organisms. Six days later, she told me her feet were improving, but she had a horrible headache every time she took a teaspoon of probiotics. After she began again more slowly, she was soon relieved of both problems.

SMALL INTESTINAL BACTERIAL OVERGROWTH (SIBO)

Small bowel overgrowth occurs when bacteria in the large intestine travel to the small intestine, often the result of poor HCl production in the stomach or an insufficient amount of pancreatic enzyme function. SIBO is a frequently overlooked contributor to health problems and often underlies such diverse health issues as irritable bowel syndrome, fibromyalgia, restless leg syndrome, and possibly interstitial cystitis.

Dr. Mark Pimentel and his research group reported that 78 percent of people with irritable bowel syndrome had small intestinal bacterial overgrowth (SIBO).

When treated with antibiotics, their symptoms were 75 percent improved or resolved. Other researchers report that about 50 percent of people with irritable bowel syndrome have SIBO. They also report that 78 percent of people with fibromyalgia have SIBO. When the infection is treated, nearly half of them no longer meet the criteria for fibromyalgia. SIBO is also commonly found in people with diabetes, scleroderma, gastric bypass surgeries, interstitial cystitis, restless leg syndrome, diverticulosis, Crohn's disease, celiac disease, strictures in the intestines, poor ileocecal valve function, poor motility, or recent stomach surgery, and it is common in elderly people. Figure 8.1 shows how stress can lead to changes in the gut mucosa, which in turn leads to changes in the balance of bacteria in the small intestine. This triggers an immune response which stimulates our enteric nervous system (digestive nervous system). All of this results in IBS-like symptoms of gas, bloating, diarrhea, constipation, and/or alternating diarrhea and constipation.

Use of proton-pump inhibitors is one cause of SIBO. If you don't have acid in your stomach protecting you from bacteria, fungi, and parasites coming in on your food, you are left wide open.

People with SIBO typically experience it as gas, bloating, diarrhea, and abdominal discomfort. Some people may experience constipation or fatigue. Some people

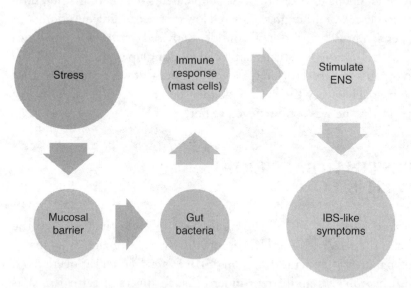

Figure 8.1   **SIBO, how it can create IBS-like symptoms.** (Adapted from Wood, Jackie D. Modified from: [2007] "Effects of Bacteria on the Enteric Nervous System: Implications for the Irritable Bowel Syndrome." *Journal of Clinical Gastroenterology*, 41, S7–S19.)

have frothy, yellow stools (called steatorrhea) and experience fat malabsorption and deficiencies of fat-soluble vitamins (A, D, E, and K). These symptoms are chronic and last for weeks and months, then years. You feel worse when eating carbohydrates and you may need to loosen your pants by the end of the day. From my experience it seems to worsen as the day goes on. What's happening is that these bacteria are fermenting carbohydrates and sugars in your belly, causing symptoms. The bacteria also produce by-products that are irritating and toxic to your intestines. This can eventually lead to leaky gut and deficiencies of fat-soluble vitamins, B_{12}, and iron. Some people lose a lot of weight as a result.

Testing for SIBO

Stool tests can help uncover whether you have a bacterial infection in your colon, but they aren't accurate at determining whether you have a bacterial infection in your small intestine. The test of choice is a hydrogen breath test, although in my experience it misses many who do have SIBO. You can also determine SIBO by using organic acid testing. Look for D lactate, Indican, and Hippuric acid. Some doctors will just look at your symptoms and treat you without doing testing. You could also experience a lot of gas and bloating from candida, lactose or other carbohydrate intolerance, or too fast a transit time. (See Chapter 11 for more information on functional testing.)

Treatment of SIBO

The current medical treatment for SIBO is antibiotics. The most common ones include Neomycin, Flagyl, Levaquin, Cipro, or Rifaxamin. Rifaxamin is an antibiotic that works locally in the digestive system, so it doesn't cause systemic problems and has fewer side effects. Dr. Gerard Mullin from Johns Hopkins is using an aggressive herbal therapy for treating SIBO. Whether herbs or pharmaceuticals are used, the goal is to kill bacteria. There are also case history reports showing efficacy of using a combination of peppermint and caraway oils. Typically treatment will resolve the issues. If the SIBO is caused from a problem with obstruction or limitations on how well the muscles in the intestines work, then the person may have to remain on antibiotics continuously.

The other most common medical treatment for SIBO is probiotics. This is in keeping with my "make love, not war" strategy of healing. While this doesn't always work by itself, it's worth trying. Probiotics are typically given in large doses, 100 million organisms one to three times daily or more, to bring the intestines back into balance. The best studied of these is VSL-3.

PARASITES

Parasites modulate our immune responses for good or ill. Parasites have evolved alongside of us and have developed strategies for surviving inside of us. In general, parasites cause us harm and we want to eliminate them from our bodies. But in some cases they can be protective and beneficial because they modulate our immune system response, much like probiotic bacteria do. For example, if you have anemia that develops from hookworm, the hookworm also helps you gain resistance to some bacterial infections. TSO pig whipworms are being used and studied to change immune response in people with inflammatory bowel disease and allergy. References in the scientific literature suggest that parasites may be the primary cause of allergies. Parasites cause damage to the lining of the digestive tract, which allows large molecules to enter the bloodstream. This provokes an antigenic response. This theory is revolutionary, and additional research needs to be done to determine just how large a role parasites play in allergies of all types. (See Chapter 9 for more information on this.) Let's focus here on parasites that make us sick.

Protozoa are single-celled microbes such as amoebas, leishmania, giardia, plasmodium, and cryptosporidium. Worms, or helminthes, are larger, and typically you can see them. Probably the most common worms in the United States include pinworms, roundworms, flukes, and, less common, tapeworms. Genova Diagnostics Laboratory routinely surveys stool samples for parasites. I had a conversation about this with Patrick Hanaway, M.D., vice president and chief medical officer at Genova Diagnostics Laboratory. In stool samples from people who had symptoms that met the diagnostic criteria for irritable bowel syndrome, parasites were discovered in 23.5 percent of 14 thousand stool samples. The most common ones were Blastocystis hominis (12.5 percent), Dientamoeba fragilis (3.8 percent), Entamoeba species (3.4 percent), Endolimax nana (2.2 percent), and Giardia lamblia (0.7 percent).

The symptoms of parasites appear to be like any other digestive problem. Chronic diarrhea is often a sign of a parasitic infection. Other symptoms include pain, constipation, bloating, gas, unexplained weight loss, fatigue, unexplained fever, coughing, itching, rashes, bloody stools, abdominal cramping, joint and muscle aches, irritable bowel syndrome, anemia, allergy, granulomas, nervousness, teeth grinding, chronic fatigue, poor immune response, and sleep disturbances. Parasites play a role in some people who have inflammatory bowel disease. Parasitic symptoms can come and go due to the life cycles of the specific parasite involved. I had one client who went through a 21-day cycle from wellness to headaches, fatigue, constipation, and diarrhea, to wellness again. If you see a cyclical pattern like this, you can suspect parasites. (See "Parasite Questionnaire" in Chapter 11.)

Pinworms

If your anus itches at night, you may have pinworms. They are most commonly found in children and parents of small children. It's fairly simple to determine whether or not you have them. When you feel the itching, put a piece of cellophane tape on your anus, and examine the tape for small, white, wiggly worms that look like white pieces of thread that move. Or, you can simply put your finger into your anus and see if you pull out any worms. With children, use tape or just look.

Parasite Testing: Ova and Parasite vs. Comprehensive Stool Testing

Many physicians request parasitology testing on random stool samples (called ova and parasite testing), but this type of testing is not very accurate. Even with repeated samples, accurate results are found only 85 to 90 percent of the time. Typically labs look under microscopes to see parasites. They may also try to culture them to grow in Petri dishes. The most accurate stool testing is usually done by labs that specialize in parasitology testing. Because of the high volume of samples, high-tech microscopes, and slow pace, their staffs have become experts in detection and recognition of parasites. Many parasites, like giardia, live farther up the digestive tract so that many labs now give an oral laxative to induce diarrhea when testing for parasites. This type of sample is called a stool purge. The newest technology in stool testing uses what's known as PCR genetic testing. By looking for the genes of parasites, they can be found more easily. (See Chapter 11, "Functional Medicine/Functional Testing," for more information on comprehensive digestive stool analysis.)

Healing Options

Prescription medication may be the most efficient treatment for most parasite infections. Within a week or two, you are parasite-free. However, these medications can be hard on the liver and are always disruptive to the intestinal flora. After using them, it's wise to take probiotics and/or to eat probiotic-rich foods to replace and rebalance the intestinal flora.

Natural options work more slowly—about a month—but can be highly effective. They generally contain garlic, wormwood (artemisia), goldenseal, black walnut, and/or grapefruit seed extract. You can find many of these in combination products. Probiotic supplements should be used after therapy is finished.

Virtually all indigenous cultures have excellent parasite cures. When I studied Hawaiian medicine, it seemed that nearly every other plant I learned was to cure parasites! Here are some common parasite remedies to try. You can find many supplements that combine several of these remedies. This helps you get the best results.

- **Take garlic.** Historically, garlic has been used for pinworms; it has antiviral, antibacterial, and antifungal properties. Allicin, the active component in garlic, has been shown to be effective against Entamoeba histolytica and Giardia lamblia. Entamoeba histolytica is an amoeba that has been used to evaluate the value of entamoeba drugs.
- **Try goldenseal or berberine.** Historically, goldenseal has been used to balance infections of mucous membranes throughout the body. It is also effective with candida infections. Berberine sulfate, an active ingredient in goldenseal, has been shown to be effective against amoebas and giardia parasites.
- **Try artemisia (wormwood).** Wormwood has been used for centuries in China and Europe for worms and parasites. It contains sesquiterpene lactone, which works like peroxide. It is believed to affect the parasite membranes, weakening them so our natural defense system kicks in. Artemisia also contains an ingredient that is effective against malaria even when it is resistant to quinine drugs. Tea of wormwood has been successfully used for pinworms and roundworms by Dr. John R. Christopher, one of America's foremost 20th-century herbalists. It's important to note that artemisia is safe when used in a tea or capsule, but pure wormwood oil is poisonous. Take ½ teaspoon powdered wormwood once or twice daily or make a tea using 2 teaspoons of fresh leaves or tops in 1 cup water. Drink 2 cups a day, 1 teaspoon at a time.
- **Try black walnut.** The juice of unripe, green hulls of black walnuts has been traditionally used for treatment of parasites and fungal infections. Black walnut is a folk remedy for ringworm, athlete's foot, and cracks in the palms and feet.
- **Try Dichroa febrifuga (saxifragaceae).** Dichroa is a Chinese herb called changshan, which is effective against malaria, amoebas, and giardia.
- **Use Jerusalem oak.** A folk medicine used throughout the Americas, the Jerusalem oak (also called American wormseed or chenopod) expels roundworms, hookworms, and tapeworms, and it is especially useful for children. More scientific studies need to be done to confirm the historical usage of this herb.
- **Eat pumpkin seeds.** Pumpkin seeds have also been used historically as a folk medicine for tapeworms and roundworms. To be really effective, enormous amounts must be eaten: 7 to 14 ounces for children and up to 25 ounces for adults. Mash them and mix with juice. Two or three hours afterward, take castor oil to clear your bowels.

BIOFILMS AND INFECTION

Biofilms are aggregate of bacteria, fungi, and other microorganisms that create communities. They can be beneficial or harmful. When we have the proper balance of bacteria, fungi, and other microbes in our microbiome, we develop healthy biofilms. Just as we live in harmony with pets, computers, cell phones, furniture, and other people, biofilms are also made of lots of types of organisms, minerals, metals, and a starchy matrix (polysaccharide). Each component takes a role and forms a cohesive force. As they mature, biofilms gain mass and influence in our bodies. They form in our mouths, respiratory system, digestive tract, and vaginas as well as inside of industrial tubing, on your contact lenses, in wounds, in catheters, on knee and hip replacement pieces, on pacemakers, in machines, on ponds, and elsewhere.

Biofilms operate like corporations. They are well organized and, if filled with a balance of microbes, are beneficial, yet when disordered they wreak havoc. It is believed that 70 percent of all bacterial infections in people are caused by biofilms. And these are hard to eradicate. They've found a cushy place to thrive at our expense and are linked to lung infections in cystic fibrosis, periodontal disease, chronic ear infections, and candida infections. Imagine, for example, that you've had a stent or pacemaker put into your heart and that it begins forming a biofilm that's loaded with candida. These biofilms can cause endocarditis, an infection inside of the heart chambers and valves. Infectious biofilms are resistant to antibiotics and can take 100 to a 1,000 times the amount of antibiotics to eradicate compared to a regular infection. If your immune system isn't functioning well, these biofilms can cause infections that become life-threatening.

Little is known about prevention and treatment of biofilms in people; research is just beginning to flourish in this field. Some of the ideas that are being researched include the following: Some researchers hypothesize that having adequate amounts of bile helps to keep biofilm formation from occurring. Others are looking at probiotic supplements to normalize biofilms. One group of researchers looked at E. coli strain Nissle 1917 and found that it helped to form healthy biofilms that pushed out disease-causing E. coli bacteria. This could be especially useful in ulcerative colitis, which has been shown to respond well to E. coli Nissle. Lactobacillus reuteri and Lactobacillus salivarius (strain: W24) also produce healthful biofilms. Other researchers report that use of prebiotics, such as inulin-type fructans such as fructooligosaccharides (FOS), support healthy biofilms and a healthy gut. One group of researchers has looked at components of oregano oil, carcavol, and thymol and found them to be effective at inhibiting biofilm formation. Chitosan, a product made from purified shrimp shells, has also been shown to break down biofilms in the heart caused by a biofilms composed primarily of a bacteria called Cryptococcus neoformans. In dental therapy use of ozone and probiotics seem to keep the gums and teeth healthy. Much more work needs to be done in this area, but common sense leads me to believe that what is healthful to overall digestive health will also prove to be healthful for prevention of disease-causing biofilms.

Lactoferrin in our eyes helps prevent infection by binding to iron, which is needed for the growth and survival of disease-causing microbes. It also appears to inhibit the development of biofilms in the eyes. In addition, lactoferrin may help control oral biofilm development and is useful in people with gingivitis. Conversely, depleted levels of lactoferrin in the sinuses increase biofilm development and recurring sinus infections. You can increase lactoferrin levels by supplementing with whey, colostrum, or transfer factor.

Dental research leads the way in the field of what works with people. Dental research shows promise with use of polyethylene glycol, chlorexidine, and sodium hypochlorite in breaking up the biofilms that develop on our teeth, in root canals, and in other oral tissues. Some integrative physicians are using chelation therapy with ethylenediaminetetraacetic acid (EDTA) to break up biofilms, although it hasn't been shown to be terribly effective in dental biofilm research.

Integrative physicians have also been experimenting with a three-step approach to eradicating disease-causing biofilms. In stage one they combine the use of enzyme products such as protein-splitting enzymes like serrapeptase, nattokinase, and proteases with oral EDTA and lactoferrin. They follow this with antibiotic treatment with either herbs or medications, and finally use insoluble fibers, charcoal, and pectin to clean up the debris. I have heard good case reports but have not seen any large-scale studies on this approach yet.

Remember that biofilms can be normal and healthy too; eradicate them only under the supervision of a clinician skilled in this area. We don't yet understand all of the ramifications of treating them.

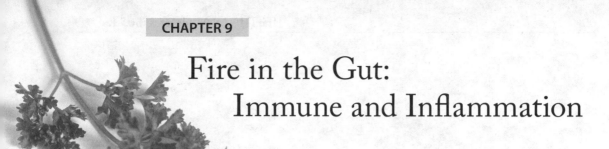

CHAPTER 9

Fire in the Gut:
Immune and Inflammation

"Our bodies respond to trauma or infection in a predictable manner, a phenomenon called inflammation. . . . Whether the stimulus is a laceration, a burn, or an inhaled speck of pollen by a person with atopic syndrome, a remarkably similar combination of signs is elicited."

—Robert Rountree, M.D.

"The gut immune system has the challenge of responding to the pathogens while remaining unresponsive to food antigens and the commensal flora. In the developed world this ability appears to be breaking down, with chronic inflammatory diseases of the gut commonplace in the apparent absence of overt infections."

—Thomas T. MacDonald and Giovanni Monteleone,
"Immunity, Inflammation, and Allergy in the Gut"

The function of the immune system is to determine what is you and what is not you: self from nonself. When exposed to a stimulus or event that your immune interprets as nonself, it begins sending warriors to the rescue. Current research indicates that 70 percent of the immune system is located in or around the digestive system. This is because of the enormous amount of food and drink that we ingest, which is "foreign" material that needs to be sorted.

Ninety-nine percent of the time, it is the immune system's job *not* to respond. We develop what is called tolerance for our environment. Otherwise each time you ate an orange or inhaled some pollen your immune system would be activated, much like the boy who cried wolf. Your body has recognition of what is similar to yourself and what's not. When you eat foods high in antioxidants, nutrients, and polyphenols (colors), your immune system sighs, "All is well." But what if we eat foods that

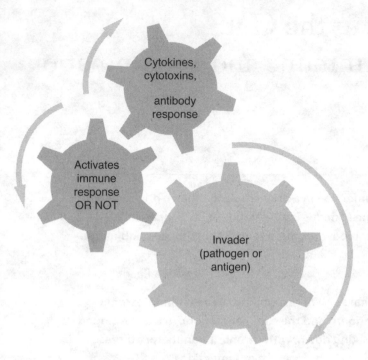

Figure 9.1   **Basic immune response.**

aren't really foods: soft drinks, trans fats, artificial colors and flavors, and other food chemicals? Immune research indicates that our reaction to these is one of "nonself," which activates the immune system. Figure 9.1 illustrates the basic mechanism of an immune response.

The external manifestation of an immune system out of balance is inflammation, which we experience as swelling, heat, and/or pain. This reaction could be triggered by hay fever, a sprained ankle, acid reflux, or eating foods that disagree with us. In fact, inflammation is now believed to be the underlying cause of obesity, high blood pressure, diabetes, atherosclerosis, Alzheimer's disease, Parkinson's disease, cancer, depression, and more.

Throughout your body, you have a continual communication that balances inflammation and healing. We are always walking a dance between just the right amount of immune surveillance and inflammation, and not feeling well. When challenged, the immune system mounts a predictable response that is proportional to the threat. (See Table 9.1.) It produces inflammatory molecules such as cytokines; interleukins; chemokines; secretory IgA; IgG, IgE, and IgM antibodies; and others.

Table 9.1 **Causes and Degrees of Immune Vigilance**

	Stuff from Inside	Stuff from Outside
Vigilance	*(Cells, Molecules)*	*(Germs, Food, Pollen)*
Too little	Cancer	Infection
Just right	Self-knowledge	Environmental knowledge
Too much	Autoimmunity	Allergy

Used with permission from Sidney Baker, M.D. Defeat Autism Now! conference, Dallas, Texas, October 2009.

IMMUNE IMBALANCES AND THE DIGESTIVE SYSTEM

When you think about inflammation and immune imbalances in the digestive system, consider pain and discomfort: acid reflux; sores in our mouths; periodontal disease; inflammatory bowel diseases, such as Crohn's and ulcerative colitis; irritable bowel syndrome; and dysbiosis. Also included are autoimmune diseases, such as type 1 diabetes, celiac disease, multiple sclerosis, lupus, Sjögren's disease, and rheumatoid arthritis. Inflammatory bowel diseases result from an exaggerated immune response to what would be normal bacteria in someone who has different genes. The main function of probiotics is to modulate the immune system. Beneficial microbes help to keep "bad" microbes in balance. (See Chapter 27, "Autoimmune Diseases.") In the chapter on probiotics, you learned that one of the main benefits of pre- and probiotics is that they modulate the immune system. When we have a balance of probiotic, commensal, and few disease-causing bacteria, there is a balance between inflammation and healing. (See Figure 9.2.) When we have a lot of disease-causing microbes and few probiotic bacteria and commensal bacteria to balance that out, it leads to inflammation, pain, and disease.

THE IMMUNE SYSTEM 1.0

Your immune system has four basic parts. Your body's first response typically is to watch and be tolerant. When something unusual occurs, the immune system has an ordered way of responding that layers your defenses from simplest to most dire and then hopefully back to health again.

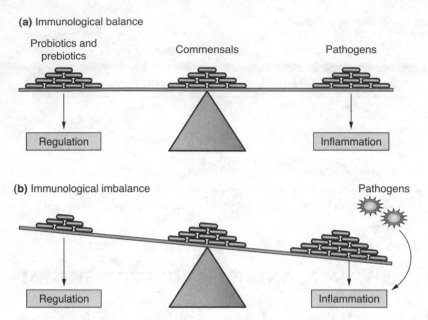

Figure 9.2 **How probiotics and prebiotics modulate the immune system.** (The original is from Mazmanian, S. K., Round, J. L., & Kasper, D. L. [2008]. "A Microbial Symbiosis Factor Prevents Intestinal Inflammatory Disease." *Nature*, 453[7195], 620–625.)

- **Innate immune system:** This is your first line of defense against things that your body generally doesn't like, such as cancer cells, mold, mildew, yeast, and viruses. It responds quickly and within minutes or hours to deal with bacteria, viruses, parasites, and other threats that can make you sick. Typically this is called a T-helper 1 cell response (Th-1 response). Some of the responses that are produced include interferon, defensins, lysozyme, complement (which activates the body to attack and kill cells), mast cells, polymorphonuclear lymphocytes, macrophages, dendritic cells, phagocytes, lactoferrin, reactive oxygen species (like hydrogen peroxide and superoxide radical), natural killer cells, and the interleukins IL-2, IL-12, and IL-18.

- **Adaptive immune system:** The second line of defense is your adaptive immune system. This is a slower response and is specific. Your body makes a more careful examination to determine whether this is a friend or foe and then develops a specific response that is appropriate. This mainly comprises allergic responses. So, perhaps the first time you are stung by a bee, it's not so bad. But then your body remembers that insult and the next time you have a huge allergic reaction.

If you are allergic to peanuts, your body produces an antigen that is specific to peanuts. Or if you have had the measles, your body will produce antibodies that are specific to measles. This is to help protect you from invaders with a long-term response. This level of immune response is also where food and environmental sensitivities reside. Typically this is a T-helper 2 (Th-2) response, where a specific response occurs to a specific challenge. Other cells involved are the antibodies IgA, IgM (memory antibodies), IgG (delayed sensitivities), IgE (allergy); T- and B-lymphocytes; and the interleukins IL-4, IL-5, IL-10, and IL-13.

■ **Immune-inflammatory response:** In this response your body overreacts and begins responding to your own tissues as if they were foreign. A combination of your own genetics plus your environmental exposures plus your overall immune balance will determine whether you trigger an autoimmune response. Increased intestinal permeability often plays a role in autoimmune conditions. For example, people with celiac disease typically have HLA-DQ2 or HLA-DQ8 positive genes. When these people are exposed to gluten-containing grains along with a leaky gut, the grain triggers an immune and inflammatory response that is celiac disease. In other diseases, such as rheumatoid arthritis (RA) and ankylosing spondylitis (AS), genes (HLAB-27) meet bacteria (proteus in RA or klebsiella in AS), which sets off the immune response. The antibodies to these bacteria, which are typically non-disease-causing in most of us, set up an autoimmune response that causes inflammation, pain, and tissue destruction in people with the "right" genes and environment. In type 1 diabetes, either a virus or food sensitivities can trigger the disease. These are typically Th-17 responses and produce the interleukins IL-1, IL-17, and IL-22 and tumor necrosis factor alpha (TNF-alpha).

■ **Regulatory system:** You also have a stop button that suppresses your immune system, called the regulatory system, which signals your body that all is well again. T cells are produced in the thymus and are called regulatory T cells (T-reg), also known as suppressor T cells, CD4, CD25, IL-10, and TGF-beta.

Of course, this all sounds nice and neat, but there is a lot of interplay and it's not all cut and dried.

THE GALT AND THE MALT

Throughout our digestive systems we have immune tissue called gut-associated lymphoid tissue (GALT). In the mucosal lining of the digestive lumen we have mucosal-associated lymphoid tissue (MALT). The MALT also encompasses your nose, your bronchia, and in women the vulvo-vaginal areas. Altogether, 70 percent of your immune system lies within the GALT and digestive MALT and it protects us from antigens and other foreign invaders. Your tonsils, appendix, and the Peyer's patches within the small intestine are examples of your GALT.

The GALT comprises two-thirds of the immune system in our bodies. It's function is to absorb nutrients. The health of the GALT and MALT correlates with our own health. If these membranes are structurally strong, then our ability to withstand the stressors of life holds true. If these surfaces are compromised, then bacteria, antigenic food particles, and other inappropriate molecules get into our blood.

Secretory IgA (sIgA) is the major way that the MALT conveys the message of immune assault. Secretory IgA is a group of antibodies in the gut mucosa that, like sentinels, are on constant alert for foreign substances. When challenged by foreign molecules, sIgA forms immune complexes with allergens and microbes. I think of immune complexes as clumps of IgA or IgG antibodies that signal the immune system to respond. If these immune complexes get deposited in organs, they can cause disease themselves. Some IgA diseases include IgA nephropathy, vasculitis, lupus, rheumatoid arthritis, scleroderma, and Sjögren's syndrome. Immune complexes signal cytokines to begin the inflammatory process designed to rid our bodies of antigenic materials, a response of the adaptive immune system. Without sufficient sIgA, the MALT cannot work properly.

Antibody reactions occur in stages. The initial response is sIgA. This is a nonspecific response. I like to think of IgA as a scout that stays outside looking for trouble. Continuing the first line of defense are the IgM antibodies. IgM antibodies are memory cells that are available for a short while. Like a temp worker, they have a memory of a specific assault and stay active until the IgG system kicks in. The secondary line of defense initiates the IgG response. IgG antibodies stay in the body for a long time or even a lifetime and are specific to foods and other molecules. They are like the guards on the castle wall and inside the gates. They respond to "enemy" molecules, while letting "friendly" molecules come inside the castle easily. Should the IgG antibodies become overwhelmed, IgE antibodies, true allergies, kick in. Evidence suggests that people don't develop true IgE allergies until all of the other systems have broken down. When food sensitivities are cleared up, often IgE allergies also partially or fully resolve.

Deficiency of sIgA is the most common immunodeficiency. Low levels of sIgA make us more susceptible to infection and may be a fundamental cause of asthma, autoimmune diseases, candidiasis, celiac disease, chronic infections, food allergies, and more. In other words, if the sentry isn't standing at the gate, anyone can come in! A study examining people with Crohn's disease or ulcerative colitis found that all of them had low levels of sIgA. It concluded that raising sIgA levels might eliminate inflammatory bowel disease. Chronic stress, adrenal insufficiencies, oral bacteria, recurring infection, leaky gut, celiac disease, Crohn's disease, viruses such as newborn rubella and Epstein-Barr, immune hypersensitivity, and anti-inflammatory drugs can lower sIgA.

High levels of sIgA are found in people who have chronic infections and whose immune systems are overloaded. It often accompanies chronic viral infections like cytomegalovirus (CMV), Epstein-Barr virus, and HIV. It has also been found in people with rare medical problems like Berger's nephropathy, dermatitis herpetiformis, gingivitis, hepatic glomerulonephritis, IgA neoplasms, parotitis, and anti-sperm antibodies. Factors that increase sIgA include acute stress, chronic infections, heavy smoking, alcoholism, periodontal disease, dental plaque accumulation, leaky gut, and throat cancer.

When microbes enter the digestive system, they are confronted with several nonspecific and antigen-specific defense mechanisms (innate immune system) including peristalsis, bile secretion, hydrochloric acid, mucus, antibacterial peptides, and IgA. This stops most microbes and parasites from infecting the body.

The mucosal surface of the gut lining is only one cell thick. Underneath this is the GALT. If the digestive system is presented with a foreign substance, an antigen, specialized cells called M-cells carry the antigen to the lining of the digestive tract. There they are "checked out," or sampled, by specialized cells called Peyer's patches in the intestinal lining. These cells in turn alert B and T cells to begin processing the antigens. The B and T cells carry the antigens back to the intestinal mucosa, where they are gobbled up by macrophages, part of the innate immune system.

We also have pattern recognition substances, lectins and toll-like receptors, that help us recognize friend from foe. The toll-like receptors (TLRs) act as gates for controlling the immune system. They are able to distinguish between disease-causing and commensal or probiotic bacteria. When the pathogenic microbes get through, the TLRs stimulate production of pro-inflammatory cytokines by activation of NF-kappaB. For example, in Crohn's disease the TLRs are altered due to changes in the NOD2 gene. This leads to an increase in inflammation from NF-kappaB and inflammatory interleukin molecules, while blocking anti-inflammatory IL-10 and defensins.

It is believed that the constant exposure to microbes in infancy and early childhood contributes to the health and responsiveness of the adult immune system. This theory is called the "Hygiene Hypothesis." In our culture, we don't challenge the immune system enough: we're too clean. We use antibacterial soaps and sponges in our obsession about microbes. As children we don't play in the dirt; we refrigerate, cook, and preserve our foods with chemicals, which lowers our exposure to bacterial and parasite contact. We have good sanitation, we take antibiotics, and we don't eat fermented and cultured foods. Children who have little challenge to microbes are at risk for allergy, eczema, and asthma, which may continue throughout a lifetime. Without these challenges our immune system doesn't develop properly.

Stress also plays a role in immune balance. Too much stress increases inflammation by modifying our gut microbiome and increases susceptibility to leaky gut.

CAUSES OF DIGESTIVE INFLAMMATION AND IMMUNE IMBALANCE

Inflammation occurs when there is damage to cells or tissues. This is part of a normal response but can get out of control. Here are several factors that play a role.

- **Genetics:** Inflammatory bowel diseases, celiac disease, and arthritic diseases often have a genetic component.
- **Translocation of bacteria:** Even correct bacteria in the wrong place can cause problems.
- **Dysbiosis:** When the balance between probiotic and commensal organisms in the digestive system is overwhelmed by disease-producing microbes. Examples include bacterial, fungal, and parasitic infection.
- **Diet:** The Standard American Diet high in refined and poor-quality foods and low in fruits, meats, vegetables, nuts, whole grains, and seeds increases inflammatory cytokines.
- **Leaky gut:** No matter what the cause, having a leaky gut leads to increased inflammation.

LABORATORY TESTING TO ASSESS GI INFLAMMATION

Calprotectin and lactoferrin are proteins found in stool. They are used to help discover whether there is inflammation in the large intestine. Calprotectin and lactoferrin are often elevated in inflammatory bowel disease, postinfectious IBS, cancer in the digestive system, some GI infections, when people have caused damage from taking too many nonsteroidal anti-inflammatory medications, true food allergy, and chronic pancreatitis. When levels are high, it is a reliable marker to diagnose inflammatory bowel disease (IBD). If you have IBD, these tests can be used to monitor the effectiveness of your chosen therapy. Stool testing is easy and is certainly less invasive than scoping of the bowels.

Calprotectin binds both zinc and protein, so when levels are high, both can become depleted in your body. Since zinc is needed for healing of inflammation and calming the immune system, being deficient in zinc gives you a double whammy. Lactoferrin levels can be falsely elevated if you are using whey protein powders or taking lactoferrin, such as in colostrums or transfer factor.

Eosinophilic protein X is another marker of GI inflammation. It can be measured in urine or stool. It helps to determine whether there are either parasites or allergies associated with your health issues. It is commonly elevated when you have parasites, allergies, asthma, or eczema. It can also be used to monitor how effective treatment is. It is neurotoxic itself, so high levels increase inflammation.

Secretory IgA can be used to look at how well your immune system is responding. Production of adequate IgA depends on a glycoprotein called a J-chain. This J-chain is needed for the formation of IgA and IgM antibodies. You can test for IgA in stool, saliva, and blood. Low sIgA levels indicate someone who has been stressed out or sick for a long time. They are low in people who have dysbiosis, small intestinal bacterial overgrowth, chronic stress, Crohn's disease, celiac disease, other autoimmune diseases such as lupus, rheumatoid arthritis, and type I diabetes. They are sometimes low in infants, in the elderly, in people with inflammatory conditions and infections, or when people have malabsorption, malnutrition, or eating disorders. Steroid medications also lower sIgA levels. Low levels open us up to chronic infections in the lungs, gut, and genitourinary tracts. If low IgA levels persist, a chronic level of inflammation can occur. These antibodies are part of the adaptive immune system.

When sIgA levels are high, it typically indicates a leaky gut, food sensitivities, or infection. It could also indicate malnutrition, malabsorption, lack of hydrochloric acid production in the stomach, allergies, liver problems, parasites, or autoimmune conditions.

Lifestyle and nutritional factors can influence sIgA levels. For example, in people with IgA nephropathy, a kidney disease, 64 percent had decreases in sIgA-containing immune complexes on a gluten-free diet. A balanced lifestyle, which encompasses our ability to nurture ourselves, environmental considerations, exercise, good food choices, and moderate stress levels can normalize low sIgA levels. Choline, essential fatty acids, glutathione, glycine, phosphatidylcholine, phosphatidylethanolamine, quercetin, vitamin C, and zinc are all required to maintain healthy sIgA levels. Detoxification programs and repair of intestinal mucosa help normalize sIgA. Saccharomyces boulardii, a nontoxic yeast probiotic supplement, has been shown to raise sIgA levels. A recent study showed that visualization and relaxation techniques significantly increase sIgA levels. Colostrum, transfer factor, fructooligosaccharides (FOS), conjugated linolenic acid (CLA), medium-chain triglycerides, Bifidobacteria longum, Lactobacillus casei, EpiCor (beneficial yeast extract), astragalus, and Korean ginseng can all increase sIgA as well.

The following can enhance sIgA production:

- **Rest and relaxation:** I often recommend that my clients rest for two hours during daylight every day. Typically within a few weeks they are beginning to feel amazingly better. Radical, I know, but effective. Rest also increases IgG and IgM antibodies.
- **Saccharomyces boulardii:** This is my favorite supplement for increasing sIgA. Typical dosage is 250 mg three times daily.
- **Vitamin A:** A typical dosage is 5,000 IU daily. Taking high levels of retinol can be toxic, so if you increase the dosage be sure to work with a health professional and have your serum retinol (vitamin A) levels monitored.
- **Bovine colostrum:** A typical dosage is 500 to 2,000 mg daily.
- **Transfer factor:** Dosage is 12.5 to 75 mg.
- **Medium-chain triglycerides (MCT oil):** A typical dosage is up to 2 tablespoons daily. You can also eat coconut or drink coconut milk or fresh coconut juice.

REBALANCING THE GUT IMMUNE SYSTEM

In nearly all cases, probiotics and prebiotics help to dial down the inflammation and promote healing in IBD. They increase our T-regulatory response and IL-10, which also reduces inflammation. They also inhibit inflammatory cytokines, including TNF-alpha and NF-kappaB. Probiotics help the membranes from becoming leaky, lessen muscle inflammation, and increase the production of mucin. (See Chapter 6 for more on prebiotics and probiotics.)

Elimination Diet
An elimination diet can reduce inflammation and pain faster than anything else. See Chapter 15.

Eat a Rainbow: Polyphenols to Heal, Soothe, and Protect
Polyphenols are chemicals found in plant foods that have anti-inflammatory and blood vessel protective properties. They are what give the rainbow of colors to our

beans, spices, fruits, vegetables, nuts, seeds, and grains. They are among the reasons we need to eat as many fruits and vegetables as possible, and among the best reasons to focus on whole foods in general and to season your food with herbs and spices. Eating just 10 cherries a day lowers inflammation. So, eat cherries, berries, and other high-polyphenol foods several times a day. Food with highest polyphenols include:

- Berries: strawberries, blackberries, raspberries, blueberries
- Fruits of all types: grapes (highest in red or purple), cherries, peaches, kiwis, apples, pears, plums
- Wine
- Tea: green (highest), black, rooibus, mint
- Chocolate
- Coffee (not a recommendation but is high in polyphenols)
- Onions, leeks
- Broccoli, cabbage
- Beans of all types, including soy
- Parsley, celery
- Millet, wheat
- Skin of citrus fruit
- Tomatoes
- Clover

More Anti-Inflammatory High-Phenol Foods and Supplements

The use of nutritional supplements has been best studied in ulcerative colitis where inflammation can roar. Curcumin from turmeric, resveratrol from red wine and red grapes, EGCG (epigallocatechin gallate) from green tea, and quercetin from maples, onions, leafy vegetables, and tea have all been shown to reduce inflammation in ulcerative colitis and throughout the body. Many high-polyphenol supplements, spices, and foods have been shown to decrease levels of NF-kappaB and to decrease inflammation. You can use many of these as foods, or you can find them singly or in combination in products that reduce inflammation.

- Curcumin (Curcuma longa): Standardized to curcuminoids 200 to 1,000 mg three times daily, or use 2 to 3 teaspoons of dried turmeric or 1 to 2 "fingers" of fresh turmeric juiced daily.
- Ginger: Drink as a tea or in fresh vegetable juice, eat crystallized ginger, use fresh or dried in cooking, or take capsules 500 to 2,000 mg daily.
- Boswellia (frankincense): 100 to 1,200 mg standardized extract daily.

- Green tea extract (EGCG): 100 to 400 mg EGCG daily, or drink many cups of green tea.
- Green tea: Standardized to catechins 100 to 300 mg three times daily, or drink green tea liberally throughout the day; decaffeinated is preferred.
- Quercetin dihydrate: 500 to 1,000 mg three times daily.
- Wheatgrass: Up to 3.5 ounces daily. If you drink too much it can cause intense nausea, so start slowly. Heidi Snyder, M.S., a nutrition consultant on faculty at Hawthorn University, suggests juicing gingerroot with wheatgrass to help the flavor.
- Bromelain: Best taken on an empty stomach to reduce inflammation; 200 to 500 mg one to three times daily.
- Carnosol: Found in rosemary leaf extract; 200 mg one to three times daily.
- Grape seed extract: 50 to 200 mg daily.
- Probiotics: 1 billion to trillions of CFU. (See Chapter 6.)
- Alpha-lipoic acid: 100 to 1,200 mg daily.
- Resveratrol: 15 to 100 mg daily.
- Vitamin D: The FDA states that 2,000 IU daily is a safe daily adult dose. If vitamin D levels are below 32, your clinician may recommend dosages up to 10,000 IU vitamin D_3 daily for a short period of time. Prescription dosages of vitamin D_2 may range between 50,000 and 100,000 IU weekly or monthly. My preference is for use of natural vitamin D_3.
- Omega 3 fatty acids: Fish oil capsules contain both EPA and DHA fatty acids. Typical anti-inflammatory dosages are between 360 and 1,260 mg of EPA and 240 and 840 mg of DHA. Check the potency of your fish oil. They vary widely. Most contain 180 mg of EPA and 120 mg of EPA. High-potency capsules can contain dosages as high as 650 mg EPA and 450 mg of EPA.
- Gamma-linolenic acid: GLA is found in evening primrose, borage, and sesame oil; 360 to 720 mg daily.
- White willow bark: 60 to 120 mg; use as needed. White willow bark may cause stomach upset for some people, but it's less likely than with aspirin or other NSAIDs.
- Devil's claw: Used as a digestive stimulant for digestive issues and pain and arthritis; 600 to 4,500 mg of powdered devil's claw daily or 200 mg of devil's claw standardized extracts up to three times daily.

Use of immune-supportive foods such as whey products, colostrum, or transfer factor may be helpful for healing. Whey can be consumed as a drink. Colostrum or transfer factor at levels of 1 to 2 teaspoons or more daily offer protective effects. Drinking raw cow's or goat's milk often can help healing for many people.

In herbal therapies, there is a group of herbs and foods called demulcents. Demulcents have a soothing effect on the GI system. Some of the most common demulcents include the following:

- Almonds
- Barley
- Borage: Available as a tea or a green
- Burdock root: A food also known as gobo root, can be found in grocery and Asian stores
- Chickweed: A spring green easy to find in yards, it is terrific in a salad
- Coconut oil
- Coltsfoot: Typically is used as a tea or in cough syrups or lozenges
- Comfrey root: Used in teas
- Fenugreek: Best as a tea
- Figs
- Flaxseed
- Hops: Available as a tea or dried in capsules
- Licorice: Available as a tea, as "real" black licorice candy, in capsule or tincture, or as a chewable tablet; overuse of licorice, if it's not deglycyrrizinated licorice (DGL), can elevate blood pressure
- Mallow: Also called malva; available as a tea
- Marshmallow: Can be found as a tea or capsules
- Mullein: Found as a tea or compress
- Oats
- Okra
- Parsley
- Pomegranate seeds
- Prunes
- Psyllium: Plain or in products such as Metamucil
- Pumpkin
- Sage: Can be cooked or used as a tea
- Sarsaparilla and sassafras: Can be drunk as a tea after simmering roots for 20 minutes in water
- Slippery elm: Can be used in teas or soups or as lozenges
- Tapioca: Use as flour, in pudding

TSO Whipworm Eggs to Reset the Immune System

Sidney Baker, M.D., promotes the idea of using beneficial whipworm eggs, called Trichurissuis ova (TSO), to calm down the immune system. These are the eggs of one of a dozen or so "innocent" worms that live in the digestive systems of pretty much all animals. There is a good body of research indicating that TSO is safe and effective. TSO treatment helps people who have conditions that involve chronic inflammation, oxidative stress, and problems with poor detoxification. Studies show dramatic remission rates in people with Crohn's disease and ulcerative colitis. TSO can also dramatically help with allergies, eczema, multiple sclerosis, asthma, hay fever, type I diabetes, and food sensitivities, and there is ongoing research in these areas. The TSO that are used therapeutically come from pigs and taste like water. The eggs hatch over a period of about 2 weeks. Then they die, since they are in a human and not a pig. To find out whether this will work for you, take more whipworms every 2 weeks for up to 14 weeks. Either you'll feel amazingly better or nothing will have occurred. Most people have no side effects. According to Dr. Baker, occasionally people can have some digestive symptoms, pungent smell to the urine, and rarely some aggravation of symptoms. To find out more about the research on TSO go to http://www.Ovamed.org. They partner with Biomonde Asia, which sells products directly to consumers. See http://www.biomonde-asia.com/.

CHAPTER 10

The Enteric Nervous System: The Second Brain

"It is always with excitement that I wake up in the morning wondering what my intuition will toss up to me, like gifts from the sea. I work with it and rely on it. It's my partner."

—Jonas Salk, M.D.

TWO BRAINS ARE BETTER THAN ONE

Do you have gut instincts? Do you get butterflies in your stomach when you're nervous? Have you experienced diarrhea from anxiety? Can a job interview cause you to have stomach cramps? These things happen because your nervous system and digestive system are intertwined. The enteric nervous system (ENS) is often called "the second brain" because it has a mind of its own.

The ENS is the nervous system that runs through our digestive system. It is connected directly to the brain through the vagus nerve, although it can work entirely on its own. (In fact, before ulcer medications revolutionized the treatment of ulcer pain, surgeons cut the vagus nerve from the brain to the stomach, and the digestive system continued to operate completely!) It makes more neurotransmitters than the brain. This nervous system is found in sheaths of tissue lining the entire digestive system. Think about the taste, texture, smell, and feel of food on your tongue; this necessitates nerves for you to sense the qualities of food. You've probably had a toothache, stomach cramp, or gas pains, so you know from direct experience that you have pain receptors and nerves in your digestive system.

Our brain talks to our gut; our gut talks to our brain. This is a two-way communication. When our behavior changes in a certain way, our brain sends a message that changes our gut bacteria, causing low-grade inflammation and possibly GI distress. Similarly, if we have dysbiosis in our gut, it can lead to behavioral changes. (See Figure 10.1.) For example, leaky gut increases the incidence of all sorts of men-

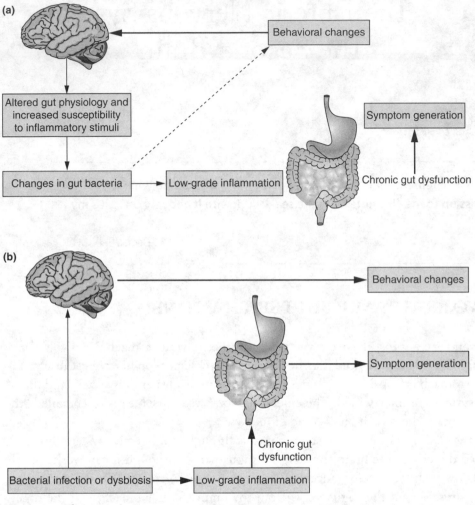

Figure 10.1 **The enteric nervous system.** (From McLean, et al. [2009]. *Gastroenterology Insights*, 1: e3.)

tal dysfunction, including depression, fatigue, confusion, poor memory, and more. In people with autism it's believed that two-thirds also experience GI issues. And 70 to 90 percent of people who have irritable bowel syndrome also experience some sort of mood or anxiety disorder, including schizophrenia, major depression, and panic disorder. And people with IBS are also more likely to experience migraines and fibromyalgia. It's estimated that about two-thirds of adults and children on the autistic spectrum have GI dysfunction. And, in the National Institutes of Health 2004 Consensus statement, ataxia, epilepsy, anxiety, depression, and migraine are all listed as associated diseases with celiac disease. In 2009, Burk and colleagues reported that in 72 people with celiac disease, 28 percent had migraines, 20 percent had carpel tunnel syndrome, 35 percent reported a history of psychiatric disease, and 35 percent had deep sensory loss. Yet the vagus nerve responds to relaxation. Mind-body therapies such as cognitive behavior therapy, meditation, relaxation techniques, biofeedback, brief counseling, and hypnotherapy can help people gain freedom from IBS.

The ENS consists of two layers in the intestinal wall, the myenteric plexus and the submucosal plexus. These two layers control muscles and secretion of neuropeptides, neurotransmitters (serotonin, dopamine, acetylcholine), and nitric oxide. In fact, we produce the same neurotransmitters that work in our brain in our gut. Neurotransmitters can have local or systemic effects. For example, 90 percent of our serotonin is produced in our digestive system to help regulate peristalsis, smooth-muscle contraction, and mucosal secretions. Serotonin is best known for its role in the brain. Without adequate amounts of serotonin we have insomnia and are depressed. Table 10.1 shows some of the common neurotransmitters, where they are produced, and their primary actions.

Table 10.1 **Examples of Neurotransmitters and Their Actions**

Neurotransmitter	Site of Release	Primary Actions
Gamma-aminobutyric acid (GABA)	Central nervous system (CNS)	Relaxes lower esophageal sphincter
Norepinephrine	CNS, spinal cord, sympathetic nerves	Decreases motility, increases contraction of sphincters, inhibits secretions
Acetylcholine	CNS, autonomic system, other tissues	Increases motility, relaxes sphincters, stimulates secretions
Neurotensin	GI tract, CNS	Inhibits release of gastric emptying and acid secretion
Serotonin	GI tract, spinal cord	Facilitates secretion and peristalsis
Nitric oxide	GI tract, CNS	Regulates blood flow, maintains muscle tone, maintains gastric motor activity
Substance P	Gut, CNS, skin	Increases sensory awareness (mainly pain) and peristalsis

Used with permission: Mahan, L. K., & Escott-Stump, S. (2008). *Krause's Food and Nutrition Therapy*, Saunders/Elsevier Pub., St. Louis, MO., p. 7.

GUT HORMONES

For the ENS to control itself, it's necessary to monitor the intestinal lumen (the inside of the intestinal tube). There aren't nerves running through it; instead, it sends messages through intrinsic primary afferent neurons (IPANS). They do this by using a system of gut hormone–producing cells called enteroendocrine cells (EC). These are distributed widely throughout the digestive system and secrete at least 16 hormones. These hormones are mainly found in the epithelium, but some are also found in the mucosal layer, neurons, central nervous system, and pancreatic islets. These are often called gut-brain peptides. These neurochemicals send messages to the gut telling it to initiate peristalsis; relax; secrete enzymes, hormones, or hydrochloric acid; or respond in some other way.

Table 10.2 shows what's currently known about enteric hormones, where they are produced in your body, what stimulates their release, and what action they promote.

GO AND STOP: STRESS, RELAXATION, AND THE SYMPATHETIC AND PARASYMPATHETIC NERVOUS SYSTEM

When you are experiencing stress or feeling fearful, anxious, or worried, the sympathetic nerves slow down GI secretions and motility. In extreme stress, they shut down digestion. Conversely, when you feel relaxed your parasympathetic nervous system signals gut secretions and peristalsis, and digestion works easily. This is probably the origin of the after-lunch siesta. On the other hand, when you are stressed, or perhaps eating on the run while you drive through traffic, your digestive capacity is compromised.

Continued stress in our body and mind affects the body's ability to heal and perform. Because the digestive tract repairs and replaces itself every few days, it is one of the first places where our bodies alert us that all is not well. Stress and emotions play a major role in many digestive problems, such as ulcers, inflammatory bowel disease, irritable bowel syndrome, constipation, diarrhea, and GERD, and these conditions often respond to stress-reduction techniques. Stress also plays a role in autoimmune issues. This happens when the nervous-immune system begins reacting to normal foods and environmental triggers as if they were dangerous. Rest and relaxation help to restore nervous-immune balance.

Deep breathing, meditation, prayer, spending time in nature, gardening, yoga, tai chi, painting, and other relaxing hobbies all tell our nervous-immune system

Table 10.2 **Enteric Hormones and Their Main Functions**

Hormone	Where Produced	Stimuli for Release	Action
Somatostatin	D cells of pancreatic islet.	Growth hormone and somatomedins, low pH	Inhibits insulin, thyroid-stimulating hormone, growth hormone, and glucagon secretion
Cholecystokinin (CCK)	Duodenum, intestinal mucosa	Partially digested fats and proteins in the duodenum	Inhibits gastrin production, slowing gastric emptying; stimulates gallbladder contraction; stimulates secretion of pancreatic enzymes; increases motility in the colon; increases satiety
Leptin	Adipose tissue, placenta, ovaries, muscle, stomach, breasts, bone marrow, long-term energy	Eating a meal, thyroid-stimulating hormone, insulin	Triggers sensation of satiety; suppresses appetite; mediates pituitary, liver balance; enhances weight loss; inhibits ghrelin
Ghrelin	Stomach, pancreas	Being hungry, not enough sleep, stress	Stimulates hunger and eating; promotes intestinal repair; promotes growth in fetuses
Gastrin	Stomach and duodenur	Peptides, amino acids, caffeine, some alcoholic beverages	Triggers secretion of HCl and pepsinogen in stomach; increases tone of esophageal sphincter
Secretin	Duodenum	Acid in small intestine	Stimulates enzyme and insulin release in pancreas; stimulates secretion bicarbonate, and enzyme secretion from pancreas; stimulates insulin release
Glucagon-like peptide (GLP-1)	Pancreas	Glucose, fat	Stimulates insulin release; inhibits glucagon
Glucose-dependent insulinotopic polypeptide (GIP)	Pancreas	Glucose, fat	Stimulates insulin release
Motilin	Stomach, small and large intestines	Gallbladder and pancreatic secretions, fasting	Promotes gastric emptying and GI motility

that all is well. We spend so much time in the outer world that taking time for our inner world brings us into better balance. Often with my clients I find that resting two hours each day during the daylight hours can do wonders for all sorts of health issues. Try it for three to four weeks and see what happens!

FOOD AND OUR BRAIN

Our relationship with food begins in the brain. We think about going to a restaurant and having a specific dish; we go to the market because we have a taste to make something specific; we begin to prepare a meal because soon we'll be hungry to eat it; we aren't hungry, but we walk by an ice cream store and soon are eating a cone. We eat emotionally because we are upset, angry, lonely, depressed, happy, celebrating, procrastinating, rewarding ourselves, and a myriad of other reasons that have absolutely nothing to do with our body's need for nutrients.

Manufactured foods are designed to stimulate our tastes for fat, sugar, and salt. Flavors are layered upon layer to "sing" to our brain a song that makes us feel rewarded and indulged. This stimulates the release of serotonin and dopamine, and then we want more of that food. So we continue to eat, even when we aren't hungry.

This emphasizes the importance of eating in a relaxed manner and appreciating the food you are about to ingest. Many people call this "mindful eating" or "gentle eating," which simply focuses our awareness of the flavors in each bite. Sounds pretty simple, yet most of the time we are eating mindlessly instead. Some people find that taking time to say grace and to look at and smell the food, as well as making a special time and place for eating, can dramatically enhance their total digestive function more completely than can enzymes, bitters, or other digestive supplements.

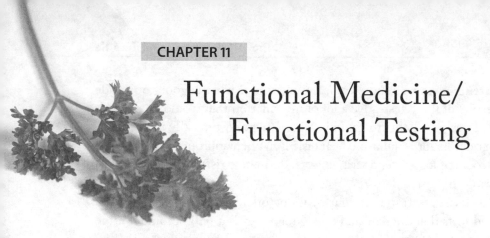

CHAPTER 11

Functional Medicine/ Functional Testing

"All truth passes through three stages: First, it is ridiculed; second, it is violently opposed; third, it is accepted as self-evident."

—Arthur Schopenhauer (1788–1860)

Modern medicine equates the absence of disease with health. Often people walk into a doctor's office feeling tired and run down, have an exam and a battery of tests that are normal, and are told that all is well. While it's good to know that there isn't anything serious wrong, they still don't feel well. This is where functional, complementary, and alternative medicines play a critical role. It's always important to treat the person and not the test. People often seek "alternative" treatment as a last resort, but the best medicine is medicine that combines what is the best of standard medicine care plus the best of functional and integrative care.

Medical disciplines and medical testing are like the ancient East Indian folktale of the six blind men touching the elephant. We test for what we "see." But each of us is "blind" because no matter how much we know, there is still so much that is unknown to us. There are hundreds, if not thousands, of possible tests that clinicians can run to help diagnose what is going on with you. The art is in knowing which specific tests may be most useful in helping you to optimize your health.

As a nutritionist, I measure improved function by how people feel. When a client comes to me with symptoms or a diagnosed medical problem, I listen carefully to what the client tells me, record the information, and ask lots of questions. I was taught that if I listened carefully my clients would tell me 90 percent of what I need to know. While I can't do that with each of you, in this chapter and throughout the book I have included questionnaires that can help you discover more about yourself, your lifestyle, and your body. These questionnaires also provide valuable information for your clinician.

Laboratory testing gives us a more complete picture of what is going on inside your body. The results of these tests give a lot of information that would be difficult to find otherwise. I ask my clients to bring in lab testing and typically refer people back to their own doctors for regular medical testing. When appropriate I will refer my clients to gastroenterologists, endocrinologists, dermatologists, or other medical specialists for testing in those fields.

This chapter discusses testing that your own doctors may not be familiar with yet. I have included tests that are new and upcoming today but will become routine in the future. The results taken in combination with how you feel, your family history, regular medical tests, and your symptoms can be a guide to putting the puzzle together to optimize your health.

There are numerous tests for functional medicine. The following are the ones I've found to be most useful for digestive problems. Most of these are laboratory tests, but a few are home tests you can perform on your own!

You can also find more resources on lab testing and specific laboratory information at http://www.digestivewellnessbook.com.

COMPREHENSIVE STOOL TESTING: A PLACE TO BEGIN

Useful for anyone with digestive problems, comprehensive digestive stool analysis (called by various labs: CDSA, CSDA, CSA, stool profile, GI-effects) is often where you can find the underlying issues. If you choose to obtain only one test, make it a comprehensive stool test in conjunction with comprehensive parasitology screening (see later in the chapter). This is a home test kit. You gather your own stool sample(s) and then ship it back to the lab. Shipping labels are included in the test kit, and the shipping cost is included in the price of the test.

A CDSA is used to assess bacterial balance and health, digestive function, and dysbiosis. It identifies the types of bacteria and fungi present and measures the levels of beneficial, possibly harmful, and disease-producing microbes. Most labs do sensitivities on any bacteria or fungi (such as candida) that are found to determine what medications or herbs will be most effective against them. These tests typically also measure calprotectin, lactoferrin, eosinophil protein X, and/or lysozyme levels to detect inflammation in the large intestine. Elevations could indicate ulcerative colitis, Crohn's disease, colon cancer, diverticulitis, or other inflammatory conditions. These markers can be used to find the inflammation without scoping, can help distinguish between irritable bowel syndrome and more serious conditions, and can also be used to monitor whether the treatment or maintenance program you are using is effective for inflammatory conditions.

In addition, a CDSA measures how well you are digesting fats, carbohydrates, and proteins; gives some indication of how well your pancreas is performing; and measures levels of butyric acid and short-chain fatty acids.

If you find candida, it gives a good clinical picture. However, if you don't see it in stool, you cannot be certain that it's not actually a problem. Organic acid testing (OAT) is the best measurement for candida and fungal infections.

There are currently two types of stool-testing procedures used. Most of the labs are using standard culturing (Genova Diagnostics, Dr's. Data, Meridian Valley Lab, Diagnostechs, etc.). The standard is culture testing: the lab technician puts samples in a Petri dish and measures what grows. When I am trying to find a specific bacterial infection, I use this type of testing. So far Metametrix Lab is the only one using newer technology using PCR genetic testing. By looking at genes of parasites, bacteria, and fungi, they can find infection at a much lower level. The problem is that this test often finds parasites and yeasts whose "taxonomy is unknown," so you don't know if this is really a problem. Currently there is no standardization of stool testing in the industry, so specific types of tests vary from lab to lab. So, when I have not been satisfied with one lab, occasionally I have used a second lab to discover parasites or other infections that weren't apparent from the initial test.

CANDIDA ANTIBODY TESTS

Many labs, including regular medical labs, offer testing for candida antibodies. These tests can help to determine whether candida/yeast overgrowth is present. Personally, I like to use Dr. Crook's yeast questionnaire, presented here, and work with yeast through diet and herbs. Many physicians will also use prescription medications to treat yeast overgrowth.

Candida Questionnaire
The following questionnaire can help you determine whether candida is a factor in your own health. A candida questionnaire for use with children is presented next.

YEAST QUESTIONNAIRE—ADULT

Answering these questions and adding up the scores will help you decide if yeasts contribute to your health problems. However, you will not obtain an automatic "yes" or "no" answer.

For each "yes" answer in Section A, circle the points that correspond to that question. Total your score and record it at the end of the section. Then move on to Sections B and C and score as indicated.

Add your three scores to get your grand total.

SECTION A: HISTORY

                                                                    Score

1. Have you taken tetracycline (Sumycin, Panmycin, Vibramycin, Minocin, and so forth) or other antibiotics for acne for one month (or longer)? 35

2. Have you, at any time in your life, taken other "broad-spectrum" antibiotics* for respiratory, urinary tract, or other infections (for two months or longer, or in shorter courses four or more times in a one-year period)? .35

3. Have you taken a broad-spectrum antibiotic drug,* even a single course? 6

4. Have you, at any time in your life, been bothered by persistent prostatitis, vaginitis, or other problems affecting your reproductive organs? 25

5. Have you been pregnant two or more times? 5

5a. One time? 3

6. Have you taken birth control pills for more than two years? 15

6a. For six months to two years? 8

7. Have you taken prednisone, Decadron, or other cortisone-type drugs for more than two weeks? 15

7a. For two weeks or less? 6

8. Does exposure to perfumes, insecticides, fabric shop odors, and other chemicals provoke:
   Moderate to severe symptoms? 20
   Mild symptoms? 5

9. Are your symptoms worse on damp, muggy days or in moldy places? 20

10. Have you had athlete's foot, ringworm, "jock itch," or other chronic fungus infections of the skin or nails? Have such infections been:
    Severe or persistent? 20
    Mild to moderate? 10

---

* Includes Keflex, ampicillin, amoxicillin, Ceclor, Bactrim, and Septra. Such antibiotics kill off "good germs" while they're killing off those that cause infection.

11. Do you crave sugar? 10
12. Do you crave breads? 10
13. Do you crave alcoholic beverages? 10
14. Does tobacco smoke really bother you? 10

Total Score, Section A _____

SECTION B: MAJOR SYMPTOMS

For each of your symptoms, enter the appropriate figure in the Score column:
   If a symptom is occasional or mild: 3 points
   If a symptom is frequent and/or moderately severe: 6 points
   If a symptom is severe and/or disabling: 9 points
   Total your score and record it at the end of this section.

                                                                        Score

1. Fatigue or lethargy .... _____
2. Feeling of being "drained" .... _____
3. Poor memory .... _____
4. Feeling "spacey" or "unreal" .... _____
5. Depression .... _____
6. Inability to make decisions .... _____
7. Numbness, burning, or tingling .... _____
8. Muscle aches or weakness .... _____
9. Pain and/or swelling in joints .... _____
10. Abdominal pain .... _____
11. Constipation .... _____
12. Diarrhea .... _____
13. Bloating, belching, or intestinal gas .... _____
14. Troublesome vaginal burning, itching, or discharge .... _____
15. Persistent vaginal burning or itching .... _____
16. Prostatitis .... _____
17. Impotence .... _____
18. Loss of sexual desire or feeling .... _____
19. Endometriosis or infertility .... _____
20. Cramps and/or other menstrual irregularities .... _____
21. Premenstrual tension .... _____
22. Attacks of anxiety or crying .... _____
23. Cold hands or feet and/or chilliness .... _____
24. Shaking or irritable when hungry .... _____

Total Score, Section B _____

SECTION C: OTHER SYMPTOMS*

For each of your symptoms, enter the appropriate figure in the Score column:

   If a symptom is occasional or mild: 1 point

   If a symptom is frequent and/or moderately severe: 2 points

   If a symptom is severe and/or disabling: 3 points

Total your score and record it at the end of this section.

                                                                          Score

1. Drowsiness .... _____
2. Irritability or jitteriness .... _____
3. Lack of coordination .... _____
4. Inability to concentrate... _____
5. Frequent mood swings.. _____
6. Headaches.. _____
7. Dizziness/loss of balance .... _____
8. Pressure above ears, feeling of head swelling .... _____
9. Tendency to bruise easily... _____
10. Chronic rashes or itching .... _____
11. Numbness, tingling .... _____
12. Indigestion or heartburn .... _____
13. Food sensitivity or intolerance.................................. _____
14. Mucus in stools .... _____
15. Rectal itching .... _____
16. Dry mouth or throat.. _____
17. Rash or blisters in mouth .... _____
18. Bad breath.. _____
19. Foot, body, or hair odor not relieved by washing .... _____
20. Nasal congestion or postnasal drip .... _____
21. Nasal itching.. _____
22. Sore throat.. _____
23. Laryngitis, loss of voice .... _____
24. Cough or recurrent bronchitis .... _____
25. Pain or tightness in chest.. _____
26. Wheezing or shortness of breath .... _____
27. Urgency or urinary frequency .... _____

---

* While the symptoms in this section commonly occur in people with yeast-connected illness, they are also found in other individuals.

28. Burning on urination . . . . _____
29. Spots in front of eyes or erratic vision . . . . _____
30. Burning or tearing of eyes . . . . _____
31. Recurrent infections or fluid in ears . . . . _____
32. Ear pain or deafness . . . . _____

Total Score, Section C _____

Total Score, Section A _____

Total Score, Section B _____

Total Score, Section C _____

Grand Total Score _____

The Grand Total Score will help you and your physician decide whether your health problems are yeast connected. Scores for women will run higher than for men, as seven items in the questionnaire apply exclusively to women, while only two apply exclusively to men.

Yeast-connected health problems are almost certainly present with scores higher than 180 for women and 140 for men.

Yeast-connected health problems are probably present with scores higher than 120 for women and 90 for men.

Yeast-connected health problems are possibly present with scores higher than 60 for women and 40 for men.

With scores lower than 60 for women and 40 for men, yeasts are less apt to cause health problems.

YEAST QUESTIONNAIRE—CHILD

For each "yes" answer, circle the points that correspond to that question. Total your score and record it at the end of the questionnaire.

Score

1. During the two years before your child was born, were you bothered by recurrent vaginitis, menstrual irregularities, premenstrual tension, fatigue, headache, depression, digestive disorders, or "feeling bad all over"? 30
2. Was your child bothered by thrush?
   Mild? 10
   Severe or persistent? 20
3. Was your child bothered by frequent diaper rashes in infancy?
   Mild? 10
   Severe or persistent? 20

4. During infancy, was your child bothered by colic and irritability lasting longer than three months?

   Mild? 10

   Severe or persistent? 20

5. Are your child's symptoms worse on damp days or in damp or moldy places? 20

6. Has your child been bothered by recurrent or persistent "athlete's foot" or chronic fungus infections of his or her skin or nails? 30

7. Has your child been bothered by recurrent hives, eczema, or other skin problems? 10

8. Has your child received:

   Four or more courses of antibiotic drugs during the past year? Or has your

       child received continuous "prophylactic" courses of antibiotic drugs? 80

   Eight or more courses of "broad-spectrum" antibiotics (such as amoxicillin,

       Keflex, Septra, Bactrim, or Ceclor) during the past three years? 50

9. Has your child experienced recurrent ear problems? 10

10. Has your child had tubes inserted in his or her ears? 10

11. Has your child been labeled "hyperactive"?

   Mild? 10

   Severe? 20

12. Is your child bothered by learning problems (even though his or her early developmental history was normal)? 10

13. Does your child have a short attention span? 10

14. Is your child persistently irritable, unhappy, and hard to please? 10

15. Has your child been bothered by persistent or recurrent digestive problems, including constipation, diarrhea, bloating, or excessive gas?

   Mild? 10

   Moderate? 20

   Severe? 30

16. Has your child been bothered by persistent nasal congestion, cough, and/or wheezing? 10

17. Is your child unusually tired, unhappy, or depressed?

   Mild? 10

   Severe? 20

18. Has your child been bothered by recurrent headaches, abdominal pain, or muscle aches?

   Mild? 10

   Severe? 20

19. Does your child crave sweets? 10
20. Does exposure to perfume, insecticides, gas, or other chemicals provoke
    moderate to severe symptoms?.. 30
21. Does tobacco smoke really bother your child?................................. 20
22. Do you feel that your child isn't well, yet diagnostic tests and studies
    haven't revealed the cause? 10

Total Score

Yeasts possibly play a role in causing health problems in children with scores of 60 or higher.

Yeasts probably play a role in causing health problems in children with scores of 100 or higher.

Yeasts almost certainly play a role in causing health problems in children with scores of 140 or higher.

Source: Used with permission from William Crook, *The Yeast Connection and Women's Health.* Garden City Park, NY: Square One Publishers, 2003.

PARASITOLOGY TESTING

Though we think of parasites as something we get from traveling in other countries, it's not true. According to the June 27, 1978, *Miami Herald*, the Centers for Disease Control and Prevention (CDC) found that one out of six randomly selected people had one or more parasites. Genova Diagnostics Laboratory routinely surveys stool samples that come into the lab for parasites. I had a conversation about this with Patrick Hanaway, M.D., vice president and chief medical officer at Genova Diagnostics Laboratory. In stool samples coming from people who have symptoms that meet the diagnostic criteria for irritable bowel syndrome, parasites were discovered in 23.5 percent of 14,000 stool samples. The most common ones were Blastocystis hominis (12.5 percent), Dientamoeba fragilis (3.8 percent), Entamoeba species (3.4 percent), Endolimax nana (2.2 percent), and Giardia lamblia (0.7 percent). More than 130 types of parasites have been found in Americans. Parasites have become more prevalent for many reasons, including contaminated water supplies, day-care centers, ease of international travel, foods, increased immigration, pets, and the sexual revolution. Most people will meet a parasite at some point in their lives. Contrary to popular myths, having parasites isn't a reflection of your cleanliness.

If you have prolonged digestive symptoms, you should really consider having a comprehensive parasitology screening. Some symptoms of parasites can appear to be like other digestive problems: abdominal pain, allergy, anemia, bloating, bloody stools, chronic fatigue, constipation, coughing, diarrhea, gas, granulomas, irritable bowel syndrome, itching, joint and muscle aches, nervousness, pain, poor immune response, rashes, sleep disturbances, teeth grinding, unexplained fever, and unexplained weight loss. Most doctors use random ova and parasite testing (O & P), which misses many parasites, so repeated testing is often necessary to get definitive results. For example, in order to rule out giardia with O & P, you'd have to do eight tests before you'd be sure.

Cryptosporidium, giardia, and Clostridium difficile can easily be tested through stool antigen tests. The most accurate testing is done by laboratories that specialize in parasitology testing. Some labs recommend inducing diarrhea with an oral laxative in order to detect parasites that live further up the digestive tract. Other parasites may be found by using a rectal swab rather than a stool sample. Still others use PCR genetic testing.

While I typically recommend natural approaches for most health issues, I recommend pharmaceutical treatment for parasites, which can be followed up with probiotics and sometimes more herbal balancing.

PARASITE QUESTIONNAIRE

Check if yes.

1. Have you ever been to Africa, Asia, Central or South America, China, Europe, Israel, Mexico, or Russia?
2. Have you traveled to the Bahamas, the Caribbean, Hawaii, or other tropical islands?
3. Do you frequently swim in freshwater lakes, ponds, or streams while abroad?
4. Did you serve overseas while in the military?
5. Were you a prisoner of war in World War II, Korea, or Vietnam?
6. Have you had an elevated white blood count, intestinal problems, night sweats, or unexplained fever during or since traveling abroad?
7. Is your water supply from a mountainous area?
8. Do you drink untested water?
9. Have you ever drunk water from lakes, rivers, or streams on hiking or camping trips without first boiling or filtering it?
10. Do you use plain tap water to clean your contact lenses?
11. Do you use regular tap water that is unfiltered for colonics or enemas?
12. Can you trace the onset of symptoms (intermittent constipation and diarrhea, muscle aches and pains, night sweats, unexplained eye ulcers) to any of the above?
13. Do you regularly eat unpeeled raw fruits and raw vegetables in salads?

14. Do you frequently eat in Armenian, Chinese, Ethiopian, Filipino, fish, Greek, Indian, Japanese, Korean, Mexican, Pakistani, Thai, or vegetarian restaurants; in delicatessens, fast-food restaurants, steak houses, or sushi or salad bars?
15. Do you use a microwave oven for cooking (as opposed to reheating) beef, fish, or pork?
16. Do you prefer fish or meat that is undercooked, i.e., rare or medium rare?
17. Do you frequently eat hot dogs made from pork?
18. Do you enjoy raw fish dishes like Dutch green herring, Latin American ceviche, or sushi and sashimi?
19. Do you enjoy raw meat dishes like Italian carpaccio, Middle Eastern kibbe, or steak tartare?
20. At home, do you use the same cutting board for chicken, fish, and meat as you do for vegetables?
21. Do you prepare gefilte fish at home?
22. Can you trace the onset of symptoms (anemia, bloating, distended belly, weight loss) to any of the above?
23. Have you gotten a puppy recently?
24. Have you lived with, or do you currently live with or frequently handle pets?
25. Do you forget to wash your hands after petting or cleaning up after your animals and before eating?
26. Does your pet sleep with you in bed?
27. Does your pet eat off your plates?
28. Do you clean your cat's litter box?
29. Do you keep your pets in the yard where children play?
30. Can you trace the onset of your symptoms (abdominal pain, distended belly in children, high white blood count, unexplained fever) to any of the above?
31. Do you work in a hospital?
32. Do you work in an experimental laboratory, pet shop, veterinary clinic, or zoo?
33. Do you work with or around animals?
34. Do you work in a day-care center?
35. Do you garden or work in a yard to which cats and dogs have access?
36. Do you work in sanitation?
37. Can you trace the onset of symptoms (gastrointestinal disorders) to any of the above?
38. Do you engage in oral sex?
39. Do you practice anal intercourse without the use of a condom?
40. Have you had sexual relations with a foreign-born individual?
41. Can you trace the onset of symptoms (persistent reproductive organ problems) to any of the above?

MAJOR SYMPTOMS

Please note that although some or all of these major symptoms can occur in any adult, child, or infant with parasite-based illness, these symptoms might instead be the result of one of many other illnesses.

■ Adults

1. Do you have a bluish cast around your lips?
2. Is your abdomen distended no matter what you eat?
3. Are there dark circles around or under your eyes?
4. Do you have a history of allergy?
5. Do you suffer from intermittent diarrhea and constipation, intermittent loose and hard stools, or chronic constipation?
6. Do you have persistent acne, anal itching, anemia, anorexia, bad breath, bloody stools, chronic fatigue, difficulty in breathing, edema, food sensitivities, itching, open ileocecal valve, pale skin, palpitations, PMS, puffy eyes, ringing of the ears, sinus congestion, skin eruptions, vague abdominal discomfort, or vertigo?
7. Do you grind your teeth?
8. Are you experiencing craving for sugar, depression, disorientation, insomnia, lethargy, loss of appetite, moodiness, or weight loss or gain?

■ Children

1. Does your child have dark circles under his or her eyes?
2. Is your child hyperactive?
3. Does your child grind or clench his teeth at night?
4. Does your child constantly pick her nose or scratch her behind?
5. Does your child have a habit of eating dirt?
6. Does your child wet his bed?
7. Is your child often restless at night?
8. Does your child cry often or for no reason?
9. Does your child tear her hair out?
10. Does your child have a limp that orthopedic treatment has not helped?
11. Does your child have a brassy, staccato-type cough?
12. Does your child have convulsions or an abnormal electroencephalogram (EEG)?
13. Does your child have recurring headaches?
14. Is your child unusually sensitive to light and prone to blinking frequently, eyelid twitching, or squinting?
15. Does your child have unusual tendencies to bleed in the gums, the nose, or the rectum?

■ Infants

1. Does your baby have severe intermittent colic?
2. Does your baby persistently bang his or her head against the crib?
3. Is your baby a chronic crier?
4. Does your baby show a blotchy rash around the perianal area?

INTERPRETATION OF QUESTIONNAIRE

If you answered "yes" to more than 40 items, you are at high risk for parasites.

If you answered "yes" to more than 30 items, you are at moderate risk for parasites.

If you answered "yes" to more than 20 items, you are at risk.

If you are not exhibiting any overt symptoms now, remember that many parasitic infections can be dormant and then spring to life when you least expect them. Be aware that symptoms that come and go may still point to an underlying parasitic infection because of reproductive cycles. The various developmental stages of parasites often produce a variety of metabolic toxins and mechanical irritations in several areas of the body—for example, pinworms can stimulate asthmatic attacks because of their movement into the upper respiratory tract.

Source: Used with permission from Ann Louise Gittleman, *Guess What Came to Dinner?* Garden City Park, NY: Avery Publishing Group, 1993.

ORGANIC ACID TEST

Organic acid urine testing provides a noninvasive window into how well your metabolism is working. Organic acids are formed as by-products of cellular metabolism, digestion of food, and by the metabolism of the gut microbes such as bacteria and yeast. I consider this test to be a general functional medicine screening and use it often. What comes out in our urine can give profound information about nutritional and immunological factors, including fatty acid metabolism, neurotransmitter metabolism, carbohydrate metabolism, oxidative damage, energy production, detoxification status, B-complex sufficiency, dysbiosis, methylation abilities, and inflammatory reactions. This is probably the best test for determining whether candidiasis is present. You can obtain this type of testing from Great Plains Lab, Genova Diagnostics Lab, Metametrix Lab, and others. It's a simple urine test, done at home and mailed back to the lab for analysis.

SMALL INTESTINAL BACTERIAL OVERGROWTH

This test differs from the comprehensive digestive stool analysis in that it tests for dysbiosis of the small rather than the large intestine. According to Pimentel 78 percent of people with IBS or fibromyalgia, and many with restless leg syndrome and chronic fatigue syndrome, have small intestinal bacterial overgrowth (SIBO). The SIBO test measures breath levels of hydrogen or methane to determine whether there is a bacterial infection in the small intestine. Small bowel overgrowth occurs when bacteria in the large intestine travel to the small intestine. To perform the test, you drink either a lactulose or a glucose drink and collect breath samples. Hydrogen is produced when lactulose or glucose comes in contact with the gut flora. A significant rise in hydrogen levels indicates SIBO. This test is currently available at large teaching hospitals, from gastroenterologists, through functional medicine labs, and at http://www.mybreathtestkit.com.

LEAKY GUT SYNDROME/INTESTINAL PERMEABILITY TESTING

The method that has rapidly become the recognized standard for intestinal permeability testing is the mannitol and lactulose test. Mannitol and lactulose are two types of water-soluble sugar molecules that our bodies cannot metabolize or use and are absorbed into the bloodstream at different rates due to their different sizes. Mannitol is easily absorbed into cells by people with healthy digestion, while lactulose has such a large molecular size that it is only slightly absorbed. A healthy test shows high levels of mannitol and low levels of lactulose. If large amounts of mannitol and lactulose are present, it indicates a leaky gut condition. If low levels of both sugars are found, it indicates general malabsorption of all nutrients. Low mannitol levels with high lactulose levels have been found in people with celiac disease, Crohn's disease, and ulcerative colitis. Your doctor can give you a test kit to collect urine samples. After collecting a random urine sample, you drink a mannitol/lactulose mixture and collect urine for six hours. The samples are then sent to the laboratory. This test is often done in conjunction with a CDSA or a parasitology test.

Although this is a terrific test, I rarely use it because it doesn't tell me why someone has the problem. I'd rather do stool testing and food sensitivity and environmental testing to discover the cause rather than just verify that increased permeability is occurring. Nonetheless, it can be useful to help monitor what's going on.

AMINO ACID TESTING

Proteins are chains of amino acids put together. The average adult has about 22 pounds of protein in his or her body. These proteins are used structurally, as enzymes, and as neurotransmitters, and they are in every cell in our bodies. Using either blood or urine testing, you can determine whether your body is able to break down food and cellular proteins into usable amino acids. If levels are low, first look at food intake of protein. Are you actually eating enough of it? Typically we need about ½ gram of protein for each pound of our body weight. Surprisingly, I often discover low amino acids in people who have low energy, in children and adults who are "failing to thrive," and in people with emotional, behavioral, learning, and mood disorders, even in people who are eating enough protein. Correcting this requires a two-point approach: first, giving free amino acids and easy-to-digest proteins from foods or medical foods, and second, trying to find the underlying mechanism for the malabsorption.

FATTY ACID TESTING

Often we eat the wrong balance of fats, and fats can modulate mood and inflammation. Testing for essential and nonessential fatty acids can be done through either standard blood testing or by a finger-prick blood test. Surprisingly, in people who have been taking fish oils for a long time, we often see people who have terrific levels of omega-3 fatty acids but low levels of beneficial omega-6 fatty acids. It's the balance of total fats in our diet that creates health and reduces inflammation.

INDICAN TEST

The indican test, or Obermeyer test, is a urine test that looks for the presence of indoles in your urine. The level of indican (a type of indole) found in urine gives information about how well you metabolize protein. People with poor digestive function, malabsorption, dysbiosis, gluten problems, and putrefaction of foods have high indican levels. Indican testing is an inexpensive, noninvasive way to screen for faulty digestion. The test won't identify where the problem begins, but it can be used to monitor whether digestion is an issue and how well the treatment plan is working. This test isn't done that often, even though it's a simple in-office test, because the chemicals are toxic.

LACTOSE INTOLERANCE TESTS

There are two ways to test yourself for lactose intolerance: You can do a home elimination or you can do a breath test. Both are detailed in this section.

Self-Test for Lactose Intolerance

This self-test requires eliminating all dairy products from your diet for 10 to 14 days. Obvious dairy sources are milk, yogurt, cheese, ice cream, creamed soups, frozen yogurt, powdered milk, and whipped cream. Less obvious sources are bakery items, cookies, hot dogs, lunchmeats, milk chocolate, most nondairy creamers, pancakes, protein-powder drinks, ranch dressing, and anything containing casein, caseinate, lactose, sodium caseinate, or whey. If you're not sure what's in a food, avoid it during the testing period. It's probably easiest to prepare all of your food at home and go to work or school with a bag lunch during the test. If you eat at a restaurant or at a friend's home for a meal, be specific about what you eat.

If lactose intolerance is causing your problems, you will probably notice that your symptoms have changed significantly and that reintroduction of dairy products triggers a return of symptoms. Most people with lactose intolerance can tolerate small amounts of dairy products or specific dairy products. I, personally, don't drink milk but do well with kefir and raw milk cheeses.

Laboratory Test for Lactose Intolerance

This simple, noninvasive, doctor-ordered test determines whether lactose intolerance is causing a digestive problem and/or contributing to another health problem. This test is ideal for people who have difficulty completing the self-test described above or are confused about their findings. First, you breathe into a bag to supply a baseline sample; then you drink a small amount of a lactose solution. You then breathe into a different bag, and finally, lab technicians measure the amounts of hydrogen and methane gas exhaled in both samples.

A normal hydrogen level is 10 parts per million (ppm), whereas levels of 20 ppm or more are commonly found in people with lactose intolerance. Normal methane levels are 0–7 ppm, and an increase of 12 ppm or more between the two samples indicates lactose intolerance, even if one's hydrogen production is normal. Measuring both methane and hydrogen considerably decreases the likelihood of a false result. Antibiotics, enemas, and laxative use are common reasons for false negative results, which occur 5 percent of the time. This test has a few false positive results, which are generally caused by eating high-fiber foods beforehand, exposure to cigarette smoke, or sleeping during testing. This test is available from gastroenterologists, or at http://www.mybreathtestkit.com.

FRUCTOSE INTOLERANCE TESTING

Diagnosis of fructose intolerance is done with hydrogen breath testing and is very similar to the test for lactose intolerance. Instead of drinking a lactose solution, you'll be given a fructose drink. To get the best results, eat a low-carbohydrate, low-fiber, non-dairy meal the night before, such as a piece of chicken or fish with a nice salad. Avoid fruit, fruit juice, soft drinks, beer, wine, and sweetened teas 24 hours prior to the test. This test can be ordered through any gastroenterologist or online or at http://www.mybreathtestkit.com.

SECRETORY IGA TESTING

You can find secretory IgA (sIgA) levels in stool, saliva, and blood; sIgA is an immunoglobulin antibody found in saliva, throughout the digestive tract, and in mucous secretions throughout the body. It provides our first line of defense against bacteria, food residue, fungus, parasites, and viruses. (It is explained more fully in Chapter 9, "Fire in the Gut.") By sitting on mucous membranes, sIgA prevents invaders from attaching to them and neutralizes them.

High levels indicate that your immune system is dealing with some stressor, such as an infection or high levels of stress. Low levels indicate that you've been fighting the stressor for such a long time that your body can't mount a response.

HEIDELBERG CAPSULE TEST

The Heidelberg capsule test is a radiotelemetry test for functional hydrochloric acid (HCl) levels. It is a simple, effective technique to determine how much HCl your stomach is producing.

In this test, you swallow an encapsulated radio transmitter that's about the size of a B-complex vitamin; the device measures the resting pH of the stomach and also the stomach's pH when administered baking soda, which is very alkaline. Then, by observing how quickly the stomach returns to an acidic condition after the baking soda challenges, the physician can determine whether or not your stomach produces adequate HCl. Unfortunately, this test is not widely available.

Self-Testing for Low HCl/Achlorhydria

Many of us have low hydrochloric acid levels. This opens us up to small intestinal bacterial overgrowth, fungal and parasitic infections, poor digestion of protein, and poor absorption of minerals. There is a simple way to test to see if you have enough HCl. However, please read the precautions carefully before doing this experiment.

Precautions

- You are taking acid. Too much will burn your stomach. *Stop* taking with any discomfort.
- Administration of HCl/pepsin is contraindicated in peptic ulcer disease.
- HCl can irritate sensitive tissue and can be corrosive to teeth; therefore, capsules should not be emptied into food or dissolved in beverages.

Self-Test Instructions

1. Begin by taking one 350 to 750 mg capsule of betaine HCl with a protein-containing meal. A normal response in a healthy person would be discomfort —basically heartburn. If you do not feel a burning sensation, at the next protein-containing meal, take two capsules.
2. If there are no reactions, after two days increase the number of capsules with each meal to two capsules.
3. Continue increasing every two days, using up to eight capsules at a time if necessary. Build slowly to a maximum of eight capsules with each meal. You'll know you've taken too much if you experience tingling, heartburn, diarrhea, or any type of discomfort, including feeling of unease, digestive discomfort, neck ache, backache, headache, fatigue, decrease in energy, or any new odd symptom. If you experience tingling, burning, or any symptom that is uncomfortable, you can neutralize the acid with 1 teaspoon baking soda in water or milk.
4. When you reach a state of tingling, burning, or any other type of discomfort, cut back by one capsule per meal. If the discomfort continues, *discontinue* the HCl and consult with your health-care professional. These dosages may seem large, but a normally functioning stomach manufactures considerably more, about 2,000 mg per meal.
5. Once you have established a dose (either eight capsules or less, if warmth or heaviness occurs), continue this dose.
6. With smaller meals, you may require less HCl, so you may reduce the number of capsules taken.

Individuals with very moderate HCl deficiency generally show rapid improvement in symptoms and have early signs of intolerance to the acid. This typically indicates a return to normal acid secretion.

Individuals with low HCl/pepsin typically do not respond as well to supplements, so to maximize the absorption and benefits of the nutrients you take, it is important to be consistent with your HCl/pepsin supplementation.

Typically I will try to wean people off of HCl supplementation over time by using digestive enzymes, bitters, umeboshi plums, acupuncture, and stress management techniques.

FUNCTIONAL LIVER PROFILE TESTING

Liver profile testing is useful for determining how well you are able to handle toxic substances. The liver is responsible for transforming toxic substances into harmless by-products that the body can excrete. It does this through the cytochrome P450 system in a variety of ways, including acetylation, conjugation, sulfation, and sulfur transferase. By examining urine or saliva, one can see how quickly the toxic materials are transformed. These tests can provide useful information about how well the body is able to detoxify a wide variety of substances.

One type of test is a challenge test. You take small amounts of caffeine, aspirin, and acetaminophen at home and then send urine samples off to the laboratory for analysis. Normal levels of cytochrome P450 are found in 50 percent of people tested. A low-caffeine clearance is found in about one-third of all people tested and indicates that your body is having difficulty detoxifying. High-caffeine clearance levels are found in people who have been recently exposed to high levels of toxins or smoke. Another way to measure liver detoxification pathways is to measure D-glucaric acid and mercapturic acid in the urine. D-glucaric acid is a general marker for phase one cytochrome P450 detoxification pathways. High levels of D-glucaric acid indicate the presence of environmental toxins such as pesticides, herbicides, fungicides, petrochemicals, and excessive alcohol intake. Mercapturic acid provides a measurement of glutathione conjugation. This test is easier on those who do not tolerate caffeine, aspirin, or acetaminophen.

ELECTRODERMAL TESTING

Electrodermal testing, computerized electrodermal screening, electrical acupuncture voltage (EAV), Voll testing, and many other devices are widely used in Europe after much positive research. Although this test has met with FDA resistance in the United States, there are many skillful professionals who use it to successfully diagnose and determine appropriate therapies.

The test measures the electrical activity of your skin at designated acupuncture points. You hold a negative rod in one hand, the practitioner places a positively charged pointer on a variety of points on your skin, and a meter measures the voltage reading between the points. The test can determine which organs are strong or weak, which foods help or hurt you, which nutrients you need or have excessive levels of, and how old patterns are contributing to your health today. It is a fast, noninvasive screening test that you do by simply holding onto a metal bar while being gently touched with a probe.

PART III

Coming Back into Balance

In this part of the book we delve into lifestyle and laboratory testing. The way we respond to everyday events and the way that we live our lives contributes to or detracts from our wellness bank account. Our lifestyle comprises the roots of our wellness tree. These roots feed our organs and body systems. The essential ingredients to build upon are represented in Figure III.1: spiritual and social connection, food, air, water, movement, a clean environment, sleep, a way to handle the stressors of daily life, and ways to balance our energetic output.

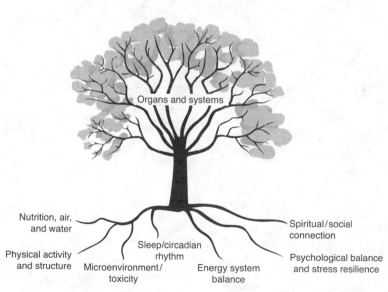

Figure III.1 **The tree of life.**

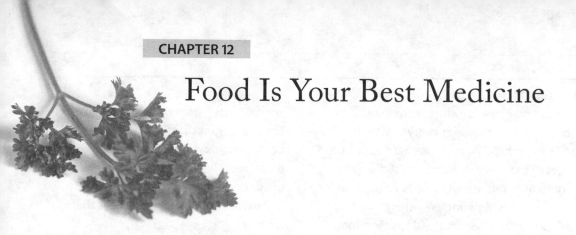

CHAPTER 12

Food Is Your Best Medicine

"Many of the things we claim to cherish—family relationships, cultural identity, ethnic diversity—were all intimately linked to the making and eating of food and now are changing as we outsource more and more of our food preparation to restaurants and industrial kitchens. Not only do we cook less than we used to, but more of us eat alone—at our desks, in our cars, standing at our kitchen counters. In America, the average family shares a meal fewer than five times a week."

—Paul Roberts, *The End of Food*

"Apprentices have asked me, what is the most exalted peak of cuisine? Is it the freshest ingredients, the most complex flavors? Is it the rustic, or the rare? It is none of these. The peak is neither eating nor cooking, but the giving and sharing of food."

—Nicole Mones, *The Last Chinese Chef*

Food is our most intimate contact with our external environment. What we eat, digest, absorb, assimilate, and excrete becomes us. You may already be eating a whole-foods, organic diet. If so, then the information in this chapter may be old news. But if you are like the bulk of the American population, you are probably overfed and undernourished. We eat more than we need to and are getting fatter and fatter. We also eat nearly half of our meals at restaurants or as takeout meals. If you are average, you eat more than half of your calories every day in highly processed, poor-quality, nutrient-poor foods. It's like fixing your home with the poorest materials possible. No wonder we are getting sicker and sicker as a nation.

The energetics of food and the way that food talks to our cells provides an additional way of looking at food. Food is information. Food interacts with our genes, regulating or disrupting normal biological pathways. Each time we eat, we produce neurotransmitters that regulate mood and behavior; polyphenols in foods send messages to our immune system telling it to sooth and calm; food also contains chemical

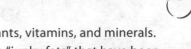

AVERAGE AMERICAN DIET

- Flour and cereal products comprise 23 percent of our calories every day, nearly all of which (89 percent) are refined, which means that they've lost most of their vitamins, minerals, essential fatty acids, and antioxidants. Refining of grains can affect blood sugar levels and lead to inflammation throughout the body.

- We eat 17 percent of our calories from refined table sugar and high fructose corn syrup. The current estimate is about 496 calories a day and more than 22 teaspoons. Of course, it takes B vitamins, magnesium, chromium, zinc, and other nutrients to metabolize and use these sugars, but there aren't any of these nutrients present in refined sugars, so your body has to steal them from somewhere else.

- Twenty-four percent of our calories come from fats and oils, most of which have been highly processed and stripped of antioxidants, vitamins, and minerals. These are "junky fats" that have been denatured, oxidized, and structurally damaged. They're found in nearly all of our packaged and processed foods and in most of the vegetable oils that we buy.

On the other hand:

- We eat only a whopping 5 percent of calories from fruits and vegetables. Less than one person in four eats at least five servings of fruits and vegetables a day (about 2½ cups), even though they protect us against heart disease, cancer, diabetes, and most other illnesses.

- The average American also eats a dearth of nuts each year, only 15 ounces, mainly on pastries. Nuts have been reported to support heart and brain health and generally be terrific for us.

messengers that tell our cells to replicate, excrete wastes, accept nutrients, and more. When we eat nutrient-dense, health-supportive foods, these messages are healthful and appropriate. But when we eat foods laden with chemicals, pesticides, and synthesized ingredients (such as food colorings and restructured fats), we aren't giving our cells the right messages. Our bodies are familiar with foods that have been eaten for centuries. Manufactured foods and genetically engineered foods give different types of messages. The standard diet is inflammatory and is damaging the health of our individual selves, our families, our communities, our schools, and even our nation. What's even more frightening is that our diet is becoming commonplace worldwide.

Once you make the decision to rely on natural foods, your body and mind will adjust so that natural foods taste more delicious than manufactured derivatives. Once your sugar taste buds calm down, fresh fruit will taste sweet again.

I use a 90-10 rule: 90 percent of your food should be excellent for your body, and 10 percent just to goof off and let loose.

Old Nutrition: Fuel	New Nutrition: Information and Fuel
Protein	Old style, plus:
Fats	Polyphenols
Carbs	Antioxidants
Vitamins	Sustainability
Minerals	Nutrigenomics
Water	Organic
	GI health

DIET = A WAY OF LIVING

The word *diet* comes from Greek and means "a manner of living" or "way of life"; the Latin root means "a day's journey." It's about everything that we ingest: our food, our thoughts, our pattern of movement, the TV shows we watch, the music we listen to, the news. Changing our food begins a process of nourishing ourselves and our families that may be the catalyst for even deeper changes.

I am less concerned about whether you are a vegetarian or a meat eater, on an Atkin's or Zone Diet, macrobiotic diet, Ayurvedic diet, Body Ecology Diet, kosher diet, or whatever your particular style of eating is than that you eat *whole foods, organically grown,* as often as possible. Good diets rely on natural, home-cooked, whole-food meals; they are devoid of artificial colors and flavors, trans fatty acids, and refined sugar; and they are loaded with phytonutrients (health-protective substances found in plant foods such as fruits, vegetables, grains, beans, nuts, and seeds), fiber, and good-quality fats.

Finding a digestion-enhancing, health-supportive diet that works for you and your family is what's important. The key is to make real changes—changes you can live with successfully on a long-term basis—in the way you approach food and your lifestyle in general.

Your Food Diary

Write down everything you eat and drink in a food diary for 7 to 14 days. If you experience symptoms or your energy drops or your mood changes, write it down. See whether you can correlate specific foods to the way you feel mentally and physically. A sample food diary shown in Table 12.1 looks like this:

Table 12.1 **Sample Food Diary**

DAY 1			
Time of day	*What did I eat?*	*Where was I?* *Who was I with?* *What was my mood?*	*How does my GI* *tract feel?*

Keep the food diary for at least 7 to 14 days. Then examine it and answer the following questions to gain insight on your eating habits—good and bad.

- Did you eat breakfast every day? "Breaking the fast" provides much-needed fuel.
- Is your digestion better or worse at specific times of the day? Timing can be a clue to causes of indigestion (what, when, where, how fast, how much, and the like).
- How often do you eat? Some of us feel best on three meals a day, others with smaller, more frequent meals and snacks.
- Do certain foods and/or beverages provoke symptoms? Eliminate suspicious foods for at least two weeks and note any differences in how you feel. (See Chapter 15 for more on elimination diets.)

- Are your mealtimes relaxed or rushed? It's important to schedule meals with enough time so you don't feel rushed.
- Do you eat at least five servings of vegetables and fruits each day? What constitutes a serving is ½ cup of fruit and most vegetables. A serving of salad greens is 1 cup.
- What percentage of your food and drinks are high sugar, low fiber, or highly processed? Replace these with fresh, wholesome foods.
- Do you consume enough high-fiber foods? Fiber is consumed in whole grains, fruits, vegetables, and legumes.
- Are you hydrated? One simple way to figure out your daily need is to take your body weight, divide it by two, and drink that many ounces. For example, if you weigh 150 pounds, divide by two and drink 75 ounces of fluids. New research indicates that tea, juice, soup, and other fluids count. Make sure that you choose healthful options and not soft drinks.

RULES TO EAT, COOK, AND LIVE BY

Here are 12 rules to help simplify healthful eating. You can tackle them all at once, or implement one at a time. Make your home a sanctuary of good eating.

1. The Life in Foods Gives Us Life

Fresh foods have the greatest enzyme activity. Enzymes are to the body what spark plugs are to the engine of a car. If we eat foods with little enzyme activity, they don't "spark" our body to work correctly. Eating foods that have natural vibrancy gives vibrant energy to our own bodies. So if it won't rot or spoil, don't eat it!

2. Plan Ahead and Carry Food with You

Planning ahead and carrying your own food are great tools for healthful eating. Planning helps you create balanced meals and saves shopping time. Carrying snacks for yourself and your kids helps keep your moods and blood sugar levels even. It also saves you money and time, and you can ensure that the snacks are healthful.

An extension of this rule is to make bag lunches. That way you have some control (or at least the illusion of control!) about what you eat at work and what your children eat at school. Just put in some leftovers or a sandwich with a salad and/or a piece of fruit, add a beverage, and you've got lunch. Lidded containers and ziplock bags simplify the process. (To save time, I often begin making tomorrow's bag lunch while putting away leftovers from dinner.)

3. Eat Small, Frequent Meals

Snacking is a great strategy for boosting and sustaining energy. Snacking keeps blood sugar levels even and facilitates digestion. People in Europe, South America, and Japan take time in the middle of the afternoon to have tea. Only American adults are "too busy" to stop for a snack—even our children have the sense to rush home from school and raid the refrigerator. Make snacking, especially in the midafternoon, a regular part of your life. You'll find that your energy level will stay more constant throughout the day and your mood will be more consistently pleasurable!

Here are a few healthy snacking ideas:

- Fruit with nuts
- Rice or corn cakes with almond butter
- Peppers with hummus or nut butter
- Pears or apples with almond or peanut butter
- ½ a sandwich
- Bowl of soup with a few whole grain crackers
- Sliced goat cheese or sheep cheese with whole grain bread or crackers
- Yogurt with fruit, sweetened with just a bit of honey or maple syrup
- Baba ganoush with cut up vegetables or pita chips
- Leftovers
- Piece of chicken
- Smoothie
- Fresh vegetable juice or green drink
- Trail mix
- Salsa with veggies and chips
- A few sushi rolls
- Stuffed grape leaves

4. Eat When You Are Hungry and Stop When You Are Satisfied

From the time babies are born, they let us know when they're hungry; they drink as much formula or breast milk as they want, and then they stop sucking when they're satisfied. As they begin eating solid foods and thereon through childhood, children know when they are hungry or full, but then we start encouraging them to just eat a little bit more or to taste something because "it's yummy," or we treat them with cookies or ice cream to reward them for eating their meals. So we learn to eat when we aren't hungry.

Emotional overeating is one of the reasons for obesity in this country. We regularly turn to food when we want love and support. Don't eat if you aren't hungry, but also don't wait until you are overhungry because that's when we lose control and eat the sweetest, fastest foods in sight.

5. Relax While Eating

Many times we don't even stop what we're doing long enough to sit down when we eat. Remember that eating is a time for rejuvenation of body and spirit and a time to connect with yourself and with those you are eating with. One way I've found to encourage peace of mind during meals is to say grace. It puts me in touch with the bounty of our earth, directs my attention to the people I am with and to my gratitude for their presence in my life, helps me thank the people who produced the food, and reminds me that we all depend on each other and community. Family meals are important. Turn the television off and have a family dinner almost every night.

6. Eat Local Foods in Season

Local produce is the freshest and has the highest level of nutrients. Ask your supermarket's produce manager and neighborhood restaurants to purchase locally grown products whenever possible. Put farm stands, community support agriculture (CSA) markets, and farmer's markets into your food-shopping routine. This has the added benefits of supporting the local economy and helping the environment by cutting food-transportation costs and consumption of fossil fuels. Act locally; think globally!

Knowing your farmers, fisheries, and what's available locally helps the food supply become more transparent. The food quality, freshness, and enzymes are most abundant in local foods eaten in season. Eating foods in season also reduces the amount of pesticide and herbicide we consume.

7. Choose Organically Grown Foods Whenever Possible

Organic foods generally have higher nutrient levels because farmers who use organic methods add more nutrients to the soil, knowing that healthy plants can better fend off pests and that the nutrients end up in the crops. Organic plants create higher levels of antioxidants and protective polyphenols. A study from Doctor's Data reported that mineral levels in organically grown apples, pears, potatoes, wheat, and wheat berries were twice as high as in their commercially grown counterparts. Italian researchers found that levels of polyphenols, which are active antioxidant nutrients, were about a third higher in organic peaches and about three times higher in organic pears. Another recent study found that wild berries had twice the antioxidant level as commercially grown berries. As consumer awareness of such benefits increases, organically grown foods are becoming more plentiful and are now stocked in many supermarkets.

Eating organically produced foods is your *only* way to avoid the genetically engineered ingredients that are found in about 80 percent of packaged foods.

Organic food production also protects soils and water, treats animals more humanely, and helps prevent antibiotic resistance. Conventionally (nonorganically) raised animals are routinely given growth-promoting antibiotics and hormones, and animal production accounts for an estimated 70 percent, or 25 million pounds, of the antibiotics used annually in the United States. When we eat nonorganic dairy, poultry, eggs, and meats, we ingest small amounts of these drugs. Antibiotics in animal feed also create the perfect environment for bacteria to develop resistance; as stronger and newer antibiotics are developed, some bacteria survive by adaptation, and these strains can then pass to humans in our food and through contact with farm animals. Conventional animal production thereby lessens the effectiveness of drugs that we so rely on.

8. Eat as Many Fruits and Vegetables as Possible

The available research on the positive benefits of eating fruits and vegetables is overwhelming. They are chock-full of vitamins, minerals, fiber, and phytochemicals (plant-produced substances) that protect us from heart disease, cancer, degenerative diseases, and other common health problems. We know this, yet only about 23 percent of us eat at least five servings of fruits and vegetables daily. And what's known is that more is even better. Shoot for 8 to 10 and make most of them vegetables!

9. Eat High-Quality Protein and High-EPA/DHA
Seafood, Organically and Sustainably Produced

If you choose to eat animal protein, such as poultry, beef, lamb, pork bison, goat, dairy products, eggs, and/or seafood, try to make sure that it is of the best quality possible.

Poultry and meat animals are raised mostly in concentrated agricultural feeding operations (CAFOs) where they receive food that isn't natural for them, and they are raised in conditions that are not conducive to their nature or optimal health. On the other hand, pasture-raised meat animals and poultry that run around on grass and soil have a healthier nutrient content. Environmentally, CAFOs are a disaster. Most water pollution is runoff from animal farming. The antibiotics given to farmed animals go into our rivers, streams, fields, crops, and bodies. The hormones they receive affect us after we eat their meat. Countries that switch from a grain-based to a meat-based economy become poorer, have more hunger and starvation, and strip their land of its natural resources.

When purchasing red meat, look for labels that tell you it has been grass fed or grass finished. If you are eating poultry, look for organic poultry. We are what we eat eats. So, if I buy the "natural" poultry in the market probably that chicken was fed genetically engineered corn and soy products. The only way I can ensure that I am not taking in genetically engineered products is by purchasing organic meats and dairy products. Some of the best products can be purchased at your local farmer's markets or directly from the producer directly at the farm.

Eat wild-caught fish that is sustainably harvested. Personally, I buy only wild-caught fish from the United States and Canada. I never eat salmon unless it's wild caught. At a restaurant, I always ask what type of salmon it is and whether it is wild caught or farmed. If it's wild caught, the chef will give a specific type of salmon, such as sockeye, king, or Chinook. Most farm-raised fish has less healthful omega-3 fatty acid and more polychlorinated bromines than wild-caught fish.

Coldwater fish are also an excellent source of the omega-3 fatty acids that are essential to our good health and promote neurological development in babies and children—hence the old saying, "Fish is brain food." The fatty acids eicosapentaenoic acid (EPA) and docosahexaenoic acid (DHA), found in all of our cells, are especially critical for the eyes, brain, nervous system, heart, and glands. Although many of us can manufacture DHA in our bodies from other fats, like flaxseeds, others lack the enzymes and nutrients (zinc, magnesium, B_6) necessary for this conversion and must obtain DHA through diet. The fish richest in EPA and DHA are salmon, halibut, tuna, mackerel, trout, sardines, eel, and herring. Lower-fat fish or fish from tropical waters are still healthful to eat, but they do not contain significant levels of EPA and DHA. Eating low-mercury and low-toxin fish such as sardines is also beneficial. To get more information on which fish are healthiest, go to the Monterey Bay Aquarium for their Seafood Watch Guides: http://www.montereybayaquarium.org/cr/seafoodwatch.aspx.

Studies show that people who eat coldwater fish twice a week have a reduced risk of heart disease and stroke. Other studies have found fish oils to be protective against, or therapeutic for, allergy, Alzheimer's disease, angina, asthma, attention deficit disorder, cancer, depression, eczema, high blood pressure, high serum cholesterol, hyperactivity, inflammatory disorders, kidney disease, lupus, migraine, multiple sclerosis, psoriasis, rheumatoid arthritis, and schizophrenia. Although supplementation with fish-oil capsules is beneficial, the best way to get these oils is to eat the fish itself.

If you like them, eat organically raised or pastured eggs. Eggs got a bad rap when they were linked to high cholesterol levels, but many researchers now believe that eating eggs has little or no effect on normal serum cholesterol. Recent studies show no significant change in the cholesterol of healthy people after six weeks of consuming two hard-boiled eggs daily, and other studies show that eating eggs can actually raise levels of "good" cholesterol (high-density lipoprotein, or HDL; "bad" cholesterol is low-density lipoprotein, or LDL). Eggs also contain high amounts of phospholipids that are integral to our cell membranes and are a precursor to the important neurotransmitter acetylcholine.

10. Eat More High-Fiber Foods

Researcher Dennis Burkitt, M.D., noticed in the 1970s that rural Africans eating a traditional diet had almost no colon cancer, constipation, diabetes, diverticular disease, heart disease, or irritable bowel syndrome, whereas Africans consuming a Western diet had a heightened incidence of these problems. In a hospital in India, he found that the incidence of appendicitis was only 2 percent of that in a similar American hospital and that there was virtually no hiatal hernia, which affects nearly 30 percent of Americans over 50 years old. After examining many factors, Dr. Burkitt concluded that the large amount of fiber in traditional diets was crucial for health maintenance.

We have since learned much more about fiber and its contributions to health:

- Diets high in soluble fiber help with Crohn's disease, hiatal hernia, irritable bowel syndrome, and peptic ulcer.
- High-fiber diets reduce the risk of heart disease, high blood pressure, and certain types of cancer, including colon cancer.
- Fiber has been shown to normalize serum cholesterol levels.
- High-fiber diets reduce the incidence of colon polyps and bowel disease.
- Dietary fiber helps prevent obesity by slowing digestion and the release of insulin and stored glucose into the bloodstream.
- Improving bowel function can help prevent diverticulosis, appendicitis, hemorrhoids, and varicose veins.

We also know that low-fiber diets lead to the digestive disorders suffered by one out of four Americans. We eat an average of 14 to 15 grams of fiber per day when adults should actually eat 25 to 30 grams of fiber daily (the same amount that Americans ate in 1850).

The richest food sources of fiber are also the four food groups that make up the bulk of a healthful eating plan: whole grains, legumes (all beans except string beans), vegetables, and fruits. (See Table 12.2.) Soluble and insoluble fibers, which work differently inside the body, are mixed in foods, so if you eat a wide variety of high-fiber foods you will get both types of fiber. As a group, beans and legumes have the highest fiber content.

Eating whole-grain products is an excellent way to increase your fiber intake. (See Table 12.3.) Think of using non-gluten-containing grains (and grainlike seeds) such as quinoa, millet, rice, wild rice, amaranth, sorghum, tapioca, corn, risotto, teff, and buckwheat. Unfortunately, many people with dysbiosis cannot tolerate gluten-containing grains (wheat, barley, rye, spelt, kamut, triticale), and some people with digestive issues cannot tolerate *any* grains. Soaking grains and beans before cooking will release minerals and make them more digestible.

11. Drink Lots of Clean Water

Our bodies are 70 percent water. If we don't adequately hydrate our cells, they cannot function properly. Moreover, the water we drink and consume in food is an essential carrier, bringing in nutrients and taking away wastes. In *Your Body's Many Cries for Water*, Fereydoon Batmanghelidj, M.D., described the numerous, even fantastic roles that water plays in the body. Good hydration can help prevent many health problems, from gout to asthma; for example, Dr. Batmanghelidj believed water is

Table 12.2 **Amount of Fiber in Selected Foods**

Food	Amount of Fiber	Food	Amount of Fiber
Fruits (raw)		**Legumes/Starchy Vegetables (cooked)**	
Apple with skin	1 medium = 4 g	Baked beans, canned	½ cup = 6.5 g
Peach	1 medium = 2 g	Kidney beans, fresh	½ cup = 8 g
Pear	1 medium = 4 g	Lima beans, fresh	½ cup = 6.5 g
Tangerine	1 medium = 2 g	Potato, fresh	1 = 3 g
Vegetables (fresh)		**Grains**	
Asparagus, cooked	4 spears = 1 g	Bread, whole wheat	1 slice = 2 g
Broccoli, cooked	½ cup = 2.5 g	Brown rice, cooked	1 cup = 2.5 g
Brussels sprouts, cooked	½ cup = 2 g	Cereal, bran flake	¾ cup = 5 g
Cabbage, cooked	½ cup = 1.5 g	Oatmeal, cooked	¾ cup = 3 g
Carrot, cooked	½ cup = 2.5 g	White rice, cooked	1 cup = 1 g
Cauliflower, cooked	½ cup = 1.5 g		
Romaine lettuce, raw	1 cup = 1 g		
Spinach, cooked	½ cup = 2 g		
Summer squash, cooked	1 cup = 3 g		
Tomato, raw	1 = 1 g		
Winter squash, cooked	1 cup = 6 g		

Table 12.3 **Nutritional Differences Between Refined Grains and Whole Grains**

Nutrient	Wheat flour, per cup			Rice, per cup		
	Whole	*Enriched*	*% loss*	*Whole*	*Enriched*	*% loss*
Protein	16 g	11.6 g	27	14.8 g	13.1 g	11.4
Fiber	2.8 g	0.3 g	89	1.6 g	0.4 g	75
Vitamin B$_1$	0.66 mg	0.48 mg	27	0.68 mg	0.86 mg	+21
Vitamin B$_2$	0.14 g	0.38 mg	+100	0.8	0.06 mg	70
Vitamin B$_6$	0.410 mg	0.066 mg	84	1.0 mg	0.3 mg	70
Biotin	6.0 mcg	1.1 mcg	82	18 mcg	5.86 mcg	67
Niacin	5.2 mg	3.9 mg	25	9.2 mg	6.8 mg	26
Vitamin B$_5$	1.32 mg	0.51 mg	62	2.10 mg	1.26 mg	40
Folic acid	65 mcg	24 mcg	63	3.2 mcg	2.0 mcg	37
Vitamin E	3.12 IU	1.87 IU	40	3.0 IU	0.7 IU	77
Calcium	49 mg	18 mg	63	64 mg	47 mg	27
Copper	0.60 mg	0.21 mg	65	0.4 mg	0.2 mg	50
Iron	4.0 mg	3.2 mg	20	3.2 mg	5.7 mg	+56
Magnesium	136 mg	28 mg	79	172 mg	13 mg	92
Manganese	3.2 mg	2.1 mg	34			
Phosphorus	446 mg	96 mg	78	432 mg	183 mg	58
Vitamin K	444 IU	105 IU	76	420 IU	179 IU	57
Selenium	77.4 mcg	21.7 mcg	72	77.2 mcg	65.1 mcg	13
Sodium	4 mg	2 mg	50	16 mg	10 mg	37
Zinc	2.88 mg	0.77 mg	73	3.6 mg	2.5 mg	28
Fat	2.4 g	1.1 g	54	3.6 g	1.5 g	58

Taken from the U.S. Department of Agriculture.

the best cure for ulcers. Drinking plenty of clean, pure water every day is one of the most promising routes to digestive wellness.

Unfortunately, any chemical we use will show up in our water supply, as groundwater is easily contaminated by runoff. The U.S. Environmental Protection Agency estimates that 1.5 *trillion* gallons of pollutants leak into the ground each year, with the highest incidence of contamination by lead, radon, and nitrates (from fertilizers). More than 700 chemicals have been found in tap water, but testing is commonly done for fewer than 200 of these, and the significance of chemicals in such low concentrations as parts per trillion is often unknown.

Many cities fail to provide good-quality water, and there is much controversy today about chlorination. The level of chlorine needed to kill water-borne bacteria is rising because of increasing bacterial resistance, but chlorine is strongly associated with elevated cancer risks. Inexpensive charcoal filters can remove chlorine and many pollutants from tap water. A pitcher with a simple carbon filter such as Brita or Pur can help purify your drinking water at little cost.

In Europe, bottled water is preferred for its high mineral content. Bottled water isn't always better than tap water, however, especially if it's just tap water that's been filtered. Water from plastic containers may also contain small amounts of plastics that are known to have hormone-disrupting effects. If you regularly buy bottled water, ask the manufacturer for information on water source, type of plastics used, mineral content per glass, and levels of toxic substances. If you rely on local tap water, find out where it originates, how it's processed, and what's been added to it, and ask your water department for an analysis. If you have a well, get a water sample tested for bacterial content and pollutants.

12. Respect Your Own Biochemical Uniqueness
The foods that are best for any person are those that agree with that person's body and unique biochemistry. You will probably need to experiment with your own diet and your family's diet to find out what works best for all of you specifically and over the long term. Whether it's the Zone, the blood-type diet, macrobiotics, a vegan diet, Ayurvedic eating, natural hygiene/food combining, or some other well-balanced program, a proper diet ought to make us feel energetic and keep our immune system strong. Our bodies run best on real foods; a natural-foods diet is the ultimate direction in eating for all of us, no matter exactly how we shape it.

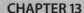

CHAPTER 13

Restorative Foods for Healing

S ometimes we are so debilitated, raw, inflamed, or compromised that we have to go back to eating basics and heal deeply before we can eat normally. Imagine what you would eat if you had the flu. If you are typical, you'll think about broths, ginger ale, flat colas, teas, and water. That's because your body needs fluids. It also needs a lot of energy to fight whatever bug you've caught. So rather than focusing on digesting food, which is also energy demanding, your appetite diminishes so that your body can deal with the infection first. The same is true with healing your body: you'll do best with simple, restorative foods. (Your mom knew what she was doing when she gave you chicken soup or beef consommé.) In previous chapters, we've discussed use of digestive enzymes, umeboshi plums, and other ways to help increase the fire in your belly. In this chapter we'll be talking about specific foods and specific diets that can accelerate healing.

HEALING FOODS DIET: NOURISH THE BELLY'S FLAME WHILE SOOTHING THE MEMBRANES

When working with clients I find myself recommending the same diet over and over for people whose digestive system is weak. You may or may not tolerate or like all of these foods. Eat what you like. Eat what works. This will be different for each person. The ideas here are all for foods that are easy for most people to utilize. They are nourishing foods. When healing, our body thrives on foods that are simple to digest. You may want to think like a sick person or like a baby when it comes to food. Yes, a baby. I've worked with many people who need to puree foods in order to utilize them. You may need to stay on this type of diet for a week or two, or even a couple of months, before your body can handle more. As you get stronger, you'll begin to want to try new foods and explore. The more success you get, the more adventurous you'll become.

Cooked Foods

You'll find that warm, well-cooked foods are easier to digest than raw and cold foods. You may love salads, but they may not love you at this moment in time. Even if you choose to eat your food at room temperature, it will be more healing if you have cooked it previously. You may want to invest in a slow cooker. With a slow cooker, you simply toss food in and it cooks all day or at night while you are sleeping.

You can also put grains and beans in a slow cooker to let them soak for a few hours before cooking. This releases the phytic acid that binds minerals and makes the food not only more nutritious but easier to digest as well.

Eat Frequently and in Small Amounts

You'll digest and use your foods best if you eat small meals and snacks throughout the day and evening. Eat something every one to three hours.

Protein

Your body needs protein to heal. I typically don't eat any red meat, but after major surgery I probably ate brisket several times a day for the first six weeks. I was like a junky who couldn't get enough. Red meat is a protein similar to my own muscle protein. My body needed it to heal. The following list offers great ways to get protein into your diet:

- Bone broths, vegetable broths, miso broth.
- Soups: You can add sea vegetables to add minerals.
- Well-cooked meats, such as brisket or stews, or chicken that was boiled.
- Bone marrow: You can take beef bones and roast them to eat the marrow. This is very nourishing.
- Stews: vegetables plus protein, perhaps some grain or potatoes or yams.
- Eggs: poached, soft-boiled. Buy organic eggs, fresh and local if possible.
- Dairy: You may or may not thrive on dairy. Try some goat's milk kefir to begin with. Try some homemade yogurt, either with sheep's or goat's milk. If raw (fresh) milk is available in your area, you may want to try drinking some raw

milk or making yogurt or kefir from raw milk. You can also make kefir or yogurt with coconut water, coconut milk, or soy milk.

- Protein powder: You can use this for snacks or to add nutrients and calories at mealtime. There are many good protein powders. Look for rice protein, pea protein, hemp protein, or whey protein. You can drink them with water or diluted juice, or use as the base for a smoothie with fruit.
- Dahl: Made with red lentils, this is typically an easy bean to digest.

Fats

Your body also needs fats. They burn slowly and also nourish and soothe your nervous and immune system.

- Healing fats: butter, ghee, coconut oil, olive oil, hemp seed, flaxseed, avocados, coconut milk, coconut water.
- Some people tolerate nuts and seeds, or seed and nut butters. Use these minimally at first. Nut butters, such as almond butter, cashew butter, and macadamia nut butter, are often tolerated in small amounts. These can even be added to a smoothie or mixed with water to make a sauce to put on vegetables. Tahini, sesame butter, can be used the same way. If you tolerate nuts well, eat them. If you soak them first, you will make them more digestible. Roasting nuts also makes them easier to digest.

Grains

Eat non-gluten-containing grains such as rice, quinoa, millet, amaranth, teff, and buckwheat. Make these well cooked, like gruel, or put into soups. You will digest these best if you soak the grains first and also if you use more water than you typically would use. Most grains require two parts water to one part grain. To make grains easier to digest, I recommend three or four parts water to one part grain. Let the grain soak in the water for a few hours before you cook it. Soaking tricks the grains; they "think" that it's spring and time to sprout, and they release precious minerals and nutrients that you'll be able to use. You'll find that the grain is easier to digest, plus the cooking time is cut in half.

Vegetables

If you look at your plate, at least half of what you eat each day ought to be vegetables. Cook these well, culture them, juice them, or eat in soups or stews. Fruits and vegetables contain excellent fibers and prebiotics, protein, minerals, vitamins, polyphenols, and carbohydrate. Here are some suggestions on what to choose:

- Well-cooked vegetables, including *all* non-starchy vegetables and root vegetables. Root vegetables have more starch in them and can be more filling and satisfying. Be brave and try new vegetables: artichoke (boiled soft), arugula, asparagus, bamboo shoots, beets, broccoli, Brussels sprouts, cabbage, carrots, cauliflower, celery, celery root (great in soup), chard, collard greens, cucumber, eggplant, fennel bulb (in soup or roasted), garlic, green beans, kale, leeks, mushrooms, mustard greens, okra, parsley, peas, potatoes (best boiled or in soup or stew), spinach, sweet potatoes, onions, winter squash, turnips, turnip greens, watercress, yams, zucchini.
- Cultured vegetables, such as sauerkraut.
- Sea vegetables. Common sea vegetables include kombu, arame, dulse, and nori. These foods provide minerals and easy-to-utilize proteins. Drop some kombu or other sea vegetable in soup while it's cooking. Use sheets of nori to wrap vegetables or grains in; buy them flaked to use instead of salt in cooking and at the table. Soak some dulse and add it to your vegetables. Add some kelp flakes to your protein powder. You typically find these in the Asian section of a health-food store or in an Asian market.
- Fresh vegetable juices prepared and used the same day. Try carrot, ginger, beet, kale, parsley, apple, watercress, cabbage, or sauerkraut.

Fruit

The amount of fruit that people can tolerate when in a weakened condition varies. Use your body to discover the right amount for you. Start with these suggestions:

- Very ripe fruit
- Cooked fruit
- Applesauce
- Diluted fruit juices

Beverages

It's important that you stay hydrated. Your body is two-thirds water. You may find that drinking teas or warm water is most soothing. Here is a list of beverages to try.

- Water, water with a bit of juice, water with lemon, water with raw apple cider vinegar
- Teas, such as mint, slippery elm, fennel, fenugreek, ginger, umeboshi, roobios, green tea
- Fresh vegetable juices
- Broths

Herbs and Spices
Use fresh or dried herbs and spices in cooking: salt, pepper, basil, oregano, dill, caraway, fenugreek, fennel, cumin, coriander, cinnamon, nutmeg, allspice, and so on. Try to avoid "hot" spices such as cayenne and chili powder unless they call out to you!

MEDICAL FOODS

If you are wasting away and cannot eat much at all, you may want to consider eating a medical food. I've found that medical foods can be life-saving for people who are literally starving. These are hypoallergenic "foods" that are composed of nutrients that are already fully digested. Proteins are presented as free amino acids. Fats are presented as fatty acids. Carbohydrates are simple. Vitamins and minerals are in basic forms that are easily utilized. Typically you would want to drink these one to six times daily to either replace or supplement your diet. There are many of these on the market today. Your physician or nutritionist may recommend one that is covered by your medical insurance plan. There are also others that are manufactured by supplement companies. Typically these are not reimbursable through your health-care plan.

SPECIALIZED DIETS FOR GUT HEALING

There are also several specialized diets that are being used for gut healing. In this section, you'll find short descriptions of the candida diet, Body Ecology Diet, Specific Carbohydrate Diet, and Gut and Psychology Syndrome Diet. What these *all* have in common is that they are low-carbohydrate diets. Bacteria and yeast feed on starches and sugars. By limiting these, you help promote a healthy gut microbiome.

- **Candida diet.** There are many variations of this diet. Typically allowed foods include vegetables that grow above the ground; protein foods such as chicken, fish, pork, beef, lamb, and bison are included. Dairy products, such as yogurt and kefir, are included, as are fats and oils. It looks much like an Atkins Diet. By restricting carbohydrates, you can starve out yeast and bacteria. I typically allow brown rice, millet, flax, psyllium, buckwheat, quinoa, and wild rice when soaked, cooked, and eaten as a whole grain. For my candida diet, go to http://www.digestivewellnessbook.com.

- **Body Ecology Diet.** I particularly like this diet. It allows for whole grains and adds fermented and cultured foods such as yogurt, kefir, sauerkraut, and kimchi. See http://www.bodyecologydiet.com.
- **The Specific Carbohydrate Diet (SCD).** Originally developed for people with Crohn's disease, this diet cuts out all disaccharides (two-sugar molecules), polysaccharides, and starches. It allows meat, fish, poultry, shellfish, hard cheeses, homemade yogurt, honey, nonstarchy vegetables, beans, peanut butter, nuts, fruit, coconut, fats and oils, tea and coffee, gelatin, mustard, and vinegar. It can be helpful for many people. See http://www.scdiet.org.
- **The Gut and Psychology Syndrome (GAPS) diet.** This diet is similar to the Specific Carbohydrate Diet. It is another low-carbohydrate diet and focuses on fresh local meats, raw dairy products, eggs, fish, shellfish, fresh vegetables, fruit, nuts, seeds, garlic, and olive oil. It works well, but I believe it is the hardest to follow. It requires the most change in your diet and the most home cooking and preparation. Nonetheless, it's the best diet for some people. See http://www.gapsdiet.com.

RECIPES

Here are a few basic recipes you may want to try. They are all nutrient laden and gut healing.

 Four-Minute Chicken Stock   Yield: 1 gallon

See the video of Liz making chicken stock at http://www.youtube.com/user/ InnovativeHealing#p/u/3/xqelGyeT14g.

Bones from poultry, fish, beef, lamb, shellfish, or whole chicken or whole carcass (remove meat when cooked— about 1 hour)

8–10 cups water

1–2 tablespoons lemon juice or vinegar

1–2 teaspoons salt

½ teaspoon pepper

2 carrots

1 onion

2 stalks celery

½ cup chopped fresh parsley, or 2 tablespoons dried parsley

1–2 teaspoons sage

1–2 teaspoons rosemary

1–2 teaspoons thyme

2–3 bay leaves

2 tablespoons raw apple cider vinegar or juice from 1 lemon

Put all ingredients into a large pot. Bring to boil. Let simmer over low heat for several hours (4–24) or in a slow cooker on low. Remove bones and vegetables. Let sit until cool, then skim off fat.

This will keep about 5–6 days in your refrigerator. You can easily freeze this and use when you are ready for it.

Uses for Broth
- Use as stock for soup.
- Drink as a warm beverage.
- Use as the cooking liquid for vegetables and grains.
- Make gravy from the fats.

Magic Mineral Broth   Yield: 6 to 7 quarts
Inner Cook notes: If you don't have time to make this from scratch, substitute Pacific or Imagine brand vegetable stock, add equal parts water, a piece of kombu, and one potato. Boil 20 minutes and strain.

Cut the following four ingredients into large chunks

6 unpeeled carrots, including 3 with tops

2 unpeeled medium yellow onions

1 leek, both white and green parts

1 stalk celery including the heart

4 unpeeled cloves garlic, halved

½ bunch flat-leaf Italian parsley

4 medium red potatoes, quartered with skins on

2 Japanese or Hannah yams or 2 sweet potatoes, quartered with skins on

1 garnet yam, quartered with skin on

1 tablespoon sea salt

1 6-inch-by-1-inch strip of kombu

2 bay leaves

12 peppercorns

4 whole allspice or juniper berries

In a 12-quart stockpot, combine all ingredients. Fill pot with water to two inches below rim, cover, and bring to a boil. Remove lid, decrease heat to low, and simmer a minimum of 2 hours. As the stock simmers some water will evaporate; add more if vegetables begin to peek out. Simmer until the full richness of the vegetables can be tasted. Strain stock using a large-mesh strainer. (Be sure to have a heat-resistant container underneath.)

Bring to room temperature before refrigerating or freezing.

Magic Mineral Broth can be frozen up to six months in a variety of airtight container sizes for every use.

Melody's Dahl   This serves 4 hungry people.

Serve this dish with rice and steamed vegetables. Use chutney and/or cultured vegetables as a condiment.

1 cup red lentils (they are actually orange)

4 cups water

1 teaspoon salt

1 teaspoon turmeric powder

1–3 teaspoons grated fresh ginger

2 tablespoons oil or butter or ghee or coconut oil

1 teaspoon powdered cumin

1 teaspoon powdered coriander

Wash red lentils and soak for 2–12 hours. Bring water and salt to a boil and add red lentils. Add turmeric powder and ginger. Turn down heat to a low simmer and cook about 30 minutes (or about an hour if you didn't have time to soak the lentils first). Stir occasionally so that dahl doesn't stick to the bottom of the pot.

Just before serving, take a small frying pan and heat oil, butter, or ghee on medium to medium-low heat. When oil is hot, add cumin and coriander. Cook 1 minute and then add to the dahl. Stir the dahl. Cook a couple more minutes and serve with rice and steamed vegetables. It's also delicious with a dab of chutney or cultured vegetables.

Bone Marrow Three Ways

1. Add marrow bones to soups and stews. The marrow will "melt" into the dish.

2. Ask the butcher to cut the bones into two- to three-inch sections. Soak these in cold water for 12–24 hours. Change the water a few times to keep the pinkish color. Boil for 20 minutes. Scoop out the marrow with a spoon. You can sprinkle this with salt and eat it or use it in soup or as a garnish.

3. Roasted marrow: Take two- to three-inch pieces of marrow bones. Place in an ovenproof frying pan or on a cookie sheet standing upright. Roast at 450 degrees Fahrenheit for 20 minutes. The marrow is ready when loose and giving. If you cook it for too long, it will simply melt away.

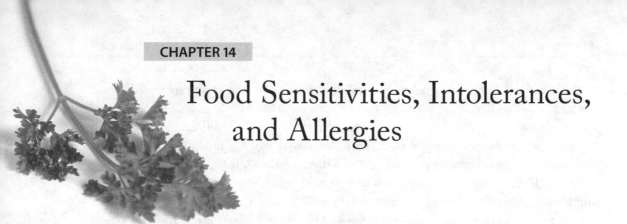

CHAPTER 14

Food Sensitivities, Intolerances, and Allergies

"The gut is a major potential portal of entry into the body for foreign antigens. Only its intact mucosal barrier protects the body from foreign antigen entry and systemic exposure."

—Russell Jaffe, M.D.

Today one out of three people say that they have a food allergy or sensitivity and change their diet to reflect this. The average American eats about 2,000 pounds of food each year, compared to a teaspoon or two of pollen that we breath in annually. Remember that two-thirds of the immune system is in the gut. Food is the main reason why: our body is deciding if it's friend or foe.

Our immune system was designed to fend off infection, so if you have reactions to food or the environment, it's a signal that your body has become less tolerant. We must build tolerance so that we can live a normal and active life. Our tolerance of our foods and other environmental exposures is based on many factors, including genetics, age, gender, intestinal permeability (or increased permeability/leaky gut), infections, and balance of gut ecology as well as the type and dose of the particular substance or antigen. It's our body's way of defending itself and coming back into balance. This can be provoked by foods, molds, pollen, chemicals, metals, and nearly any other substance.

TRUE FOOD ALLERGIES

True food allergies—those that trigger IgE reactions—are rare, affecting only 0.3 to 7.5 percent of American children and 1 to 2 percent of adults. The foods that most often trigger true allergic reactions are eggs, cow's milk, nuts, shellfish, soy, wheat, and white fish. Allergy to peanuts has doubled within the past five years in children under the age of five. Peanut allergy can be so severe that a child may react if someone else recently ate peanuts or peanut butter in the room the child is in—that's why peanuts are no longer served on many airplanes and why all nuts are not allowed in many schools. Physicians diagnose food allergies through the use of patch skin tests and RAST (radioallergosorbent test) blood testing, which are great for detecting food allergies but do not accurately determine food sensitivities. IgE antibodies attach to mast cells in mucous membranes and in connective tissues, stimulating the release of inflammatory cytokines and histamines. The resulting allergic response produces symptoms a few minutes to two hours after the food is eaten. Common symptoms include closing of the throat, fatigue, tearing, hives, itching, respiratory distress, watery or runny nose, skin rashes, itchy eyes or ears, and sometimes severe reactions of asthma and anaphylactic shock.

FOOD SENSITIVITIES

It is estimated that 10 to 20 percent of us have food sensitivities. Food sensitivity reactions, also called delayed hypersensitivity reactions and in the past called "serum sickness," occur when IgA, IgG, and IgM antibodies are triggered in response to foods, chemicals, and bacterial toxins. The most common antibody reactions are IgG to mold and foods; exposure to molds and foods is quite high compared to pollens. These IgA, IgM, and IgG responses are called "delayed" sensitivity reactions because the symptoms they cause can take from several hours to several days to appear, which makes it very difficult to track down the offending food or substance.

When antibodies bind to antigens, as in delayed food sensitivity reactions, they form "immune complexes," which are clumps of molecules that the immune system disposes of. Large ones are eaten up by macrophages, the Pacman of the immune system. Smaller immune complexes, however, can bind to tissues, causing problems. Use of protein-digesting enzymes (also called protease enzymes or proteolytic enzymes) can help to clear the bloodstream of circulating immune complexes.

It is estimated that 95 percent of all food allergy is of this delayed type. IgM antibodies circulate temporarily, about three months, until IgG antibodies are mobilized to take over the fight. IgG antibodies are longer lasting, and we keep producing them as long as we eat the offending foods or are exposed to chemicals, bacterial toxins, or other foreign substances (antigens) that are challenging the immune system.

Although almost any food can cause a food sensitivity reaction, beef, citrus, dairy products, egg, corn, pork, and wheat provoke 80 percent of them.

Food sensitivities can underlie a huge variety of symptoms (see box). It's important to discover which foods you are reacting to and also to see what the underlying cause may be, such as parasites, candidiasis, bacterial or viral infection, pancreatic insufficiency, enzyme deficiency, medications, or poor lifestyle habits.

SENSITIVITY SYMPTOMS

Professional evaluation is necessary to determine whether the following symptoms, which can be caused by many health conditions, are due to food and/or environmental sensitivities:

- **Head:** Chronic headaches, migraines, difficulty sleeping, dizziness
- **Mouth and throat:** Coughing, sore throat, hoarseness, swelling or pain, gagging, frequently clearing throat, sores on gums, lips, and tongue
- **Eyes, ears, nose:** Runny or stuffy nose, postnasal drip, ringing in the ears, blurred vision, sinus problems, watery and itchy eyes, ear infections, hearing loss, sneezing attacks, hay fever, excessive mucus, dark circles under eyes, swollen, red, or sticky eyelids
- **Heart and lungs:** Irregular heartbeat (palpitations, arrhythmia), asthma, rapid heartbeat, chest pain and congestion, bronchitis, shortness of breath, difficulty breathing
- **Gastrointestinal tract:** Nausea and vomiting, constipation, diarrhea, irritable bowel syndrome, indigestion, bloating, passing gas, stomach pain, cramping, heartburn, GERD, ulcers
- **Skin:** Hives, skin rashes, psoriasis, eczema, dry skin, excessive sweating, acne, hair loss, irritation around eyes

- **Muscles and joints:** General weakness, muscle and joint aches and pains, arthritis, swelling, stiffness
- **Energy and activity:** Fatigue, mental dullness and memory lapses, difficulty getting your work done, apathy, hyperactivity, restlessness
- **Emotions and mind:** Mood swings, anxiety and tension, fear, nervousness, anger, irritability, aggressive behavior, binge eating or drinking, food cravings, depression, confusion, poor comprehension, poor concentration, difficulty learning
- **Other:** Overweight, underweight, fluid retention, insomnia, genital itch, frequent urination, bed-wetting

In addition to the symptoms previously listed, children with food and/or environmental sensitivities may have:
- Attention deficit disorder
- Behavior problems
- Learning problems
- Recurring ear infections

Children with these problems will often benefit from a dietary evaluation and environmental sensitivity testing.

FOOD INTOLERANCES

Some people have intolerances to sugars or specific carbohydrates in certain foods. This means that they lack the enzymes that are needed to digest them. The most common ones include gluten intolerance, lactose intolerance, and fructose intolerance.

Lactose intolerance is common, affecting 25 percent of Americans and 75 percent of people globally and is highly prevalent in African Americans, Asian Americans, Caucasian Americans of Mediterranean and Jewish descent, Hispanics, and Native Americans. Lactose intolerance is not a milk allergy, which is the inability to digest milk proteins such as casein. Lactose intolerance is caused by a deficiency in lactase, an enzyme that digests lactose, which is a sugar naturally found in milk and milk products. After the age of two, our lactase production gradually tapers. Lowering of our ability to digest lactose can also occur from infections (bacterial, viral, parasitic, fungal), foods, and other substances that can injure the lining of the gut. Lactose intolerance causes a wide variety of symptoms, including abdominal cramping, acne, bloating, diarrhea, gas, eczema, headaches, and nausea. Often when dysbiosis is balanced, lactose intolerance becomes less of a problem.

Most people who are lactose intolerant can tolerate some dairy products, which makes figuring this out less obvious than one would think. Often it's a matter of amount; sometimes it's a matter of which type of dairy product. I, personally, can eat kefir and raw milk cheeses but cannot drink milk. Other people have told me that they can eat low-fat yogurt but not full-fat yogurt; and others just the opposite. Eliminating dairy completely from your diet for two to four weeks or doing a hydrogen breath test will give you a good idea whether dairy is for you.

A hereditary form of fructose intolerance occurs in 1 in 10,000 people and generally shows up when children are small. They naturally dislike sweets, juices, and foods that have fructose because it makes them sick.

But we can acquire fructose intolerance because of the high amount of fruit and sweeteners we eat. The average person eats more than 140 pounds of processed sugars a year, pushing many of us above the threshold that we can tolerate. Fructose is found in highest conentrations in table sugar, apples, pears, fruit juices, dried fruit, watermelon, honey, high fructose corn syrup, corn syup solids, agave nectar, sorbitol, xylitol, and sweet wines. So, drinking sweetened teas and soft drinks is a big no-no!

Typically people with fructose intolerance are diagnosed with irritable bowel syndrome. Common symptoms include loose stools or diarrhea, constipation, alternating diarrhea and constipation, gas, bloating, cramping, indigestion, depression, sometimes belching, nausea, and occasional vomiting. Testing for fructose intolerance is also done with breath testing.

If you have fructose intolerance, you'll want to avoid all foods that contain high amounts of fructose. You may also want to avoid foods with high fructan content including artichokes, asparagus, leeks, onions, and wheat products.

See Chapter 11, "Functional Medicine/Functional Testing," for more information on lactose, fructose, and gluten testing.

LECTINS

Lectins are found everywhere in nature. They are found in high amounts in all beans, peas, lentils, and peanuts, and in smaller amounts in edible snails and wheat. Plants produce them to protect themselves from being eaten, and they are involved in germination. In our own bodies lectins play a role in the immune system by recognizing carbohydrates that don't belong. On the other hand, they can wreak havoc if we don't have the enzymes to digest them: They bind to carbohydrate molecules in all tissues and cause them to clump together. They bind to the GI mucosa, which weakens it and allows it to become permeable (leaky). They degranulate mast cells, which causes them to produce IgE antibodies and set off allergic reactions.

Lectins, when not properly digested, can connect two IgE molecules, which triggers the release of histamines and begins an allergic reaction, mimicking food allergies. The digestive system and nervous system are especially sensitive to lectin reactions. This can appear as irritable bowel syndrome, arthritis, or nearly any inflammatory condition. The people whose arthritis responds to elimination of the nightshade family of foods (potatoes, eggplant, tomatoes, peppers) probably have lectin sensitivities.

By cooking beans for long periods of time or in a pressure cooker, we can destroy most of the lectins. Taking digestive enzymes can also help.

FOOD CRAVINGS AND EXORPHINS

Oddly enough, about half of people with food sensitivities and intolerances crave the foods that make them sick. This is because many foods, such as wheat and dairy products, produce protein molecules that are really similar to our natural endorphins, called exorphins. Endorphins and their mimics, exorphins, lessen pain and help generate a general sense of well-being in our world. So, even if we are intolerant of lactose, we crave it and even feel better when we drink milk . . . temporarily, that is. And then we crave some more.

ENVIRONMENTAL ILLNESS

Environmental sensitivities are another type of enzyme deficiency, but this one is a lack of liver detoxification enzymes. (See Chapter 18 for more on detoxification.) Chronic exposure to food additives, household chemicals, building materials, contaminated recirculating air, and impure water can so depress and weaken a person's immune system that eventually exposure to even a small amount of a toxin can make one acutely or chronically ill. This condition, called environmental illness or multiple chemical sensitivities, is becoming more and more common. Two recent studies put its incidence at 12.9 percent and 15.9 percent in adults.

If blood testing shows that you have environmental allergies, or if you know that specific substances make you ill, it is essential that you avoid these substances. Malic acid taken supplementally can be helpful in neutralizing some of the reactions. Unfortunately, many people look fine and are treated as if they are depressed or psychotic. This is a serious illness and if you suspect environmental illness, it is also important to work with a health-care provider who is educated in this area. Look for an M.D. who specializes in environmental medicine (http://www.aaemonline.org).

LABORATORY TESTING FOR SENSITIVITIES AND ALLERGIES

Allergy testing for true IgE allergies is straightforward. It is most often done with scratch testing, but it can also be done with a simple blood test called modified RAST testing.

Testing for food and environmental *sensitivities* is less clear-cut. One problem is that there is little standardization of non-IgE-mediated laboratory testing. That means labs use a variety of methodologies, and results don't compare well between methods; however, they can compare well when the same methods are used. Some labs test for generalized inflammation to various foods by measuring inflammatory markers. Other labs test for specific antibodies, mainly IgG, while some labs test for IgA, IgM, or IgG4 antibodies. And some of these labs also test for IgE, true allergies, at the same time.

Table 14.1 offers a comparison of laboratories that test for food allergies. This table gives specifics on what each laboratory is measuring, which may include specific antibodies (IgA, IgE, IgG, IgG4, IgM), type III immune complexes, or type IV cell activation.

Table 14.1 Comparison of Laboratories for Delayed Food Sensitivity Reactions

	Alletess Medical Lab	Elisa Act	Genova Diagnostics	Great Plains Lab.	Immuno Laboratories	Metametrix Clinical Lab	Meridian Valley Lab	US Biotek Laboratories	Alcat (Antigen Leukocyte Cellular Antibody Test)	LRA (Lymphocyte Response Assay) Medical Lab	NuTron/NOVO Immogenics	MRT/LEAP Testing (Mediator Release Testing/Lifestyle Eating and Performance)	Sage Medical Lab (Complement Testing)
Specific IgG or IgG4 (memory)	X							X					X
Specific IgE (allergy)	X												
Specific IgA (mucosal)								X					
Specific IgM (current)								X					
Type III immune complex								X					X
Type IV cell activation									X				

Environmental screening panels measure antibody reaction to chemicals commonly found in our homes, yards, workplaces, and public places. People often test positive to household cleaning supplies and petroleum-based chemicals. Several laboratories perform antibody testing for foods, dusts, environmental chemicals, heavy metals, molds, and pollens.

What I find is that although the results differ, all of these labs can give information that will give you good results. None of the labs finds all sensitivities; yet they all find enough to lower your overall load to help you feel better. These labs are listed in the Resources section at http://www.digestivewellnessbook.com.

HEALING OPTIONS FOR SENSITIVITIES AND ALLERGIES

With a holistic treatment program, you can become increasingly less sensitive to foods and environmental antigens over time. Begin by avoiding all substances you are sensitive or allergic to. Using the probiotics, anti-inflammatory nutrients, and herbs listed in this section will speed the process. Eating organically grown, nutrient-rich, natural foods promotes the body's self-repair. An exercise program and stress management also play a part in recovery.

Do at least the first five of these recommendations for best results:

- **Avoidance:** Avoid all substances that cause you to have a sensitivity or allergic reaction, for a period of four to six months. To substitute for these, check out a health-food store's plethora of special foods for people with food allergies. If chemical sensitivity is an issue, use natural household-cleaning products (it's good to use them anyway!). Some people also react to mattresses, gas stoves, paints, carpeting, and upholstery, which can make avoidance difficult. Consult a health-care professional who can help with the details.
- **Try an elimination diet:** See Chapter 15 for instructions.
- **Glutamine:** This is an amino acid that will help heal the intestinal tract. Take 500 mg once daily up to 15 grams daily, mixed in juice or water.
- **Probiotics:** Ones such as lactobacilli and bifidobacteria (see Chapter 4) protect the digestive tract's mucosal lining and limit damage caused by pathogenic bacteria. Take 10 billion to 50 billion CFU daily with food.
- **Enzymes:** Digestive enzymes and proteolytic enzymes (protein-splitting enzymes) are very useful in helping normalize allergies. They are gentle and help in several ways. The digestive enzymes help the foods to be more fully digested.

The proteolytic enzymes are taken between meals and break up immune complexes. Take one to two capsules of digestive enzymes with each meal and snack, or one capsule of proteolytic enzymes at bedtime and upon rising.

- **Quercetin:** This bioflavonoid reduces pain and inflammatory responses and controls allergies. Take 250 to 1,000 mg one to four times daily.
- **Herbs:** Examples include milk thistle, dandelion root, and burdock, and they support the liver. These herbs can be used singly or in combination in tea or tinctures or capsules. Typical dosage for tea is 1 to 3 cups daily. For tinctures and capsules, use as directed on label.
- **Vitamin C:** This helps flush toxins. Take 500 to 3,000 mg or more of buffered ascorbate or Ester-C daily.
- **Mineral salts:** These contain bicarbonates of calcium, magnesium, and/or potassium (for example, Alka-Seltzer Gold) to alkalize the stomach and to help minimize reactions. Use as directed on label.
- **Malic acid:** This acid naturally occurs in fruits and can be used to stop or slow reactions if you have eaten something questionable. Use as directed on label.
- **Four-day food-rotation diet:** This is helpful if you are sensitive or allergic to a large number of foods and food families. Someone who is sensitive to a wide variety of foods often becomes sensitive to more and more foods. A four-day food rotation prevents an ever-widening set of food issues. In this protocol, you avoid eating any foods to which you had strong antibody reactions, and eat the remaining foods in a four-day pattern that helps prevent the development of sensitivity to those foods as well. We basically trick the body into being more tolerant by rotating our foods. When we eat a specific food that we are sensitive to, we begin to produce antibodies against that food over the next 24 hours. If we eat the food again the next day, we have symptoms from it. If we don't eat it again for several days, those antibodies, which were ready for a fight, disappear as if it were a false alarm. When we restart the rotation and resume eating the food, the antibody-production process begins again, but we don't develop symptoms in response to the food because the antibodies are never present at the time you eat the food. Most labs supply customized rotation diets along with your results. *Allergy Recipes* by Sally Rockwell, Ph.D., and *The Rotation Diet* by Trish Blascak are two good books on the topic. (See a sample rotation diet at http://www.digestivewellnessbook.com.)

CHAPTER 15

The Elimination Diet, or How to Feel Remarkably Better in Two Weeks

"If the patient has been to more than four physicians, nutrition is probably the medical answer."

—Abram Hoffer, M.D., Ph.D.

If we had a drug that worked as effectively as an elimination diet, it would be the bestselling drug of all time. Food can be inflammatory; food can be healing. An elimination diet is simple: you take away foods that potentially cause inflammation and eat only foods that have a low possibility of provoking a reaction. This is also called a low-antigen diet. You eat this way for a minimum of two weeks to a maximum of three months and then begin adding foods back into your diet to see what provokes symptoms. Often the foods we are sensitive to are the ones that we *least* want to live without. When I hear someone say "I just couldn't live without dairy," then I'm pretty sure that's one of the foods that may be hurting that person at the moment.

There are many types of elimination diets. The one in this chapter will work for about 80 percent of people. Yet there isn't one perfect diet for all needs. In Chapter 13, you'll find information on some of the other diets that work when the elimination diet doesn't. If you have candidiasis or small intestinal bacterial overgrowth often a low carbohydrate diet will work better for you than the elimination diet. That's why I recommend that you work with a nutrition professional if you aren't sure.

To enhance this process, you may also want to have a blood test for food sensitivities. While many foods may be unmasked during the elimination-provocation challenge, others may remain hidden. Upon testing I often find foods that we just didn't suspect.

If you suspect that chemicals, molds, or pollens are causing problems, you should also be screened for them. (Labs offer these tests either separately or as part of a complete screening package.) Sensitivities are rated from normal to severe reactions. In addition to a detailed readout documenting your personal reactions, most laboratories also include a list of foods that are hidden sources of the offending foods, a rotation menu, and other educational material to help you in the healing process.

DETOXIFY WHILE DOING THE DIET?

Sometimes I recommend using a rice-based medical food while doing this elimination diet. It allows the diet to work more deeply and effectively. It's not for everyone; read more about it in Chapter 18, "Cleansing and Detoxification."

ELIMINATION-PROVOCATION DIET

This diet is used to determine whether or not you have food allergies that may be causing some or all of your symptoms. During a period of two to three weeks you eliminate foods from your diet that are the most likely culprits. If your symptoms improve during the three-week period, you'll carefully add foods back into your diet one at a time to see which foods may be triggering symptoms. You may want to keep dairy, eggs, and gluten-containing grains out of your diet for up to three months to get the best result. Make sure to read all labels carefully to find hidden allergens. Eat a wide variety of foods and do not try to restrict your caloric intake. If you find no improvement within three weeks either you do not have any food allergies or you have food allergies but there is yet another factor complicating the picture. There are no magical answers here; this is a journey of self-exploration and discovery. (At http://www.digestivewellnessbook.com you will find shopping lists, recipes, and more.)

Allowed Foods
Please read all ingredients carefully. You want to eat only those ingredients that are specifically allowed.

- **Rice:** All types of rice are allowed, as are 100 percent rice cakes, 100 percent rice crackers, rice noodles, dry cereals (puffed rice cereal), rice milk (read all ingredients and do not use if it has corn or other prohibited ingredients), Crispy Brown Rice, 100 percent rice bread, and plain rice protein powder.

- **Additional grains:** If desired you can add these specific grains: quinoa, buckwheat, millet, amaranth, teff, tapioca, and potato flour.
- **Fruits:** All fruits are allowed except for citrus fruits. Avoid oranges, lemons, grapefruits, tangerines, tangelos, and any other citrus. Use fresh fruit or canned fruits in their own juices; you can also cook or poach fruits. You can drink diluted fruit juices. You can use a limited amount of dried fruit (unsulfured only). If you suspect candidiasis or small intestinal bacterial overgrowth, limit fruits or avoid them completely during these initial three weeks.
- **Vegetables:** Use a wide variety. All vegetables except corn are allowed. If you have arthritis, you may want to also eliminate the nightshade family foods: tomatoes, peppers (green, red, yellow, chilies, cayenne, chili powder), eggplant, and potatoes. You can use vegetables any way you like: steamed, raw, juiced, roasted, in salads, stir-fried, and grilled.
- **Fish:** All fresh, wild fish are OK. Canned fish is OK; for canned tuna choose a type that is packed in water. Avoid shellfish, swordfish, shark, tile fish, and king mackerel.
- **Poultry:** Use organic chicken, turkey, duck, pheasant, lamb, quail, wild game birds, and so forth.
- **Nuts and seeds:** Coconut, pine nuts, and flaxseeds are allowed.
- **Oils and fats:** Choose sunflower, coconut, olive, flax, ghee. Use cold-pressed or expeller-pressed, or virgin olive oils only.
- **Sweeteners:** Use sparingly; brown rice syrup, honey, agave, stevia, fruit sweetener, blackstrap molasses.
- **Beverages:** Water is the best beverage. Also allowed are carbonated water (no flavorings), mineral water, seltzer, pure fruit juices without sugar or additives (dilute 50 percent with water), and herbal teas without caffeine. (Sometimes if it's a deal breaker, I'll allow black coffee, or black or green tea.)
- **Dairy substitutes:** Rice milk and hemp milk are allowed.
- **Spices and condiments:** Use salt in moderation, pepper, all herbs and spices either fresh or dried (without preservatives, citrus, or sugar).

If you are a vegetarian, replace fish with legumes. If not, please eliminate all beans for at least three weeks.

Examples of legumes include lentils, navy beans, black beans, split peas, and string beans. Dried beans should be soaked overnight. Pour off the water and rinse before cooking. Canned beans often contain added sugar or other potential allergens. If you want to use canned beans, look to health-food store brands.

What to Expect and How to Ease the Transition

- The first two to three days are the hardest. It's important to go shopping to get all of the foods you are allowed to have. Plan your meals and have a pot of rice available. Make a pot of vegetable soup. Make a large salad. Have planned leftovers.
- Keep it simple.
- Avoid any foods that you know or believe you may be sensitive to, even if they are on the "allowed" list.
- Eat regular meals. You may also want to snack to keep your blood sugar levels normal. It is important to keep blood sugar stable. Carry food with you when you leave the house to avoid straying from the plan.
- Try to eat at least five servings of fresh vegetables each day. Choose at least one serving of dark green (for example, broccoli, kale, spinach, collards) or orange (carrot, winter squash) vegetables, and if you can digest it, eat at least one salad daily.
- Vary what you eat.
- Generally, eat grains as whole grains rather than as flours in breads or crackers.
- Don't eat too many sweets. Replacing regular cookies with gluten-free cookies may not get you the results you are looking for, especially the first couple of weeks.
- Buy organic produce when possible.
- This is *not* a weight-loss program. If you need to lose or gain weight, work with your practitioner on a program.

POSSIBLE PROBLEMS

Most people feel better and better each day during the allergy elimination diet. However, if you are used to using caffeine, you may get withdrawal symptoms the first few days, which may include headaches, fatigue, irritability, malaise, or increased hunger. If you find your energy lagging, you may need to eat frequently to stabilize your blood sugar levels (for thinking and energy). Be sure to drink plenty of water. If you lose too much weight on this diet, stop and find a clinician to help you troubleshoot.

TESTING INDIVIDUAL FOODS

Once you have completed two to three weeks on the elimination diet you can begin to add foods back into your diet. *Keep a journal of all foods eaten and all symptoms.* Be sure to add foods one at a time, one every four days. Be sure to test foods in a pure form: for example, test milk or cheese or wheat, but not macaroni and cheese that contains milk, cheese, and wheat! Eat the test food at least twice a day and in a fairly large amount. Often an offending food will provoke symptoms quickly—from 10 minutes to 12 hours. If this occurs, do not continue to eat the food. Many times you will eat a food one day and feel fine, but the second day you will notice that you are reacting to the food. Signs to look for include headache, itching, bloating, nausea, dizziness, fatigue, diarrhea, indigestion, anal itching, sleepy 30 minutes after a meal, flushing, and rapid heartbeat. If you are unsure, take the food back out of your diet for at least one week and try it again.

THE RESULTS

When you avoid symptom-provoking foods and take supportive supplements to restore gut integrity, most food allergies or sensitivities will resolve in four to six months. This means that in most cases you will then be able to again eat foods that formerly bothered you. In some cases, you will find that the allergy doesn't go away. In this case either you must wait longer for it to heal or it is a "fixed" allergy that will remain lifelong.

AFTER THE TESTING

It is advisable to return to your health practitioner for a follow-up visit to determine next steps. If you find allergies in too many foods, you may want to explore a four-day food rotation diet, described in Chapter 14.

You can find a more complete Elimination Diet with shopping lists and recipes at http://www.digestivewellnessbook.com.

CHAPTER 16

Managing Stress and Finding Balance

"To the ego, the present moment hardly exists. Only past and future are considered important. This total reversal of the truth accounts for the fact that in the ego mode the mind is so dysfunctional. It is always concerned with keeping the past alive, because without it—who are you?"

—Eckhart Tolle, *The Power of Now: A Guide to Spiritual Enlightenment*

"In Sri Lanka, we often compare human life to a river. When river water falls down the hills, it creates a beautiful waterfall. When it crashes on rocks, white foam is created, expressing its incredible hidden beauty. When the river silently flows through the valleys, it becomes mysterious and magical. These different things that happen to the river water along its path are all manifestations of its beauty. So, too, if we are to make meaning out of our odyssey as human beings on this planet, we have to accept that whatever happens on our way adds to life's beauty."

—Bhante Wimala, *Lessons of the Lotus: Practical Spiritual Teachings of a Travelling Buddhist Monk*

It is the meaning we attach to our experiences that makes them stressful or stress-free. Last week we had torrential rain here in Asheville. I loved the rain. The sound of it reminded me of the heavy rains of my childhood in the Chicago suburbs. The creek below my house grew and I could hear it in the mornings from my bedroom. I settled in and took life a bit more slowly. The foliage developed a deep green hue that felt nurturing and satisfying. The land needed the rain. All of this fit my mood. But when I mentioned this to two people, the responses that I got were: "I hated the rain. I'm sensitive to mold and couldn't breathe" and "It's a good thing it stopped raining; otherwise we would have had flooding in a few days." It is our perspective and beliefs that shape whether something is stressful or pleasurable. To me, the rain was a delicious treat. To others, something dreaded. Our attitude can affect how severe our digestive issues are as well.

From the time we are small, we attach meaning to events. When you first spilled milk from your glass and got yelled at for it, you attached: "not good enough" or "less than" to that spill. This happens to all of us, and we carry these meanings and conditioning around as adults, deeply held even though we aren't even aware of it. In my clients, I often find that I can go only so far by trying to balance biochemistry. Often, emotional and spiritual blockages prevent healing from occurring on a deep level. Once these are released, more healing takes place. Working with a therapist, co-counselor, coach, energetic healer, acupuncturist, bodyworker who incorporates emotional release, or others can help to facilitate release of the emotional issues that keep your healing stuck. One of my favorite of these personally was many years ago when I took a workshop called "The 12 Stages of Healing" with Dr. Donald Epstein. The second stage of healing is in releasing "stuck" energies in our bodies. When we found "stuck" places we shouted out "I'm stuck" to help release these. A group of crazy people to be sure, but we felt amazingly shifted after the weekend was over.

We experience stress on four levels: physical, environmental, mental/emotional, and spiritual. In preceding chapters we've talked a lot about physical and environmental stress, so here we will focus on the mental, emotional, and spiritual aspects. We all have stressful periods in our lives. Most of us have overly busy lives with to-do lists that can never be completed. We can't eliminate stress, but we can learn to flow more easily. It's finding peace in "what is" rather than looking outside to find peace.

THE ONLY CONSTANT IS CHANGE

From the moment we are born, we begin to change, and this continues until we take our last breath. Our body changes; our ideas change; our desires change. This is the nature of life. And all changes around us too. People come and go; jobs come and go; babies are born; loved ones die; we travel; we move houses; we leave for college; we retire; and so on.

Fear of change motivates behavior in some people. To keep life steady and predictable we often box ourselves in so that we have control. This is an illusion. No matter how hard we try to protect ourselves from change, change happens. (See Figure 16.1.) No matter how hard we try to control our lives, change happens. We'd be just as likely to control the seasons.

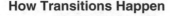

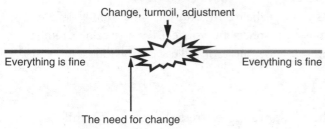

Figure 16.1 **How transitions happen.**

Change often happens in an instant. We're moving along and suddenly our life gets derailed by losing our job, getting sick, finding out our spouse is having an affair, an earthquake, planes crashing into the World Trade Towers, finding out that you'll be doing another tour of duty in the military, having a traffic accident, finding out that company is coming, and so forth. When we live in the present moment and accept what is, we are relieved of a great burden. Think of yourself flowing down a river toward the ocean. Sometimes you'll meander; sometimes you'll work hard to keep your head above water because the flow is so quick. Other times you'll be stuck in an eddy, going nowhere. Our lives are exactly this way. We are just flowing down the river of life. We don't control the river's flow. We just bob along trying to keep our head above water and enjoying the scenery.

STRESS OR OPPORTUNITY?

Though we mainly think of stress as a negative thing, it does have a positive side. The stress of going to college, getting married, having children, or earning a promotion provides opportunities and challenges that force us to change, grow, and strive to fulfill our potential. When I was younger I took a self-defense course to become more streetwise living in Chicago. My instructor said a very wise thing: "If you have enough time to be afraid, you have enough time to think about solutions." This statement has rung true for me many times in my life. Rather than spending my thoughts on fear or worry, I can be creative to see what solutions are available. And not to be Pollyanna-ish but sometimes what appears as the very worst thing possible at the moment, in retrospect seems like one of the best things that could have happened.

ANYTIME ABDOMINAL BREATHING EXERCISE

Take 10 deep breaths through your nose. As you inhale, feel your belly expand; feel the inhalation spread until it fills your lungs to the top. Exhale by letting your lungs gently deflate. Notice how you feel. If you're calmer, remember this tool and use it as needed.

But even positive stress can overwhelm us, causing distress. When we bite off more than we can chew, we feel stressed out. In many instances, we have little control over stressors, like illness, loss of a job, financial worries, and death. But even in these circumstances we have control over our thoughts and behavior. This is where stress management offers many benefits. Studies have shown that people who have emotional hardiness handle distress more easily than people with less resilience. Hardy people take on a challenge, make a commitment, take control, and see what happens. If success comes their way, it encourages them to try new things. If they fail, they pick themselves up and try again, recognizing that experience gained from "failure" adds to life's perspective. Fortunately, it's possible for anyone to learn hardiness skills.

Mental stress is one of the greatest challenges to our immune systems, putting pressure on nearly every organ and system in the body. When we feel stressed out, our bodies react with an increased heartbeat, shallow and rapid breathing, a release of adrenaline, and raised blood sugar levels and oxygen rates. Our muscles tense so we can move quickly. An increased blood supply is sent to our brain and major muscles, with decreased blood flow to our extremities. Even our pupils dilate and we sweat more. Our bodies react this way because our minds tell us there is a dangerous situation that requires quick thinking and movement. Historically, this might have been a bear on our path, a forest fire, or the exhilaration of the hunt. Today, it can be anything from a near car collision, to three phone lines ringing at once, to burnt toast! Because our first reaction is to unconsciously hold our breath and breathe shallowly, deep-breathing exercises are an excellent stress-management tool. Breathing deeply brings more oxygen to our tissues while waste products are excreted. It slows us down, so we feel more balanced and centered and can make clearer decisions. Deep abdominal breathing is something you can do anywhere, and no one can tell!

How do you know when you're under too much stress? Your body will usually tell you before your mind does. You may get a neck ache, backache, or headache, a sick feeling in your stomach, hives, fatigue, or a myriad of other symptoms. But even though your body is telling you to stop, you keep on going. Our culture rewards this type of behavior. But we owe it to ourselves to listen to our own needs more carefully

SIGNALS OF STRESS

Emotional	*Physical*	*Behavioral*
Moodiness	Muscle tension	Overuse of drugs/alcohol
Worry	Aches and pains	Overeating
Irritability	Fatigue	Forgetfulness
Hostility/anger	Sleep disturbances	Clumsiness
Bad dreams	Diarrhea	Depression
Lassitude	Digestive symptoms	Tension
Defensiveness	Headaches	Poor eating
Difficulty concentrating		

and to respond to them in kind. Pain and discomfort is our body's way of asking us to pay attention, now!

We can tune into these signals, or we can choose to ignore the messages and carry on with our activities. If we ignore them, the symptoms may go away, or they may blast louder and louder until we are forced to pay attention or our bodies break down. Being attentive to small signals allows us to gently get back on track without experiencing major upheavals in our lives.

The most important component of a good stress-management program is to have a plan with reasonable and realistic goals. If you need to, get a buddy or professional who will support you. Think of the ways in which you might slip or lose your way and prepare for them. Once your goals and support system are in place, you can forge into action.

SELF-RENEWAL

Do you take time each day for self-renewal and nurturing yourself? Getting restful sleep, taking time to exercise, spending time doing things you enjoy, and eating healthful foods are the foundation of a healthy lifestyle. How do you nurture yourself? How do you renew?

Exercise
The best stress-management tool is exercise. When I ask people to describe the benefits of their exercise program, they tell me they have more energy, have higher

self-esteem, and feel more relaxed. Exercise makes us stronger and more flexible and increases our balance, which helps keep us injury free. Regular exercise helps control blood sugar levels so our energy is more sustained, and being fit lowers the risk of heart disease. In addition, our bodies release endorphins, morphine-like molecules in the brain, which make us feel happy and reduce pain!

Positive Thoughts

Positive thinking is an important part of stress management. If you could tape the conversation in your brain for an hour or two, you might find you had a lot of self-criticism or self-doubts. With practice we can easily learn to "flip" these negative images and turn criticism into a positive thought or plan of action. When we catch ourselves playing a negative tape, we need to eject it and put in a new tape. Instead of thinking "My ulcerative colitis will get worse and worse until I need surgery," you can flip the image and say, "So far I haven't licked this problem, but if I am persistent, I can improve my health."

Get Restorative Sleep

Essential to healing is getting enough sleep. As a culture, we are sleep deprived. Set your schedule so that you get at least seven to nine hours of sleep every night. This is where your body heals and recenters. Without adequate sleep, it is nearly impossible to heal. It is beyond the boundaries of this book to discuss sleep hygiene and tips and tools for sleeping better, but here are just a few tips.

- At least one hour before bed, turn off your computer. Now it's time for a bath or reading, listening to calming ideas, or relaxing with some music.
- Go to bed at the same time each night; wake up at the same time each day. Our parents knew something when they regulated our bedtime!
- Take calcium and magnesium before bed. This helps to relax your nerves and muscles.
- You may find teas that contain chamomile, hops, valerian, and/or passionflower to be calming and restful.
- Some people find that taking 1 to 3 mg melatonin, or 5-hydroxy-tryptophan (5HTP) at doses of 50 to 200 mg help with sleep.

Remember to rest when your body is tired. It is not culturally normal to nap unless we are in preschool or are elderly. Yet in many cultures, napping is considered to be an essential habit. Rather than pushing yourself when you've run out of steam, take time to rest or nap. You'll find that this is restorative.

"THE GREATEST HITS" OF YOURSELF

Close your eyes for a minute, and think of all your most wonderful attributes. Compliment yourself freely. Take some time to appreciate your good points and achievements. Think about times in your life when you helped someone, fell in love, were in a beautiful place, made someone happy, and really felt good about yourself. Now quickly write down all of your best attributes. Don't be shy: overstate!

This is your "Greatest Hits" list. It's OK if you repeat yourself. Some of your attributes are worth repeating!

If you'd like to, keep this list somewhere so you'll be reminded of how terrific you are and how many blessings fill your life. Liking ourselves also helps our view of others and the world around us.

FINDING BALANCE

Prioritizing helps us find the balance point in our lives. Balance is hard to achieve and maintain, but it is an honorable goal. Like many people, if something really interests me, I take on new responsibilities and enjoyable events until I become overwhelmed. Then I make a list of all of my commitments and prioritize them to see what I can let go of responsibly. Soon my life is back in balance—until the next exciting possibility comes along and I'm overcommitted again. Be assertive: Learn to say no! (Liz, are you hearing this?)

Many years ago I read *The Goddess Within Us* by Dr. Jean Shinoda Bolen. My big aha was that we expect ourselves to play many roles perfectly—wife/husband/mate, daughter/son, mother/father, businessperson, athlete, spiritual being, homemaker, cook, artist, and civically dedicated citizen, both locally and globally. Yet the Greek and Roman gods and goddesses were excellent at only one thing. So why do we put such unreasonable and unrealistic demands on ourselves? A Buddhist saying is: "Expectation is the root of all suffering." If we can be easier on ourselves and in our relationships, we can find more love, contentment, and peace.

Most of us invest a lot of energy in our work, home, family, and friends. We begin with a barrel filled with apples. If we keep giving our apples away, soon our barrel is empty. We all need time to fill back up to rejuvenate. Sometimes I ask my clients to take two hours during the middle of the day to rejuvenate themselves. The usual response is: "That sounds terrific, but you know it's never going to happen." But inside they know they really need to do this, so they figure out a way to make it happen.

Your prescription: Take an hour or two every day to recharge your batteries. It's not important what you do. Each of us finds renewal in different things. Here are

COMPARTMENTALIZATION EXERCISE

Imagine you are sitting before a roll-top desk with pigeonholes in it. In each hole is a scroll tied neatly with a ribbon. See yourself opening one scroll at a time, examining it, putting it back in its proper place, selecting another, and repeating the process. Do this for several minutes. Find a way to use these pigeonholes in your daily life to help you accomplish tasks step by step. Practice this exercise to help you create closure between tasks and events in your life.

some ideas: read something for fun, play a musical instrument, listen to music, garden, exercise, be outdoors, build something, have a date with a friend, write a letter, keep a journal, enjoy a hobby, take a class, go to church/temple, read holy scriptures, meditate. Vacations are an important way to put our lives in perspective, to value what is truly important. When was the last time you took a vacation? If it's been more than a year, see if you can create the space to take one . . . even if it's just for a few days.

On the other hand, many people never grab for the ring, and they watch the world go by because they're worried about taking a risk. Because we are afraid, we box ourselves into worlds that are small, hoping to gain control of the chaos "out there." Fear is also stressful. Break out of your box. Act! Oh, to have loved and lost is way better than never to have loved at all.

OVERCOMING OVERWHELM

Compartmentalizing thoughts is a useful tool. Since we can think about or act upon only one responsibility at a time, it helps to put each one in a "compartment." The pearl here is to be able to be 100 percent present and focused on each task while you are doing it. This frees the mind and calms the spirit.

Quick Ideas for Stress Management
- Eat healthy foods.
- Develop better communication skills; learn to really listen.
- Exercise regularly.
- Spend time outdoors.
- Make time for yourself each day for pleasure or relaxation.
- Meditate or learn self-hypnosis or visualization techniques.

- Realize that you don't have to be perfect.
- Think creatively.
- Go at your own pace.
- Think of solutions, not problems.
- Prioritize.
- Keep journals.
- Live one day at a time.
- Play and laugh.
- Spend time with friends and family.
- Be flexible.
- View your problems as an opportunity for growth.
- Plan for chaos in your daily schedule.
- Set clear priorities and stick to them.
- Breathe deeply.
- Plan ahead: wake up 15 minutes earlier each morning, keep your car in good working order, put a duplicate car key in your wallet, and so on.
- Learn to say "No!"
- Turn off your phone or let your voice mail pick up the calls.
- Take a bath, shower, steam, or Jacuzzi.
- Make lists.
- Keep a calendar or appointment book.
- Reduce your driving speed by 10 miles per hour.
- Take one day a week to relax.
- Honor the Sabbath.
- Believe that people have good intentions and are doing the best job they can.
- See the world through a "loving" filter.

If you begin with just one or two of these stress-management techniques, you'll find more peace and balance in your life. Find what works for you and make it into a habit. If you want to truly heal your body, you will find that exploring your emotional and spiritual self speeds up the process.

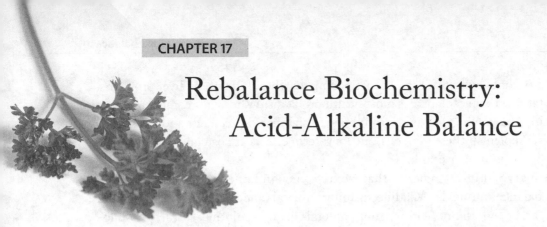

CHAPTER 17

Rebalance Biochemistry: Acid-Alkaline Balance

"Metabolic acidosis underlies chronic disease and makes people more likely to be resistant to treatment and to feel helpless and hopeless."

—Russell Jaffe, M.D.

Our acid-alkaline balance is regulated by the body's mineral management. Our bodies strive to maintain our blood pH between 7.3 and 7.5, which corresponds to a urinary pH of about 7.0. Our metabolism, enzymes, immune system, and repair mechanisms work most effectively within this narrow pH range. The body is very sensitive to changes in blood pH, so that always has to stay fairly constant or else we are rushed to the emergency room. To balance blood pH, minerals are drawn from elsewhere in the body. Sodium and potassium are pulled into the bloodstream from the reservoirs of fluid outside of our cells (extracellular fluid); when these extracellular stores have been used up, the body then resorts to pulling calcium, magnesium, and other alkalizing minerals from the bones and illnesses can occur.

ACID WOES

Imagine how much harder it would be for us to function if the air were filled with sulfuric acid; the more caustic the environment, the more detrimental it would be to our health. Similarly, our cells react to an acidic internal environment by becoming sluggish and unable to function properly. A change of 0.1 in either direction outside of the optimal blood pH range of 7.3 to 7.5 can produce up to a 10-fold reduction in enzyme activity. This happens for *each* 10th of a point, so the more out of line pH is, the less cellular activity occurs. Wastes build up, toxins aren't excreted, cellular messages aren't sent, and nutrients aren't properly utilized—it's kind of like a labor strike!

Acidity contributes to disease, constipation, diarrhea, kidney and liver problems, and the fatigue that accompanies most health problems. What's more, most of us are continually "borrowing" minerals from bone to stabilize our cellular and blood pH. If we don't replenish these minerals, the long-term effects are osteoporosis, osteoarthritis, and overall poor health.

A urinary pH of 7.0 indicates that we have enough buffering (alkalizing) minerals to balance our acids. Alkaline-forming minerals include sodium, potassium, calcium, and magnesium. Acid-forming minerals include chlorine, sulfur, phosphorus, and iodine. Many of us are deficient in potassium, calcium, and magnesium, although we do get plenty of sodium chloride (salt). Optimal cellular health and resistance to bacterial infections are promoted by all of these minerals, but especially by abundant supplies of sodium and calcium.

Why Are We Acidic?

Most of us unknowingly have a slightly acidic body environment. An excess of carbon dioxide and carbonic acid is created and accumulated in our blood through:

- Eating an acid-forming diet
- Stress
- Toxins
- Immune system reactions
- Metabolic regulatory mechanisms that create acid by-products

It's essential that our foods contain buffering minerals to offset this naturally acidic internal state. Fruit, vegetables, seaweed, and some other foods help alkalize our systems—but we don't usually eat enough of these. Unfortunately, the standard American diet contributes to our overall acid load, as proteins, fats, sugars, grains

SOFT DRINKS DEMINERALIZE BONES AND TEETH

One 12-ounce can of cola contains enough phosphoric acid to dramatically change our pH. The pH of the cola is between 2.8 and 3.2, but the kidneys cannot excrete urine that is more acidic than about 5.0; in order to dilute this can of cola to an appropriate urinary pH, you'd need to produce 33 liters of urine! So, the body turns to its stores of alkalizing minerals. If there aren't enough reserves of potassium and magnesium in the extracellular fluid, then calcium will be taken from bone. The amount of minerals needed for this particular task is equivalent to the buffering capability of four Tums!

(generally speaking), and refined foods are acid producing. Stress, alcohol, and cigarettes further compound the problem.

When our diet is high in protein and low in fruit and vegetables, as is often the case today, we have a greater need for buffering minerals. (Eating a high-protein diet temporarily causes an "alkaline tide," but the net result is not alkalizing.) When we are under stress, we have a greater need for buffering minerals. And when we drink soft drinks, we *really* need more buffering minerals; see the accompanying box for an eye-opening example.

An acidic internal environment is also a microbe's playground, in which bacteria, fungi, and parasites flourish and replicate with abandon; but when this overacidity is neutralized, these organisms cannot thrive. Many health-care practitioners recommend killing parasitic, fungal, and bacterial infections with medications and herbs. Nutritionists often find, however, that simply rebalancing internal pH can achieve the same antimicrobial effect without using any drugs.

MONITORING YOUR pH LEVEL

Getting your pH properly balanced is an important accompaniment to other healthful dietary changes. It's easy and inexpensive, and you can do it at home—even as a fun "experiment" for the whole family's participation and benefit.

Reading the Morning pH Paper
Purchase a packet of pH test paper with a testing range of 5.5 to 8.0 (available at most health-food stores; see also Resources at http://www.digestivewellnessbook.com). You can then perform the test by simply dipping a two- to three-inch strip of pH paper into your first morning urine stream and reading it by matching the color of the test strip with the color chart on the back of the package. Optimally, urinary pH will be between 6.5 and 7.5, which is fairly neutral. The pH of water, 7.0, is best. Any number below 7.0 indicates that your urine is on the acidic side. The lower the number, the more acidic, and the pH scale is logarithmic; that is, 6.0 is 10 times more acidic than 7.0, and 5.0 is 100 times more acidic than 7.0. You can use Figure 17.1 to record your urinary pH.

Rebalancing Your pH
If your readings fall consistently below 6.5, begin to make dietary changes to bring your urinary pH back into the optimal range (6.5–7.5). Be sure to include lots of fresh fruits and vegetables in your meals and snacks. Use Table 17.1 to identify alkalizing

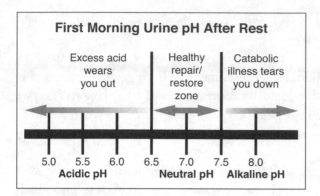

Figure 17.1 **First-morning urine pH, after rest.** (Used with permission: Jaffe R., & Mani J. *The Joy of Food: The Alkaline Way Guide*, (2009) Elisa Act Biotechnologies, LLC.)

foods; the further to the left on the chart, the more alkalizing the foods are. Take a mineral supplement daily and use a fully buffered vitamin C-mineral ascorbate to promote alkalinity.

In addition to nutrition, incorporate stress-reducing habits in your routine to normalize your pH: meditating, spending time outdoors, gardening, playing catch with friends, and taking gentle walks around the block or in the woods. At bath time, dissolve ½ cup each of baking soda and Epsom salts in your bathwater to alkalize, gently detoxify, and relax the body as they cleanse the skin.

What should you do if your urinary pH is *above* 7.5? An occasional reading of 7.5–8.0 is acceptable. Readings that are typically between 7.5 and 8.0, however, likely represent a "false alkalinity" that may indicate an active inflammation or other health issue; if this occurs, see your health-care practitioner.

Foods Affect the Body's pH

Many people assume that if the pH of a specific food, say lemons, is acidic, the food will be acid-producing in the body—but this assumption is inaccurate. In the 1920s and 1930s, scientists with the U.S. Department of Agriculture (USDA) began burning foods and measuring the pH of the ash residue. Later, realizing that this technique didn't yield sufficient information about what occurred inside the body, the USDA performed tests to see what would happen if someone ate only a specific food for 14 days. (How would you like to eat only carrots for two weeks?)

Subsequently, Russell Jaffe, M.D., a former researcher for the National Institutes of Health, found a way to calculate the body's net response to a food by using a formula based on that food's mineral, sugar, fat, and amino acid composition. Dr.

APPLE-CIDER VINEGAR IS ALKALIZING!

Use apple-cider vinegar in salad dressings, mix it into sweet juices (such as apple juice), and drizzle it over vegetables, chicken, or fish. It helps promote healthy digestion, increase blood oxygen levels, prevent intestinal putrefaction of food, regulate calcium metabolism, reduce frequent urination, and regulate menstrual cycles. Along with many essential enzymes and minerals, it also contains malic acid, which helps neutralize toxins. Always buy organic apple-cider vinegar; it's most beneficial raw, unfiltered, and unpasteurized.

Jaffe's formula correlates with the results of the USDA's few mono-diet studies. (It is the most accurate system I have seen for predicting the effect on pH of eating a particular food.)

If you are healthy and have a urinary pH of 6.5 to 7.5, eat 60 percent of your foods from the alkalizing side of Table 17.1 and 40 percent from the acid-producing side of the chart. If you need to rebuild health, have a chronic ailment, or have a urinary pH consistently lower than 6.5, eat 80 percent alkalizing foods and 20 percent acid-producing foods. Eating fruits and vegetables in abundance helps maintain a healthful acid-alkaline balance. And avoid brown-colored soft drinks! Lemon or lime juice in water makes a refreshing and alkalizing drink, as does ginger tea with rice syrup and lemon. Fresh vegetable juices flood the body with alkalizing minerals.

Additional Tips for Healthful Eating

- Switch to quinoa, oats, and wild rice as your main grains.
- Use sucanat, molasses, and rice syrup as your main sweeteners.
- Eating daikon radish and steamed greens daily is strongly recommended.
- Lentils, miso soup, and yams are extremely alkalizing.
- Use lemon, lime, and vinegar to flavor your foods.
- Drink fresh vegetable juices.

Table 17.1 Food and Chemical Effects on Acid-Alkaline Body-Chemical Balance

Food Category	Most Alkaline	More Alkaline	Low Alkaline	Lowest Alkaline	Lowest Acid	Low Acid	More Acid	Most Acid
spice/herb	baking soda	spices/cinnamon valerian licorice *black cohosh agave	*herbs (most): amica bergamot Echinacea chrysanthemum ephedra feverfew goldenseal lemongrass aloe vera nettle angelica	white willow bark slippery elm artemesia annua	curry	vanilla stevia	nutmeg	pudding/ jam/jelly
preservative	sea salt			sulfize	MSG	benzoate	aspartame	table salt (NaCl)
beverage	mineral water soda yeast/hops/malt	*kambucha	*green or Mu tea	ginger tea	Kona coffee	alcohol black tea	coffee	beer
sweetener		molasses	rice syrup	*sucanat	honey maple syrup		sacchann	sugar cocoa
vinegar		soy sauce white/acetic vinegar	apple cider vinegar	*umeboshi vinegar	rice vinegar	balsamic vinegar	red wine vinegar	

therapeutic	*umeboshi plum *psychotropics*	*antibiotics*		*sake	*algae. blue green			*antihista-mines*
processed dairy				*ghee (clarified butter)	cream/ butter	cow's milk	*casein	*processed cheese* milk protein cottage cheese
cow/human		ice cream			human breast milk	yogurt	aged cheese	new cheese
soy							soy cheese	soy milk
goat/sheep							goat/sheep cheese	goat milk
egg				*quail egg	*duck egg	chicken egg		
meat					gelatin/ organs	lamb/ mutton	pork/veal	beef
game					*venison	boar/elk *game meat	bear	
fish		shellfish (processed)			fish	mollusks shellfish (whole)	*mussels/ squid	*lobster

* Indicates therapeutic, gourmet, or exotic item.
Italicized items are NOT recommended.

(continued)

Table 17.1   Food and Chemical Effects on Acid-Alkaline Body-Chemical Balance (continued)

Food Category	Most Alkaline	More Alkaline	Low Alkaline	Lowest Alkaline	Lowest Acid	Low Acid	More Acid	Most Acid
fowl					wild duck	goose/ turkey	chicken	pheasant
grain/cereal/ grass				oat "grain coffee"	*triticale millet	buckwheat wheat	maize barley groat	barley processed
flour				*quinoa wild rice amaranth japonica rice	kasha brown rice	*spelt/teff/ kamut farina/ semolina white rice	corn rye oat bran	
nut seed/sprout oil	cottonseed pumpkin seed hazelnut	poppy seed cashew pepper	primrose oil sesame seed chestnut almond *sprout	avocado oil seeds (most) cod liver oil olive/maca-damia oil linseed/ flax oil	pumpkin seed oil grape seed oil coconut oil pine nut canola oil	almond oil sesame oil sunflower oil tapioca *seltan or tofu	pistachio seed chestnut oil safflower oil pecan palm kernel oil	oil/meat lard walnut Brazil nut fried food
bean vegetable	lentil brocoflower *seaweed nori kombu wakame hijiki	kohlrabi parsnip/taro garlic asparagus	potato/bell pepper mushroom/ fungi cauliflower cabbage	Brussels sprouts beet chive/ cilantro celery/ scallion	spinach fava bean kidney bean black-eyed pea	split pea pinto bean white bean navy/red bean	green pea peanut snow pea	soybean carob

legume pulse root	onion/miso *dalkon/ taro root *sea vegeta- bles (other) dandelion greens *burdock/ *lotus root sweet potato/ yam	kale/parsley endive/ arugula mustard green Jerusalem artichoke gingerroot broccoli	rutabaga *salsify/ ginseng eggplant pumpkin collard greens	okra/ cucumber turnip greens squash artichoke lettuce jicama	string/wax bean zucchini chutney rhubarb	aduki bean lima or mung bean chard	
citrus fruit	lime	grapefruit	lemon	orange	coconut		
fruit	nectarine persimmon raspberry watermelon tangerine pineapple	cantaloupe honeydew olive *dewberry loganberry mango	pear avocado apple blackberry cherry peach papaya	apricot banana blueberry pineapple juice raisin, currant grape strawberry	guava *pickled fruit dried fruit fig persimmon juice *cherimoya date	plum prune tomato	cranberry pomegran- ate

* Indicates therapeutic, gourmet, or exotic item.
Italicized items are NOT recommended.

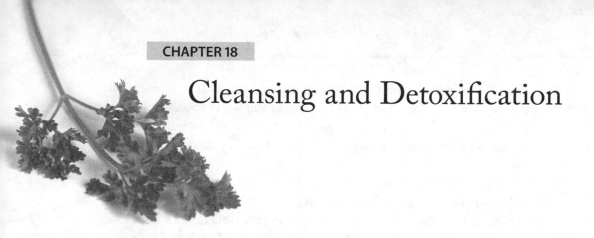

CHAPTER 18

Cleansing and Detoxification

"It can be strongly said that the health of an individual is largely determined by the ability of the body to detoxify."

—Joseph Pizzorno, N.D., and Michael Murray, N.D.,
Encyclopedia of Natural Health

"Brushing, clipping, combing, cutting, shampooing, picking, scratching, shaving, washing, scrubbing, sweating, blowing, breathing, coughing, sneezing, clearing, burping, defecating, flatulating, discharging, dripping, draining, menstruating, spitting, sweating, urinating, vomiting, wiping, methylating, acetylating, glucuronidating, sulfating, glutathionylating, glycinating. . . . Ridding oneself of unwanted stuff is a lot of work. The serious part of this work is synthetic, and unlike the items in the first part of my list, requires the lion's share of daily energy requirements involved in making new molecules."

—Sidney Baker McDonald

We are exposed to toxins everywhere—from the air we breathe to the foods we eat, even as a result of metabolism. These toxins cause irritation and inflammation throughout our bodies. People have always been exposed to toxic substances, but today's exposure to contaminants far exceeds that of previous times. Each week, approximately 6,000 new chemicals are listed in the Chemical Society's Chemical Abstracts, which adds up to more than 300,000 new chemicals each year. Annually, we consume, on average, 14 pounds of food additives, including colorings, preservatives, flavorings, emulsifiers, humectants, and antimicrobials. In 1990, the EPA estimated that 70,000 chemicals were commonly used in pesticides, foods, and drugs. Between January of 2007 through June of 2008, the EPA received a total of 1,724 new chemicals to review for approval. More than one billion tons of pesticides are used in the United States every year.

It's estimated that the average person is exposed to 100 synthetic chemicals daily. You probably say, "Not me!" But think about it: shampoo, deodorant, cleaning products, gas for your car, hair dye, cosmetics, lotions, potions, dishwashing soap, pesticides, phthalates found in plastics and inside of cans. . . . The list goes on and on and on.

Our body normally produces toxins as a by-product of metabolism. We call them endotoxins, which means they come from within us. If not eliminated, these endotoxins can irritate and inflame our tissues, blocking normal functions. Endotoxins formed by bacteria and yeasts can be absorbed into the bloodstream. Antibodies formed to protect us against the harmful effects of these endotoxins often trigger a systemic effect, causing an autoimmune reaction, so our body begins fighting itself. By assisting your body in removal of stored toxins through detoxification programs, your body can more easily heal itself.

Some of the many functions of the liver are to act as a filter, to let nutrients pass, to "humanize" other substances if possible, and to transform toxins into safe substances that can be eliminated in urine and stool. When the liver enzymes fail to break down these toxins, they are stored in the liver and fatty tissue throughout our bodies.

TRADITIONAL CLEANSING

Throughout time and in various cultures, people have seen the need for periodic internal cleansing. Native Americans and Mexicans use sweat lodges. Ancient Roman bathhouses had rooms for bathing in steam, warm water, and cold water. Jewish women have used ritual mikvah baths to cleanse both body and spirit. Most Swedish people have home saunas, and our own health clubs have saunas, steam baths, hot tubs, and Jacuzzis. People "take the waters" in Europe and parts of the United States. Hawaiians use steam and a form of massage, called lomilomi, where they scrub people clean with the red Hawaiian dirt and sea salt. In fact, mud and clay have been used worldwide to draw toxins from the body while simultaneously providing essential nutrients.

Fasting is an important part of many religious holidays and customs. Both Jesus and John the Baptist fasted to gain mental and spiritual clarity. During Ramadan, an important Muslim holiday, people fast during daylight hours for a month. Jewish people fast on Yom Kippur. Indigenous people of many cultures use fasting as a way to clarify thought and provoke visions.

Removal of waste material—detoxification—is essential to the healthy functioning of our bodies. This is shown in the many different ways the body cleanses itself. Skin is our body's largest organ. In addition to being a protective organ, it is also an organ of elimination through perspiration. Sneezes clear our sinuses. Lungs breathe out carbon dioxide, and even the breath allows for removal of some wastes. Kidneys filter wastes from the bloodstream. Stool is the residue from the digestive process. The liver filters the substances that are absorbed through the digestive barrier into the bloodstream. White blood cells gobble up bacteria and foreign substances, and the lymphatic system clears the debris from circulation. During a cleansing program, your body more rapidly recycles materials to build new cells, take apart aged cells, and repair damaged cells.

HOW YOUR LIVER DETOXIFIES

Your liver detoxifies in a two-phase system, called the cytochrome P450 system. In phase one your body pulls stored fat-soluble toxins from tissues throughout your body. These are stored in fat, nerves, brain, kidneys, and other tissues. We packed these away because they were toxic, and now they are floating in our bloodstream, which makes them more dangerous than when they were in our tissues. In phase two, we prepare these substances so that they can be excreted from the body. Adding a water-soluble molecule to each of these fat-soluble chemicals allows them to be taken out of the body.

How well the cytochrome P450 system works is determined by your genetics, how well nourished you are, and how toxic you are. I often have clients who are poor phase two detoxifiers. When they take a drug or supplement or are exposed to a chemical, they are slow to convert it. It stays in their system longer than for most people, so the doses they need for supplements and medications are typically less. I recognize it because when they try to cleanse or take medications or supplements, they are extremely sensitive to them. The cytochrome P450 process is energy demanding and requires many nutrients to function properly. In Figure 18.1 you can see which nutrients are required in phase one, phase two, and between phases. Since many of us lack antioxidants and other nutrients, this process cannot work optimally.

Common medications can inhibit the liver's ability to adequately process toxins. For example, acetaminophen (Tylenol) causes liver damage when used in combination with alcoholic beverages. Cimetidine, an ulcer medication, limits the liver's ability to detoxify foreign substances.

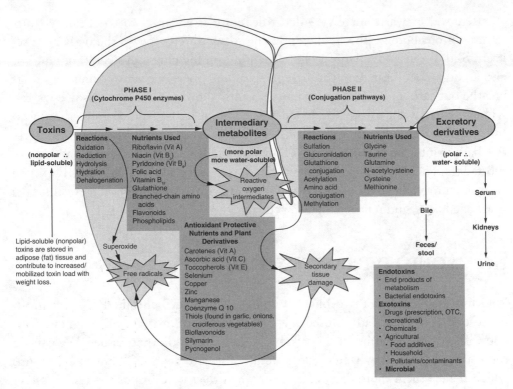

Figure 18.1 **Liver detoxification pathways and supportive nutrients.** (Used with permission of the Institute for Functional Medicine.)

FOOD AND DETOXIFICATION

Food can effect the way our liver detoxifies too. Naringinen and other molecules in grapefruit juice slow down phase one detoxification pathways. Many people are told not to drink grapefruit juice because it changes the dosages of medication they need. The catechins in red wine and the piperine in black pepper also slow down metabolism of drugs. Several studies indicate that eating a diet high in animal protein increases the level of intermediary metabolites. This is not seen in people eating a vegetarian diet. Eating more fruits and vegetables helps the liver to detoxify better. Polyphenols in foods such as red wine, green tea, turmeric, ginger, and spices have been shown to reduce rates of cancer and most other illnesses. Glucosinolates in cruciferous vegetables also help us detoxify and lower cancer risk.

Your body's ability to detoxify through the cytochrome P450 system can be measured in several ways. See Chapter 11 for more on this topic.

It is best if you follow a detoxification program under the supervision of a medical or health professional who can guide you through the process. Toxins released too quickly can make you feel worse than when you began and can aggravate your symptoms.

WHO BENEFITS FROM A CLEANSE OR DETOX?

I do a liver cleanse once or twice a year. Generally I do one of three things: implement an elimination diet, use a rice-based protein powder along with an elimination diet, or make up a variation on the elimination diet, and add a lot of fresh vegetable juices and green drinks. We're all exposed to an average of 100 chemicals daily, so I think that nearly everyone ought to cleanse. Complete the following questionnaire to compare your "before and after" results. See what symptoms improved.

MEDICAL SYMPTOMS QUESTIONNAIRE (MSQ)

Name: _____ Date: _____

Rate each of the following symptoms based on your typical health profile for:

☐ Past 30 days ☐ Past 48 hours

Point Scale

0: *Never* or *almost never* have the symptom
1: *Occasionally* have it, effect is *not severe*
2: *Occasionally* have it, effect is *severe*
3: *Frequently* have it, effect is *not severe*
4: *Frequently* have it, effect is *severe*

Head

_____ Headaches
_____ Faintness
_____ Dizziness
_____ Insomnia
Total _____

Eyes

_____ Watery or itchy eyes
_____ Swollen, reddened/sticky eyelids
_____ Bags, dark circles
_____ Blurred or tunnel vision *(does not include near- or far-sightedness)*
Total _____

Ears

_____ Itchy ears
_____ Earaches, ear infections
_____ Drainage from ear
_____ Ringing/hearing loss
Total _____

Nose

_____ Stuffy nose
_____ Sinus problems
_____ Hay fever
_____ Sneezing attacks
_____ Excessive mucus
Total _____

Mouth/Throat

_____ Chronic coughing
_____ Gagging, throat clearing
_____ Sore throat, hoarseness
_____ Swollen/discolored tongue,
        gums, lips
_____ Canker sores
Total _____

Heart

_____ Irregular/skipped beats
_____ Rapid/pounding beats
_____ Chest pain
Total _____

Skin

_____ Acne
_____ Hives, rashes, dry skin
_____ Hair loss
_____ Flushing, hot flashes
_____ Excessive sweating
Total _____

Lungs

_____ Chest congestion
_____ Asthma, bronchitis
_____ Shortness of breath
_____ Difficulty breathing
Total _____

Digestive Tract

_____ Nausea, vomiting
_____ Diarrhea
_____ Constipation
_____ Bloated feeling
_____ Belching, passing gas
_____ Heartburn
_____ Intestinal/stomach pain
Total _____

Joints/Muscle

_____ Pain or aches in joints
_____ Arthritis
_____ Stiffness/limited movement
_____ Pain or aches in muscles
_____ Feeling of weakness or
        tiredness
Total _____

Weight

_____ Binge eating/drinking
_____ Craving certain foods
_____ Excessive weight
_____ Compulsive eating
_____ Water retention
_____ Underweight
Total _____

Energy/Activity

_____ Fatigue, sluggishness
_____ Apathy, lethargy
_____ Hyperactivity
_____ Restless leg
_____ Jet lag
Total _____

Mind

_____ Poor memory
_____ Confusion, poor
           comprehension
_____ Poor concentration
_____ Poor physical coordination
_____ Difficulty making decisions
_____ Stuttering or stammering
_____ Slurred speech
_____ Learning disabilities
Total _____

Emotions

_____ Mood swings
_____ Anxiety, fear, nervousness
_____ Anger, irritability,
           aggressiveness
_____ Depression
Total _____

Other

_____ Frequent illness
_____ Frequent or urgent urination
_____ Genital itch or discharge
_____ Bone pain
Total _____

Grand total _____

©2009 Institute for Functional Medicine

DETOXIFICATION AND CLEANSING PROGRAMS

Most detoxification programs focus on the liver or colon. The liver is, in my opinion, the most overworked organ of the body. It has responsibility for manufacturing 13,000 different enzymes, producing cholesterol, breaking down estrogen, regulating blood sugar, filtering blood, manufacturing bile, breaking down old red blood cells, and detoxifying harmful substances. When the liver loses its ability to easily perform these functions, we begin to feel ill, with many systems out of balance.

Detoxification techniques such as fasting, modified fasting, metabolic cleansing, colonic irrigation, steaming, mud packs, saunas, herbal detoxification programs, and hot tubs all have therapeutic benefits. When choosing a detoxification program, it must meet specific criteria: it needs to (1) work with your life and your values, (2) be thorough, and (3) be gentle and nurturing to your body.

During the past several years, I have personally and professionally relied on three main detoxification programs that are effective and gentle: fruit and vegetable cleansing, metabolic cleansing, and low-temperature steams and saunas. I also recommend vitamin C flushes between cleansings. Other professionals may prefer fasting programs or colonic irrigation, which in the right hands can be powerful tools for healing. Because there are many fine books on fasting and colonic irrigation, I have not included information about them here.

THE ELIMINATION DIET

The elimination diet outlined in Chapter 15 works well as a gentle cleanse. See Chapter 15 for more information.

FRUIT AND VEGETABLE CLEANSING

The first cleanse that I ever used was simply fruits and vegetables for 7 to 10 days. Typically you'll eat between 8 to 12 cups daily of produce.

I used this cleanse as a jump-start for many of the weight control groups I facilitated. While this works amazingly well, some may not feel that it provides enough food to keep blood sugar levels even. So, if it doesn't feel right to you, don't do it.

In this gentle cleanse, you may eat all you want of fruits and vegetables, and use olive and sunflower oils, salt and pepper, and other herbs for 7 to 10 days. Fresh fruit and vegetable juices are an excellent source of easily assimilated nutrients and alkalizing minerals and can enhance the detoxification pathways. You can have raw, steamed, juiced, grilled, stir-fried, and cultured vegetables. You can have raw, juiced, cooked, frozen, or dried fruit. You can use canned fruit if it's packed in its own juice. You can make smoothies. Eat large salads every day. Make salad dressings with lemon or lime and olive oil, salt, pepper, and fresh herbs. Make pots of vegetable soup. Make a batch of roasted or baked root vegetables for something hearty to eat.

It's important to eat every two to three hours to keep your blood sugar levels normal. The major benefit of this detox method is that you can do this on your own without professional supervision. Of course, if you are under a doctor's care or taking medication of any kind, you'll need to let your physician know of your plans. The first few days may require mental and physical adjustments to your new regimen, but most people feel a sense of general well-being. You may notice that many of your outstanding symptoms have disappeared or become less aggravated.

You may also experience some discomfort during the first three or four days. Headaches, bad breath, skin breakouts, and changes in bowel habits are fairly common and may be the result of withdrawal from caffeine, sugar, alcohol, or other substances. They are an indicator that toxins are being flushed out or that your body is going through withdrawal. To facilitate this, drink a lot of water, diluted juices, and all herbal teas except those containing caffeine. Dandelion tea is especially useful.

Some people develop rashes or pimples as the skin works hard to eliminate toxins. Taking saunas, steam bathing, and massaging your skin with a soft, dry brush or loofa can help your skin. If you are constipated, make sure you eat enough fiber-rich fruits and vegetables (apples, broccoli, pears, sweet potatoes, peas, brussels sprouts, corn, potatoes, carrots, greens, blackberries, bananas, strawberries, raspberries, and spinach). Constipation opens up a chance for toxins to be reabsorbed into your bloodstream, causing symptoms such as headaches and nausea, so add a fiber supplement if needed; psyllium seeds or psyllium seed husks work well. Begin with 1 teaspoon in water, and drink quickly before it turns into a gel. Aloe vera juice may also help regulate your bowels.

After the cleansing, slowly reintroduce healthful foods such as beans, tofu, chicken, and fish. Then add healthful grains, nuts, seeds, and cultured dairy products.

METABOLIC CLEANSING

Metabolic cleansing is a gentle yet deep method of detoxification, and it is the best, most thorough program I have used. The foundation of this program is a hypoallergenic-sensitive, rice-based protein and nutrient drink that is designed specifically to assist with phase one and phase two liver detoxification. There are many companies that make this type of product. You can find them in the resource directory at http://www.digestivewellnessbook.com.

Use of liver detoxification protein drinks has been researched for its health benefits. These drinks have been reported to be of enormous benefit in people with fibromyalgia, chronic fatigue syndrome, arthritis, weight loss, and other conditions.

I use this product along with the elimination diet that is outlined in Chapter 15. If you know that you are sensitive to bananas, melons, or other foods that are allowed on the plan, then avoid them as well. It is possible for people to continue their normal daily routine while on this program.

Typically I begin people with two scoops of the detoxification drink once daily for several days; then increase to two scoops twice daily for several days; then finally continue with two scoops three times daily until they are ready to complete the cleanse.

This program is administered only through health professionals who can monitor your progress, determine when you should quit, and help you adjust if you have any difficulties. Most people find a dramatic alleviation of symptoms and a distinct improvement in energy levels. The high levels of nutrients found in the rice protein drink and in the fruits and vegetables help the liver activate its detoxification pathways and move unwanted materials out of the body. The intention here is to allow your digestive system to rest, relax, and heal itself.

Once you have completed the cleansing, it is important to slowly reintroduce foods back into your diet. Being a food sleuth takes a lot of patience; it's not always apparent which foods cause adverse symptoms. But with persistent detective work you can discover many of them. Keep a running record of everything you eat and of your symptoms. Food sensitivities often display delayed reactions, so it may take up to 48 hours to feel the effect of a newly introduced food.

You may want to have testing done for food allergies and sensitivities at this time. If you have uncovered a problem, these tests can further pinpoint which foods and substances are making you ill.

VITAMIN C FLUSH

I learned this technique from Russell Jaffe, M.D., and am indebted to him for this protocol and many other things. It's something that I personally use and used with my children. Over the past 20 years, I've used this flush with many clients. Although it's a bit harsh on some people, others say that after the first or second time they feel better than they've felt in years. A good-quality ascorbate can be utilized by the body to produce energy. Because of that, I often hear that energy levels have dramatically improved after a vitamin C flush.

Vitamin C has been well researched for its ability to help detoxify bacterial toxins, drugs, environmental toxins, and heavy metals from our bodies. Its gentle and potent detoxification counteracts and neutralizes the harmful effects of manufactured poisons.

High levels of vitamin C help detoxify the body, rebalance intestinal flora, and strengthen the immune system. The vitamin C flush can be used between metabolic cleansing therapies or at the first sign of a cold or infection. If your immune system is weak or you've been exposed to a lot of toxins, you may want to do a vitamin C flush once a week for a month or two. On days when you are not doing a vitamin C flush, take a minimum of 2,000 to 3,000 mg. Humans are one of the only animals that do not produce their own vitamin C, so we need to replenish our supply daily.

To do a vitamin C flush, you take vitamin C to the level of tissue saturation. You'll know you've reached it because you will have watery diarrhea. You'll need to purchase powdered mineral ascorbate C, which is more easily tolerated by most people because it doesn't change your pH balance. The amount you take varies depending on your personal needs that day. Many of us require about 5,000 mg; others need 15 or 20 times that much. For instance, if you're coming down with a cold, have chronic fatigue syndrome, or are under excessive stress, you'll probably need a lot more.

To do a vitamin C flush, take ½ teaspoon, about 1,500 mg, of vitamin C powder, mix with water or fruit juice, and drink. Repeat in 15 minutes. Keep taking ½ teaspoon of ascorbate every 15 minutes until you have watery diarrhea. It's like you are urinating out of your backside. It will have a brown, green, or yellow color. As soon as you see this, stop taking the ascorbate.

Do not stop with just gas. Rapidly adding vitamin C helps prevent bloating and cramping. Stop once you get diarrhea. Keep track of how much vitamin C you take. This will help you determine your optimal dosage. In divided amounts, take daily one-half to three-quarters of the amount it takes to produce a vitamin C flush.

Over time your needs may increase but then substantially decrease as repair occurs.

LOW-TEMPERATURE SAUNAS AND STEAMS

"If the sauna, schnapps, and tar don't help, then the illness is fatal."
—Old Finnish adage

Low-temperature saunas or steambaths are useful to eliminate fat-soluble chemicals from our systems. They are commonly used to help detoxify those who have had high exposure to pesticides, solvents, pharmaceutical drugs, and petrochemicals. Slow, steady sweat encourages the release of fat-soluble toxins through the skin from their storage sites in our tissues. Saunas increase our peripheral circulation; decrease circulation to our muscles, kidney, and organs; increase our metabolism; and increase oxygen utilization, blood pressure, and heart rate. In the process, we lose sodium, potassium, and chloride via our sweat, so remember to rehydrate and replenish with vegetable juice or diluted fruit juice. Taking saunas increases hormones such as cortisol, adrenaline and noradrenaline, growth hormone, thyroid-stimulating hormone, and prolactin. It ultimately opens up our lungs, relaxes our muscles, makes us more flexible, and thins synovial fluid in our joints. It also gives us a good cardiovascular workout, similar to doing moderate to vigorous walking.

Saunas help us to release xenobiotic toxins from our fat cells. Many compounds have been reported to be released, including minerals, urea, drugs, and polychlorinated bromines (PCBs). In addition, hyperthermia is well known to help with cancer treatment and is being used in some oncology centers in the United States and Europe.

Most saunas and steam baths are set at temperatures too high to accomplish the full detox potential, so be sure a dry sauna is set between 110 and 120 degrees Fahrenheit and a steam bath is at 110 degrees Fahrenheit so you can stay in for at least 45 minutes without getting too hot or chilled. It is best to spend 30 to 60 minutes in a sauna or steam three to five times a week. Releasing toxins cannot be accomplished with higher heat or shorter amounts of time. The object is to sweat slowly and steadily.

After you are done sweating, you must shower immediately, using a glycerin-based soap such as Neutrogena. It will wash away the toxins and keep you from reabsorbing them.

Precautions

Saunas are contraindicated in women who are at high risk for pregnancy and for people with aortic stenosis, unstable angina, and recent heart attack. If you have extreme toxicity from environmental chemicals, you'll need to detox under the supervision of a physician. The temporary release of toxins into your circulation can be quite severe and debilitating. Some clinics specialize in using saunas for medical detoxification. In her excellent book *Poisoning Our Children*, Nancy Sokol Green describes her experience in a detox clinic in depth: "On the fourteenth day of detox, I started experiencing allergic symptoms, such as eyelid swelling, while I was in the sauna! . . . I was actually beginning to reek of the pesticides that had been sprayed in my home. . . . Several of the patients at the clinic who were sensitive to pesticides had to stay away from me as I triggered adverse reactions in them."

Saunas are a useful detoxification therapy when used preventively and therapeutically. If you are using a sauna therapeutically, do so under the supervision of a physician who can guide you through the process. And next time you get into your car that's been warmed by the sun, spend a few minutes basking in the glory of the heat. You have your own infrared sauna!

Natural Therapies for Common Digestive Problems

"Hope cannot be said to exist, nor can it be said not to exist.
It is just like the roads across the earth.
For actually there were no roads to begin with,
But when many people pass one way a road is made."

—Lu Hsun, 1921

Maya Angelou said, "I did then what I knew how to do. Now that I know better, I do better." I hope that these pages will help you to know better so that you can do better.

Part IV provides a comprehensive list of self-care ideas for the most common digestive problems. We start our journey at the mouth and move south. Some of the following ideas alleviate symptoms, while others work to help your body heal the underlying cause. The remedies are mostly nutritional and herbal because those are the fields I know best; I have included other modalities whenever possible. The most important ones are listed first. Read each section that applies to you, find the remedies for your symptoms, and try those recommended more than once first. Also try the remedies that make the most sense intuitively.

In all cases begin with the DIGIN model for optimal healing then look for specifics in these chapters.

Each herb or nutrient is listed separately, but often they can be found in combination supplements. You'll notice that specific recommendations are repeated for many problems. Although each health condition has its own unique properties, many have similar characteristics that respond to similar treatment programs. You'll probably want to work with a health professional to tailor a program that will best suit your needs.

Health care is both a science and an art. You may need the science in the form of lab testing, diagnosis, and evaluation of your needs. Your clinician will order the customary lab work. I have included information about functional lab tests that are most likely to reveal new information; these tests will probably be unfamiliar to your physician. You will find a resource directory of suggested laboratories and supplement companies online at http://www.digestivewellnessbook.com.

The art of healing comes into play when determining which paths to follow, which ideas have the most merit, and which dosages are appropriate. Healing often happens in layers. Sometimes you try the right thing at the wrong time. Later, you try it again with great results because the initial obstacle has been removed. If the first program you try doesn't work or works only partially, try another. You can feel better when you are persistent and patient. Remember, our symptoms are our body's way of telling us to pay attention, that something is out of balance. By listening, we often have the inner wisdom to know exactly what we need.

Begin your program by taking a multivitamin and mineral supplement. Think of a multivitamin with minerals as inexpensive health insurance, and arm yourself with an excellent supplement. Your diet is likely to be deficient in several nutrients that supplements can provide. Because minerals are bulky, you'll find yourself taking anywhere from two to nine pills daily. Read the ingredients on the label carefully. If a product contains artificial colors, preservatives, shellac, or carnauba wax, put it back on the shelf and keep looking. Also, look for an expiration date and batch number. Although I love food-based supplements, if you have a lot of food sensitivities or allergies, think twice about taking one. It's likely that one of the foods that's in the supplement may be one that you react to. Look for a multivitamin and mineral supplement that contains at least the following:

Recommended Multivitamin with Minerals
- 1,000 mg of calcium
- 400 to 600 mg of magnesium
- 400 IU of vitamin D
- At least 100 IU of vitamin E
- At least 250 mg of vitamin C
- 200 mcg of chromium
- 200 mcg of selenium
- 5–10 mg of manganese
- At least 15 mg of zinc
- At least 400 mcg of folic acid
- At least 10 mg of each B vitamin

If you do this, the rest of the nutrients will be in line.

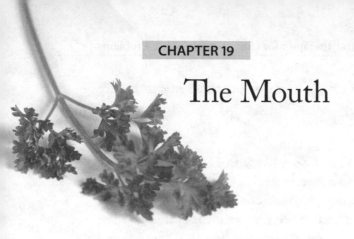

CHAPTER 19

The Mouth

The health of our teeth, tongue, and gums is integral to the health of the rest of the digestive tract. Digestive enzymes in saliva begin the process of carbohydrate digestion, and chewing sends signals to the brain, which in turn sends signals to the stomach that food is on the way. Thorough chewing of food can help with indigestion.

Irritation and inflammation in the mouth can be signs of food or chemical sensitivities or allergies. The mouth is our first contact with ingested allergens. Careful investigation of the mouth area can give information about a person's nutritional status. Bleeding gums indicate the need for vitamin C and bioflavonoids. Receding gums indicate bone loss, so bone nutrients are needed. Deep pockets in gums indicate the need for vitamin C, bioflavonoids, and coenzyme Q10 (CoQ10).

BAD BREATH OR HALITOSIS

Using mouthwash for bad breath is like putting a Band-Aid on a broken leg. First, consult a dentist to see if it is caused by poor dental hygiene, periodontal disease, or tooth infections. Halitosis is typically caused by dental issues. If so, follow your dentist's advice, and also look in the section on gum and tooth health that follows. But also look deeper: halitosis often signals digestive imbalances lower down in the digestive tract. Bad breath can signal an infection of some sort: H. pylori, chronic tonsillitis, chronic sinusitis, or digestive dysbiosis. Other contributors include low

HCl levels in the stomach, GERD, poor flora, liver disease, pancreatic or kidney disease, respiratory infections, and constipation.

Healing Options

- **Check for infection.** Halitosis has been associated with H. pylori, a bacteria involved in stomach infection. Ask your doctor to check you for H. pylori. H. pylori was found in 15 percent of people with periodontal disease. See the sections on GERD and gastric ulcers in Chapter 20 for treatment options.
- **Eliminate constipation.** See the section on stool transit time in Chapter 2 and do the self-test. See also the section on constipation in Chapter 25.
- **Try a probiotic supplement.** Take one or two capsules of acidophilus and bifidus between meals.
- **Consider possible lactose intolerance.** Lactose intolerance can cause bad breath, other digestive symptoms, and headaches. The simplest way to discover if you have lactose intolerance is to avoid all dairy products and dairy-containing food for two weeks, then see if your symptoms have improved.
- **Look for other causes if the problem persists.** If you continue to have problems, you might be fermenting rather than digesting your foods. First, check out your HCl levels. (See Chapter 11.) Second, ask your doctor to run a comprehensive digestive stool analysis (CDSA) with parasitology evaluation. You may have dysbiosis, parasites, or a helicobacter infection (the bacteria implicated in ulcers). A CDSA can help you find out what's amiss.

CHEILOSIS, OR CRACKS IN THE CORNERS OF THE MOUTH AND LIPS

Our skin is continuously replacing itself, and the places where our skin folds need to be replaced even more often. B-complex vitamins, particularly vitamins B_2 (riboflavin) and B_6 (pyridoxine), assist in formation of new skin. Cracks at the corners of our lips, called cheilosis, are most often associated with these nutrient deficiencies. They can easily become infected by yeast (Candida albicans). If they do not respond to nutritional therapy, have a physician look for other causes.

Healing Options
Take B-complex vitamins. Try 50 to 100 mg one to three times daily in trial for four weeks.

GINGIVITIS AND PERIODONTAL DISEASE

Gingivitis is an inflammation of the gums that, if left alone, often progresses to periodontal disease, an inflammation of the bone around the teeth. Although the inflammation is in the mouth, it's well established that people with inflammation in their gums have increased risk of heart disease. A Scottish study with more than 11,000 participants demonstrated that people who brushed their teeth less than twice daily had a 70 percent higher risk of having heart disease than people who brush twice daily. This was also demonstrated with higher levels of inflammatory markers such as C-reactive protein and fibrinogen. Seems like a pretty easy thing to do: brush twice a day and floss once a day.

Periodontal disease increases with plaque buildup, age, long-term use of steroid medications, and in diabetics, people with systemic disease, and smokers. The presence of silver fillings, which contain 50 percent mercury, has also been found to predispose people to periodontal disease. One study showed that when silver fillings were removed, 86 percent of the 125 oral cavity symptoms being studied were eliminated or improved.

Gingivitis and periodontal disease are complex problems that have complex solutions. Periodontal disease will affect 9 out of 10 Americans during their lifetimes, and 4 out of 10 will lose all their teeth. Regular dental care is essential. Follow your dentist's advice and practice consistent oral hygiene: brush and floss daily.

Nutrition plays a critical role in dental health. One recent study looked at gingivitis, plaque adhesion, and calculus deposit with regard to the eating habits of teenagers. They concluded that teenagers with diets adequate in nutrients had better oral health than teenagers with diets that contained fewer nutrients.

NUTRIENTS AND OUR TEETH

Teeth are made of bone material and need the same nutrients for rebuilding as other bones. It has long been considered that receding and inflamed gums were a sign that people brushed too hard, causing damage to the gums, but new theories propose that gums recede because bone throughout the body, including the teeth, is demineralizing. If other bones need 19 nutrients to remineralize, the same goes for teeth. Calcium alone cannot reverse the problem. Stress and fast-paced living can cause bone loss by making the body more acidic. To compensate, the body takes alkaline materials from bones and teeth. Read and follow the section on acid-alkaline balance in Chapter 17.

Vitamin C deficiency causes bleeding gums and loose teeth and contributes to gingivitis. Bleeding gums is one symptom of scurvy, a vitamin-C-deficiency disease. We rarely see outright scurvy in our population, but we often see people with bleeding gums. Vitamin C is also important for bone formation and collagen synthesis and is essential for gum repair. Vitamin A is also necessary for collagen synthesis and formation of gum tissue.

Other researchers look to zinc deficiency or a low zinc-to-copper ratio as the culprit in gum disease. Zinc is integral to maintenance and repair of gum tissue, inhibits plaque formation, and reduces inflammation by inhibiting mast cell release of histamine. It also plays a role in immune function.

Vitamin E has been used clinically for periodontal disease. Bacterial plaque, long known to be a culprit in tooth decay and gingivitis, produces compounds that weaken and irritate the gum tissue. They include endotoxins and exotoxins, free radicals, connective tissue–destroying enzymes, white blood cell poisons, antigens, and waste products.

Antioxidant nutrients and CoQ10 have been associated with improved gum health, reduced periodontal pocket depth, and decreased tooth movement. Bioflavonoids make the tissues stronger, reduce inflammation, and cross-link with collagen fibers, making them stronger. Because bioflavonoids work synergistically with vitamin C, bleeding gums often respond to vitamin C and bioflavonoid supplementation. My favorite bioflavonoid is quercetin.

Folic acid, a B-complex vitamin, is important for maintenance and repair of mucous membranes. The need for extra folic acid was first noted for pregnant women, while subsequent studies have shown that it plays an important role for gingival health in all people.

When I interviewed John Cannell, M.D., of the Vitamin D Foundation, he mentioned that taking vitamin D strengthened his gums. There's no published research on this, but it's worth getting your vitamin D level checked.

Healing Options
- **Brush your teeth twice daily.** Brush your teeth twice a day and floss once a day. Your dentist may also recommend some sort of oral wash that is used with an oral irrigator. It may have hydrogen peroxide, peppermint, or other herbs in it.
- **Make dietary changes.** Focus on fresh fruits, vegetables, whole grains, and beans. Foods rich in flavonoids are beneficial: blueberries, blackberries, and purple grapes.

- **Take a multivitamin with minerals.** Because you are depleted in many nutrients, arm yourself with an excellent multivitamin with minerals. Because minerals are bulky, you'll probably take anywhere from two to nine pills daily. In the introduction to Part IV, you'll find my recommendations on what to look for in a multi-vitamin with minerals.
- **Try coenzyme Q10.** Take 75 to 200 mg daily for a trial period of three months.
- **Take antioxidants.** Vitamins C and E, selenium, glutathione, N-acetyl cysteine (NAC), superoxide dismutase (SOD), beta-carotene, and other antioxidant nutrients are depleted in diseased gum tissues. Supplementation can facilitate repair. For ease of use, purchase an antioxidant supplement. Use as directed for three months.
- **Take vitamin C.** Try 500 to 1,000 mg one to three times daily. For maximum benefits, use until your tissues are saturated. See Chapter 18 for information on a vitamin C flush.
- **Try bioflavonoids.** Use quercetin, bilberry (blueberry), grape seed extract, or Pycnogenol for their anti-inflammatory and antioxidant effects.
- **Try myrrh.** Myrrh has been used since biblical times. It has soothing and antiseptic properties for mucous membranes.
- **Use a folic acid mouthwash.** Use of a 0.1 percent folic acid mouthwash can be quite effective. Be sure to have your blood tested for pernicious anemia first, because folate supplementation can cause nerve damage in people with vitamin B_{12} deficiencies.
- **Try fish oil capsules.** In a controlled placebo trial, it was found that MaxEPA fish oil capsules significantly reduced gingival bleeding and reduced inflammatory factors. Take 2 to 4 g EPA/DHA daily.

MOUTH ULCERS OR CANKER SORES

Mouth sores are common. Most of us have experienced mouth ulcers, canker sores, or cold sores, but some have chronic problems. Usually found inside the mouth, canker sores, called aphthous stomatitis or aphthous ulcers, are the result of poor intestinal flora, food sensitivities or allergies, stress, hormonal changes, and nutritional deficiencies. High-sugar and high-acid foods, such as pineapples, citrus, and tomatoes, sometimes trigger canker sores.

If you have recurring canker sores, thoroughly investigate the possibility of food sensitivities. Also, make sure your toothpaste, mouthwash, and floss aren't causing the problem. A study showed that use of Piroxicam, an NSAID, caused mouth ulcers that resolved when the patient was taken off the medication. If you have mouth sores that don't resolve after several weeks, let your doctor or dentist examine you.

Healing Options

- **Investigate allergies and sensitivities.** Cigarettes, toothpaste, mouthwash, and flavored dental floss can cause irritation. Make sure they are not the source of your problem. Food sensitivities often are. Rule them out carefully with an elimination-provocation diet or food allergy or sensitivity blood testing.
- **Try a probiotic supplement.** Lactobacillus acidophilus is often beneficial in prevention and treatment of canker sores. Take capsules or powdered probiotic supplement as directed on the label. Products vary in dosage.
- **Take B-complex vitamins.** Deficiencies in vitamins B_1, B_2, B_6, B_{12}, and folic acid have been associated with recurrent canker sores. People with B-complex deficiencies showed significant improvement of mouth ulcers during three months of supplementation with B-complex vitamins.
- **Consider gluten sensitivity.** Gluten is a protein fraction found in wheat, rye, spelt, barley, and oats. A considerable amount of research has been done on the connection between gluten intolerance and mouth ulcers because people with celiac disease (also called sprue) often have recurring mouth sores. About 25 percent of people with chronic canker sores have elevated antibodies to gluten, which indicates a specific sensitivity. When they avoid gluten-containing grains, their mouth sores go away.
- **Address iron-deficiency anemia.** Iron deficiency is associated with canker sores. If you get recurrent canker sores and are anemic, you may respond to iron supplementation. People who are not anemic will not benefit. Ask your physician to test you for anemia. Take 30 to 75 mg of elemental iron daily. Because iron tends to be constipating, a slow-release iron, like Feosol or generic equivalents, may be helpful. Floradix, an herbal iron supplement, is gentle and works well. Cooking in cast-iron pots and pans is another way to gain iron from your diet.
- **Practice stress-management skills.** Ask yourself if stress plays a significant role in your canker sores. If so, work on your stress-management skills.
- **Take zinc.** Zinc deficiencies have been linked to mouth ulcers. Zinc plays an important role in healing wounds and immune system function. In one study, zinc supplementation helped heal canker sores 81 percent of the time in people with low zinc levels or a low zinc-to-copper ratio.

Topical Remedies

- **Use ice.** Ice compresses dry up canker sores quickly. Apply ice directly to the sore for either 45 minutes once a day or for 5 minutes several times a day. You'll still have a scab that needs to heal, but the sores won't be painful.

- **Try licorice root.** Licorice root is soothing to the mucous membranes of the digestive tract, and chewable licorice can help reduce inflammation and pain from mouth ulcers. Licorice promotes healing of mucous membranes by stimulating production of healing prostaglandins. Just be sure to buy deglycyrrhized licorice (DGL), which means it has had the glycyrrhizins removed. Glycyrrhizins can raise blood pressure and lower serum potassium levels. Chew two licorice tablets between meals as needed up to four times daily, or eat real licorice, such as Panda brand. Most licorice is made with anise, not licorice.

- **Try myrrh.** Myrrh is an herb that has been used since biblical times to soothe mucous membranes. It has antiseptic properties and can be used in a variety of ways. Chewing gum with myrrh can be temporarily soothing, and a glycerin tincture can be used topically to soothe the sores. It can be combined with the herb goldenseal in tea, paste, or tincture.

- **Try goldenseal.** Goldenseal is soothing to mucous membranes and also has antiseptic properties. It can be taken internally in a tincture, as a tea, in capsules, or dabbed directly on the sores.

- **Try castor oil.** An old Edgar Cayce remedy is to soak a cotton swab in castor oil and apply to the canker sore.

THRUSH

Thrush is a yeast infection in the mouth and throat. It has a white, cottage-cheesy look and is common after use of antibiotics. Thrush can be treated with either prescription or natural medicines. If it persists, you must treat yourself systemically. It is of primary importance to use probiotic supplements of acidophilus and bifidobacteria to reestablish normal mouth-throat flora. Natural remedies such as garlic, grapefruit seed extract, pau d'arco, and mathake tea, along with dietary changes, can make your body inhospitable to candida. Follow the protocols for candida infections. In one study, one-third of people with thrush were found to have folic acid, vitamin B_6, or vitamin B_{12} anemia, so it's worth having your doctor check you for anemia and B-vitamin status.

TONGUE PROBLEMS

Tongue problems can arise from systemic illness, so celiac disease, diabetes, Behcet's disease, anemia, and syphilis should be ruled out by your physician. More often, tongue problems are indicators of nutritional needs or mouth irritants, such as smoking or other chemicals.

Glossitis is an inflammation of the tongue, which can be extremely red and smooth, like a bald tire. Studies have found that glossitis is a sign of protein calorie malnourishment, nutritional deficiencies, or marginal nutritional deficiencies of several vitamins and minerals. Glossitis affects 5 percent of our elderly. It most often signals the need for increased B-complex vitamins and iron. You will often find a reddened tongue with pellagra, which is caused by a deficiency of niacin (vitamin B_3).

Other people may also develop what's called a geographic tongue, where the center of the tongue looks like a miniature Grand Canyon. Look in a mirror, look at your friend's and family's tongues, and you'll probably find one. Cracks down the center of the tongue are an indication of the need for increased B-complex vitamins, especially folic acid and B_{12}, and possibly zinc and iron. A bald or pale tongue may be associated with deficiencies of folic acid, B_{12}, B_2, or iron. A tongue with scalloped edges has been associated with grinding one's teeth (bruxism), temporomandibular joint issues (TMJ), or a niacin or B_{12} deficiency.

BURNING TONGUE

I've worked with several people who have burning tongues. I've found that it's often associated with candida issues, although the research on it is mixed. Take a look at the section on candida and yeast overgrowth in Chapter 8 to find out if it can help you. Burning tongue is also associated with cadmium overload. Sources of cadmium include denture paste, cigarette smoke, and some white flour products. Research also reports that this can be associated with menopause and hypothyroid, so think about hormone therapies. Use of lipoic acid can help. Lipoic acid is a powerful antioxidant. Stress, anxiety, and depression are all associated with burning tongue syndrome. I, too, would be anxious if my tongue burned all the time, but do look at stress factors in your life that may be contributing.

Healing Options
- **Take B-complex vitamins.** The most important B vitamins for tongue health are riboflavin (B_2), niacin (B_3), vitamin B_{12}, and folic acid. Choline is found in

B-complex vitamins and also plays a vital role in tongue health. Take 50 to 100 mg of B complex one to three times daily for a trial period of four to six weeks.

- **Address iron-deficiency anemia.** Iron-deficiency anemia can also cause a sore and inflamed tongue. Have your physician check to make sure your iron status is normal. Thorough testing would include hematocrit, hemoglobin, ferritin, TIBC, and transferrin.
- **Take zinc.** Zinc is important for healing. Take 25 to 50 mg daily.
- **Investigate food sensitivities.** Check for food sensitivities using an elimination diet or other method found in Part III.
- **Take vitamin E.** One study of elderly people with glossitis found that they had lower serum levels of vitamin E. It is not known if vitamin E is just a marker or if it will help therapeutically, but vitamin E has low toxicity and is worth trying. You should take 400 IU every day.
- **Try lipoic acid.** In one study 26 percent of people benefited from lipoic acid. Begin with 100 to 300 mg daily.

CHAPTER 20

The Esophagus and Stomach

The most common problems in the esophageal area are belching, medically called eructation; heartburn, also called gastric reflux; and Barrett's esophagus.

BELCHING OR ERUCTATION

Belching is a symptom of gas in the upper part of the digestive tract. Air trapped in the stomach can be painful, and belching is a safety valve that relieves the pressure. It is a release of trapped air from the stomach and usually comes from swallowed air. Just as a baby needs to be burped if she swallows air, we also burp if we swallow air— it's normal. Other than being culturally embarrassing, it's usually without problem.

Foods and drink that contain air contribute to belching. Without fail, when I have a carbonated drink, I burp. Whipped cream and egg whites can have the same effect on many people. Gulping drinks and food causes us to take in more air, while eating slowly prevents us from swallowing air. People also swallow air during exercise, while chewing gum, and while sucking on pipes, straws, or cigarettes. If you are overweight, you are more likely to belch from exercise.

On the other hand, if you are someone who belches a lot, figure out why. Typically I find that people who belch too much have issues with low hydrochloric acid levels. Some have H. pylori infections.

Functional Laboratory Testing

- **H. pylori infection:** Sometimes H. pylori infection can cause belching, with or without other digestive symptoms. Ask your doctor to test for H. pylori.
- **The Heidelberg capsule:** This test measures your ability to produce hydrochloric acid when challenged with alkaline substances. See Chapter 11 for complete details.

Healing Options

- **Make lifestyle changes.** Eat slowly and chew your food well. Avoid carbonated beverages. If you smoke, stop. Be glad you have such a benign reason to stop. Reach and maintain ideal body weight. Stop chewing gum or sucking on candy. As an alternative, you can suck on or eat umeboshi plum, or you can make it into a tea. These salty, fermented plums are highly alkalizing and aid in digestion.
- **Do a self-test or do a Heidelberg capsule test to see if you have enough hydrochloric acid.** I often find that taking betaine HCl capsules eliminates belching in my clients. (See Chapters 3 and 11 for more information.)
- **Try charcoal tablets.** These can absorb toxins, make breath smell better, and calm an overexcited digestive system.
- **Check your supplements.** Some supplements, such as fish oils, can cause belching. Try any of the remedies for heartburn, gastric reflux, and hiatal hernia.

HEARTBURN, GASTROESOPHAGEAL REFLUX DISEASE (GERD), AND HIATAL HERNIA

Hiatal hernia occurs when a portion of the stomach gets pushed through the diaphragm and into the thoracic cavity where it doesn't belong. Hiatal hernias may or may not cause symptoms, but the most common symptom is heartburn; they can also be a cause of GERD. Hiatal hernias are found in about 20 percent of all middle-aged Americans. Dr. Dennis Burkitt, called the father of fiber, hypothesized that hiatal hernia was a contemporary problem and the result of a modernized diet. Straining with bowel movements is one cause. Chiropractic adjustment can gently put the stomach back in place, and in many cases only a single adjustment is necessary.

Gastroesophageal reflux disease (GERD), also known as heartburn, is caused by stomach acid backing up into your esophagus. It's not that you necessarily have too much acid but rather acid that is in the wrong place. The esophageal sphincter is supposed to keep the stomach contents in place, but if the sphincter relaxes, acid can push up into the esophagus. The most common symptoms are heartburn, regurgitation, and trouble swallowing. Less common symptoms include coughing, chest pain, wheezing, excessive salivation, belching, and a sour taste in the mouth.

GERD is alarmingly common: 44 percent of us have heartburn monthly, 10 to 20 percent weekly, and 10 percent daily. Another 3 to 7 percent suffer from Barrett's esophagus, an esophageal illness caused by acid reflux that results in scarring, constriction of the esophagus, swallowing disorders, and an increased risk for esophageal cancer.

For most people, heartburn is a mild, self-limiting problem, yet for 20 percent of those affected it becomes a serious health problem. Stress plays a huge role. Figuring out how you can simplify your life and relax more can go a long way to solving the problem. Sensitivities to gluten and other foods can also trigger symptoms. I have several clients whose GERD has vanished after they stopped eating gluten-containing grains, eggs, or other foods.

Lifestyle plays a role in GERD. Other triggers include wearing tight-fitting clothes, lying down, bending over, and eating large meals or specific foods. If you experience heartburn in the middle of the night, be sure to eat your last meal at least four hours before going to bed. Heartburn is common among pregnant women whose organs are squashed in a most peculiar way. Some drugs can also cause heartburn or reduce the tone of the lower esophageal sphincter. The most common are NSAIDs, aspirin, steroids, birth control pills, diazepam, nicotine, nitroglycerine, progesterone, provera, and theophylline.

There are several categories of medications that are used to decrease hydrochloric acid production. Heartburn sufferers commonly take antacids, such as Tums, Rolaids, Maalox, and Mylanta, for temporary relief. H2 acid blockers such as Tagamet, Pepcid, Axid, and Zantac have been used for a long time and partially block acid production. Proton-pump inhibitors (PPIs), such as Prilosec, Prevacid, and Nexium, are also used to block production of stomach acids completely. PPIs are huge money makers and as a group generate the third-highest sales of all drugs sold worldwide.

Once you begin taking acid blockers your doctor will probably want you to stay on them indefinitely. These medications were originally approved for 12 weeks. Joel E. Richter, FACP, chair of the department of gastroenterology and hepatology at the Cleveland Clinic, recommends using them for four to six months. This allows the inflammation to heal. About half of people taking them would like to stop. The good news is that 60 percent of people who stopped stayed symptom free a year later. Research indicates that there is a rebound in many people who stop taking PPIs. They stop and they have rebound symptoms of GERD, which encourages them to stay on the medication. Weaning off of the medications slowly can help prevent this. Rather than weaning off of the PPIs and moving to H2 blockers or antacids, try the suggestions included in this chapter.

There are other repercussions of taking antacids. A recent study looked at 155 healthy people who had been using antacids for heartburn over long periods of time. The study found that 47 percent had erosion of the esophagus and 6 percent had Barrett's esophagus, a more serious condition. People with Barrett's esophagus who take PPIs to prevent further development of cancer have high levels of leaky stomach (gastric hyperpermeability). People on PPIs have been shown to have decreased levels of calcium, magnesium, and zinc; iron deficiency; vitamin B_{12} deficiency; and increased risk of developing osteoporosis, depression, irritable bowel syndrome, pneumonia, and Clostridium difficile infectious diarrhea. Blocking stomach acid increases your risk of developing small intestinal bacterial overgrowth. The parietal cells respond to these medications by making more acid. Eventually the parietal cells get exhausted, so over the long term, antacids cause the parietal cells to make less HCl and intrinsic factor, which is necessary for absorption of vitamin B_{12}. People who stay on PPIs long term have an increased risk of developing gastric polyps and atrophic gastritis, which both increase risk of developing stomach cancer.

People on these medications often have poor digestion. There is also evidence that pancreatic enzymes aren't activated without proper stomach acid. HCl is needed for proper digestion of protein. Symptoms can present as bloating, pain, and diarrhea.

People on PPIs also have higher levels of IgE antibodies after three months of usage. Women over the age of 50 who take PPIs for more than a month increase the risk of hip fracture due to poor mineral absorption. The longer women take PPIs, the higher the risk of hip fracture. Use of the older H2 blockers does not increase risk.

Functional Laboratory Testing
- H. pylori test
- Heidelberg capsule test
- Food sensitivity testing
- Celiac testing

Healing Options
- **Try osteopathic care and chiropractic adjustment.** Seek chiropractic care for hiatal hernia. Cranial-sacral adjustments can often correct gastric reflux, especially in children. Chiropractic or osteopathic adjustment is often all the therapy you need for these problems.
- **Try acupuncture.** Acupuncture treatments can be effective for GERD.

- **Make dietary changes and try an elimination diet.** Late-night eating can trigger GERD. Offending foods are individual—you need to discover what yours are. I've seen people respond to a gluten-free diet and others respond to an egg-free diet. The National Institute of Diabetes and Digestive and Kidney Disease recommends eliminating the following foods and food groups to discover which ones contribute to your GERD: citrus fruits, chocolate, caffeinated drinks, fatty and fried foods, garlic, onions, mint flavorings, spicy foods, and tomato-based foods like spaghetti sauce, salsa, and pizza. Eating a whole-foods diet rich in vegetables and fruits can often help.

- **If you are overweight, lose weight.** One of the contributors to GERD is being overweight. If you lose weight, it can help.

- **If you smoke, stop.** GERD is high in people who smoke than in nonsmokers.

- **Drink plenty of water.** Some people find that increasing water consumption up to a gallon of water a day resolves acid reflux. Dr. F. Batmanghelidj popularized the water cure for GERD and ulcers in his book *Your Body's Many Cries for Water*.

- **Place a six-inch beam under the head of your bed.** If you suffer from nighttime heartburn, raising the head of your bed can alleviate symptoms. Although you might think that raising your bed would feel strange, the difference is barely noticeable, and the heartburn improves.

- **Consider possible H. pylori infection.** H. pylori is a bacteria that has been implicated in gastric and duodenal ulcers. In some cases, it is also involved in gastric reflux. Treatment with antibiotics and bismuth-containing supplements or drugs can eradicate the bacteria.

- **Try hydrochloric acid supplements.** Heartburn has traditionally been treated with antacid therapy, but often it responds well to supplementation with hydrochloric acid pills. Often, the symptoms of excess stomach acid and decreased stomach acid are the same. (See sections in Chapter 3 and 11 for more information on HCl.)

- **Drink cabbage juice.** Cabbage juice is a long-standing folk remedy for heartburn. Its high glutamine content is probably the key to its success. Cabbage juice has a strong flavor, so dilute with other vegetable juices.

- **Try slippery elm bark.** Slippery elm bark has demulcent properties, and it's gentle and soothing to mucous membranes. It has been a folk remedy for both heartburn and ulcers in European and Native American cultures and was used as a food by Native Americans. It can be used in large amounts without harm. Drink as a tea or chew on the bark. To make a tea, put 1 teaspoon of slippery elm bark in 2 cups of water. Simmer for 20 minutes and strain. Sweeten if you want, and drink freely. You can also purchase slippery elm lozenges at health-food stores and some drugstores.

- **Use lobelia.** Massage tincture of lobelia externally onto the painful area and take two to three drops internally. This remedy is recommended by Dr. John Christopher, one of the greatest American herbalists of the 20th century.
- **Use ginger.** This root can provide temporary relief in a tea. Steep ½ to 1 teaspoons of powdered ginger or a few slices of fresh ginger per cup of boiled water for 10 minutes and drink. If you like, sweeten it with honey. Use freely.
- **Try meadowsweet herb.** Also a demulcent, meadowsweet soothes inflamed mucous membranes. To make a tea, steep 1 to 2 teaspoons of the dried herb in 1 cup of boiled water for 10 minutes. Sweeten with honey if you like. Drink three cups daily.
- **Repair your gut with soothing nutrients.** Taking healing nutrients will repair the damage in your esophagus. Use zinc (especially carnosine), glutamine, fish oils, gamma oryzanol, turmeric, and ginger. Eat okra.

BARRETT'S ESOPHAGUS

Barrett's esophagus is an esophageal illness caused by long-term acid reflux (GERD) that results in scarring and constriction of the esophagus, and swallowing disorders. It affects between 3 and 7 percent of adults in the United States. It's hard to know exactly how many because 25 percent of people who have Barrett's have no symptoms. It is more common in men than in women, and especially in people who are white or Hispanic. Smoking, getting older, and obesity increase your risk.

Barrett's itself may or may not cause any symptoms. Barrett's does not cause cancer, but it often precedes it. The risk of developing esophageal cancer is 30 to 125 times higher in people who have Barrett's esophagus than those who don't. The incidence has risen more than 350 percent since the mid-1970s. People with known Barrett's esophagus should be frequently monitored for early detection of cancer. Only 5 percent of people who develop esophageal cancer knew that they had Barrett's prior to being diagnosed with cancer, so people who have chronic GERD ought to be seen by a gastroenterologist for an evaluation. Barrett's esophagus can occur in people without gastric reflux, but it is three to five times more common in people who do have it. Treatment with acid-blocking drugs sometimes improves the extent of the Barrett's, but it doesn't correlate with a reduction in cancer rates. Production of peroxynitrite, a damaging free radical, contributes to Barrett's esophagus. Vitamin C, glutathione, and folic acid are known to help reduce the formation of damaging peroxynitrites. Barrett's is diagnosed by doing an upper GI endoscopy and biopsy.

The following healing options may help with the symptoms of Barrett's esophagus. They may also help prevent cancer of the esophagus, which is the long-term problem to be concerned about. Very little literature about this is available, but I am working with what is known in other areas of the digestive tract and personal experience with clients. It is necessary to continue to have medical testing and to be vigilant about this illness. You may also benefit from the many suggestions in the section on heartburn and gastric reflux.

Healing Options

- **Eat a diet high in folate.** Folic acid, found in a huge variety of foods, prevents esophageal cancer and colon cancers. Research on giving folic acid supplements, on the other hand, has been mixed. Giving folic acid supplementation *may* actually increase the risk of developing esophageal cancer. It remains to be seen how genetics play a role; people who have variations in the MTHFR gene have different needs for folic acid than people with normal MTHFR expression. Nonetheless, you will do well to eat high folic acid foods, such as brewer's yeast, black-eyed peas, rice germ, soy flour, wheat germ, liver, soy beans, wheat bran, legumes of all types, asparagus, lentils, walnuts, spinach, kale, nuts, greens of all types, peanuts, broccoli, barley, brussels sprouts, and more.

- **Increase antioxidant nutrients.** Several studies indicate that free radical damage helps initiate Barrett's esophagus. Antioxidant nutrients are useful in nearly every condition. Selenium levels in people with Barrett's esophagus are lower than in controls. Glutathione levels are reduced, while malondialdehyde and NF-kappaB levels are increased. It is prudent to increase levels of antioxidant nutrients such as vitamin C, carotenoids, vitamin E, selenium, N-acetyl cysteine (NAC), lipoic acid, folic acid, and others. You can begin with a combination antioxidant supplement with 200 to 400 mcg selenium. Add an additional 1,000 IU of vitamin E, 1,000 to 2,000 mg NAC, and at least 1,000 mg vitamin C. You may want to use the vitamin C flush described in Chapter 13.

- **Try probiotics and digestive enzymes.** No published research on the use of probiotic bacteria or on the use of digestive enzymes in Barrett's is available, but it would make sense to give each a trial.

- **Try gut-healing herbs and nutrients.** The use of supplemental glutamine has not been studied in people with Barrett's esophagus, but it has been shown to be effective in preventing radiation-induced damage and weight loss in people undergoing radiation treatment for small-cell lung cancer.

DGL licorice, slippery elm, marshmallow, gamma oryzanol, turmeric or curcumin, fish oils, and other herbs and supplements that are used to reduce inflammation make sense to try. (See Chapter 9.)

EOSINOPHILIC ESOPHAGITIS

Eosinophilic esophagitis (EE) is a chronic inflammatory condition of the esophagus that is characterized by high levels of eosinophils in the blood. Eosinophils are typically elevated when people have allergies or parasites. Officially identified in 1993, this disease is emerging in many developed countries, including the United States, England, Japan, Spain, Australia, Switzerland, and Italy. It first came to medical attention in children, but now that physicians are looking, they are finding EE in adults as well. An article from Cincinnati Children's Hospital suggests that EE is becoming the most common inflammatory digestive condition, more common than Crohn's disease or ulcerative colitis. Despite this explosion, very little information on the disease is available, and much of the research on EE so far has gone into simply figuring out what the problem is and how to recognize it. Because the symptoms are similar to those of heartburn and gastroesophageal reflux disease, many people are incorrectly diagnosed and treated for those other conditions instead. The disease is diagnosed by an endoscopy, an examination using a scope down the esophagus, followed by a biopsy, to look at the tissue.

Symptoms of EE include nausea or vomiting, diarrhea, failure to thrive in children (poor growth or weight loss), stomach or chest pain, regurgitation, GERD, painful or difficult swallowing, poor appetite, bloating, anemia, blood in the stool, malnutrition, and difficulty sleeping. People will often have food allergies, eczema, or asthma. Children may not want to eat because it hurts. In addition, scarring from untreated EE can make it difficult to swallow, so some of these children are shorter and weigh less than they should because they fail to eat enough. Many children with EE have white specks or plaques in the esophagus, which tend to occur when the condition is severe.

One study found asthma in one-third of children with EE; EE is being called "asthma of the esophagus" because allergic reactions to foods and also environment allergens such as mold, dust, and pollen appear to play a big role. People with EE are advised to go on a diet that eliminates all foods to which they are allergic. Physicians also encourage the use of an elemental diet, using medical foods that are hypoallergenic. Often people who eat only this product for several months show great improvement in symptoms and at repeat endoscopy and biopsy.

One study showed an atypically alkaline esophageal environment in nine out of nine children with EE. More research on this subject is needed, but it would seem that if esophageal pH is low, you may wish to try increasing your level of stomach acid to see whether this relieves the symptoms.

I have worked with several children who have EE. One toddler began having problems immediately after an immunization, a story commonly heard from parents of autistic children. A different parent I've worked with began working with an autism trained physician and used biomedical approaches to heal her son's EE. You will remember from the DIGIN model that no matter what the diagnosis, we always use the same principles to treat digestive issues.

I hypothesize that children with EE may have detoxification problems like children with autism do, but they manifest a different set of symptoms. The theory that heavy metals such as mercury play a role in this problem will either be validated or tossed out as it is put to the test.

EOSINOPHILIC GASTROENTERITIS

Eosinophilic gastroenteritis (EG) is similar to EE, but it takes place in the stomach and small intestine rather than in the esophagus. It is characterized by severe infiltration of eosinophils into the stomach, small intestine, or both. It is also called eosinophilic gastritis (when just in the stomach) and eosinophilic enteritis (when just in the small intestine). It was first discovered in 1937 by a researcher named Kaijser.

Half the children who have EG have a history of eczema, asthma, or food allergies. Many children and adults with EG also have more typical allergies to dust, pollen, and mold. Typical symptoms of EG include abdominal pain, diarrhea, and pain with swallowing. Often a child will refuse to eat because it hurts. Cramping and abdominal pain may be accompanied by nausea and vomiting.

As with children with EE, it is essential to test them for food allergies and sensitivities, especially to gluten and dairy products.

Dr. DicQie Fuller had a baby daughter, Colleen, who suffered from eosinophilic gastritis. Her daughter was failing to thrive, and she was told that her daughter would simply die. In an effort to save her daughter's life, Dr. Fuller began giving her daughter enzyme supplements. She used digestive and proteolytic (protein-splitting) enzymes. It not only saved her daughter's life, Colleen is now in her 40s and has been living healthfully since.

TREATING EE AND EG

Treatments for EE and EG may include steroids, but they aren't often used due to the long-term side effects. At this time, medical treatments aren't that promising and the long-term implications of having EE or EG are uncertain. This leads one to really use more of an integrated approach when working with these diseases. Begin with the DIGIN model.

One resource is the American Partnership for Eosinophilic Disorders: http://www.apfed.org.

Laboratory Testing for EE and EG

If EE or EG is suspected, I recommend exploring gut health with comprehensive testing because there is little understanding of the disease's cause. Regular IgE scratch testing or a modified RAST will reveal the true allergies but will not discover the contributions from foods that have delayed hypersensitivity reactions. Tests to consider include the following:

- Food-allergy testing/IgE
- Food-sensitivity testing/IgG and, if possible, IgM and IgA
- Urine provocation test for heavy metals
- pH test, quantitative fluid analysis, or the Heidelberg capsule test

Healing Options for EE and EG

Drugs currently used for EE include steroid medications, cromolyn sodium, and leukotriene inhibitors. Initial research shows that even with medication, restriction of allergy-inducing foods is still necessary to achieve the full benefit. The other natural healing options presented herein are my own ideas, as no research has been conducted on natural therapies for EE and EG.

- **Elimination-provocation diet.** See Chapter 15 for instructions.
- **Quercetin.** It will diminish, relieve, and prevent allergy symptoms and protect esophageal tissue. Quercetin is very effective when combined with grape seed extract or Pycnogenol. Adults can take 500 to 6,000 mg. A child can take 200 to 1,000 mg three to six times daily, depending on the child's size and symptom severity.
- **Probiotics.** This will balance gut ecology and immune system function. See Chapter 6 for dosages and types.

- **Consider heavy-metal toxicity.** See Chapter 18. Children with EE and EG fit the profile for children who have impaired detoxification pathways. This can be tested for or observed. In addition you may want to ask for porphyrin testing to determine exactly what your child might be reacting to.
- **Digestive enzymes.** Use these to enhance complete digestion of foods so that they don't become allergens. Take one capsule each time you eat.
- **DGL licorice.** This will soothe inflammation and stimulate repair. Take one to three tablets, chewables, or capsules before meals. You could also consider using the demulcent herbs marshmallow, meadowsweet, and slippery elm.
- **Folic acid.** This will protect mucous membranes from inflammation elsewhere in the gastrointestinal tract. Take 800 mcg daily.

GASTRIC HYPOFUNCTION OR HYPOCHLORHYDRIA

Hypochlorhydria (low stomach acid) has been associated with many common health problems. (See Chapters 3 and 11.) Stomach acid is used to begin the process of protein digestion. Stomach acid also provides our first defense against food poisoning, H. pylori, parasites, small intestinal bacterial overgrowth, and other infections. In addition, without adequate acid we leave ourselves open to indigestion, decreased immune resistance, mineral deficiencies, and vitamin deficiencies. A normal stomach acid level is a pH of 1.5 to 2.5. As we age, the parietal cells in the stomach lining produce less hydrochloric acid. Use of acid-blocking medications increases stomach pH to 3.5 or higher.

Common symptoms of low stomach acidity include belching or burning sensations immediately after meals, bloating, a feeling that the food just sits in the stomach without digesting, and an inability to eat more than small amounts at any one sitting. Poor HCl levels have been associated with childhood asthma, chronic hepatitis, chronic hives, diabetes, eczema, gallbladder disease, lupus erythematosus, osteoporosis, rheumatoid arthritis, rosacea, under- and overactive thyroid conditions, vitiligo, and weak adrenals.

Stomach acid is also necessary for absorption of many minerals, so mineral depletion may occur with use of these medicines. Minerals that can become depleted include iron, calcium, magnesium, zinc, and copper. Adequate HCl is necessary for the absorption of vitamin B_{12} from food. B_{12} deficiency causes weakness, fatigue, and nervous system problems. Most B-complex vitamins require normal levels of stomach acid for proper absorption. Vitamin C levels are also low in people with poor stomach acid. Acid is critical for the breakdown of protein bonds in the stomach.

Hypochlorhydria may be caused by the following: pernicious anemia, chronic H. pylori infection, long-term treatment with proton-pump inhibitors (PPIs, such as Prilosec), autoimmune gastritis, and mucolipidosis type 1V; it is also common in autoimmune diseases.

Functional Laboratory Testing

- Heidelberg capsule test
- Self-test for HCl adequacy

For healing options, see Chapter 3.

DYSPEPSIA AND GASTRITIS

Dyspepsia is a general term that means "bad digestion" in Latin. About 40 percent of us complain of bad digestion. It's typically self-limiting and goes away on its own. If you have two or more of the following factors, it's time to see your doctor: being over age 50, loss of appetite, feeling full even though you haven't eaten much, trouble swallowing, blood in your stools or in phlegm, or abdominal masses.

Gastritis is a general name that describes any inflammation in the stomach that doesn't involve an ulcer. This could be a chronic issue or something that's acutely painful. The most common symptoms are gnawing or burning ache or pain in your stomach that gets better or worse with food, loss of appetite, bloating, belching, hiccups, indigestion, nausea, vomiting, vomiting of blood, dark stools, feeling full even if you haven't eaten much, and weight loss. It's typically found when a gastro-enterologist does an endoscopy. It can be caused by alcohol, infection such as with H. pylori, taking NSAIDs (such as aspirin), smoking, chronic stress, bile reflux, drinking poisons or caustic substances, and autoimmune disorders.

Other causes include corticosteroids, cancer drugs, and antibiotics; excessive coffee consumption; organ failure; and severe stress or trauma. It is common in the elderly, affecting 20 percent of people between the ages of 60 and 69 and 40 percent of people over age 80. The lack of hydrochloric acid secretion in the elderly allows for bacterial growth, such as H. pylori; however, when treated with antibiotics, symptoms improve.

Long-term effects of gastritis include poor vitamin B_{12} status in all people. Signs of B_{12} deficiency often mimic those of senility. Many people have B_{12} deficiencies with normal serum levels. Tests for B$_{12}$ status include methylmalonic acid and trials with B$_{12}$ injections or sublingual B$_{12}$.

Gastritis is usually treated with H2 blockers or proton-pump inhibitors (PPIs). However, there are natural solutions that don't have the long-term effects that H2 blockers and PPIs have. Looking at triggers such as stress, medications, and poor HCl production is also an important step toward prevention.

GASTRIC ULCERS

Gastric ulcers occur in the stomach and the duodenum (the first section of the small intestine) where gastric juice has burned a hole in the lining. It hurts! Gastric juice is so acidic it would burn your hand if you spilled some on it. A mucous layer protects the stomach tissue from being eaten away by pepsin (a protein-splitting enzyme) and the gastric juices. Secretions of bicarbonate (baking soda) from the stomach lining are mixed into the mucus, buffering the acid. This makes an effective barrier to keep the stomach lining from harm. Pepsin, the real villain in this story, slowly digests this mucus layer, and if the mucus isn't replaced, gastric juices come into contact with the stomach lining and ulcers occur.

About half a million Americans have ulcers. About 10 percent of us will develop ulcer disease at some point in our lives. Each year 6,000 American people die from ulcers, half from peptic ulcers and half from duodenal ulcers. Since the discovery and screening of H. pylori infections in 1982 the incidence of ulcers has been decreasing. Eighty percent of ulcers are caused by H. pylori infections, 10 percent are caused by the use of NSAID medications, and another 10 percent are of unknown origin.

Symptoms include abdominal pain that is frequently described as burning. This pain can radiate to your back and typically occurs one to five hours after you've eaten. You may feel better if you eat, take antacids, or vomit. All of this typically is in a daily pattern that is specific to you. As if this isn't enough to alert you to see a doctor, if you have bleeding, are anemic, have unexplained weight loss, feel full even though you only ate a little bit, have increasing trouble swallowing or painful swallowing, suffer recurrent vomiting, or have a family history of GI cancer, see a doctor now. If you have sharp and sudden severe stomach pain that persists, bloody or black stools, bloody vomit, or vomit that looks like it has coffee grounds, seek immediate medical help.

On the other hand, if you are slowly burning a hole in your stomach from over-use of NSAIDs like aspirin, Motrin, Aleve, and prescription pain relievers, you may not notice a thing until you begin to see bleeding or have anemia. Continued use of these therapies has been widely shown to cause ulcers and hospitalizations. It's estimated that up to 30 percent of regular NSAID users have ulcers. NSAIDs block pain but also block healing and repair to the stomach lining by decreasing beneficial prostaglandins and cyclooxygenase. It has been estimated that 107,000 people are hospitalized each year because of NSAID complications, and at least 16,500 NSAID-related deaths occur each year among arthritis patients alone.

Ten percent of people with ulcers and gastritis do not have H. pylori infection, nor have they used NSAID medications. For these people, the cause of ulcers and gastritis is still a mystery. Looking at stress, diet, and lifestyle may yield important clues. Stress plays a significant role in ulcers and gastritis. While low-grade stress probably won't cause an ulcer, severe stress has been shown to cause ulcers in both animal and human studies. Psychological stress increases stomach acid and causes the mucus to become more fragile, making it easier for ulcers to form.

There are simple blood, stool, and breath tests that detect H. pylori. In a breath test, you swallow a capsule, drink a liquid, or eat a pudding that contains urea that's been tagged with carbon. You then breathe into a container, and if the carbon atom is present, it signals high amounts of urease and you are diagnosed with H. pylori infection. Blood tests are done to discover if you have elevated H. pylori antibodies. Stool testing looks at antigens to H. pylori. If you've been having severe symptoms or bleeding, your doctor may order an endoscopy.

H. pylori infection is common even in those of us without ulcers. There is debate about whether treating people who are without symptoms will be of benefit or not. Is this a bacteria that can become detrimental in the wrong environment but is harmless in others? H. pylori has also been associated with increased risk of duodenal and gastric cancers, chronic gastritis, cirrhosis, and chronic indigestion. On the other hand, it appears to protect much of the world's population by preventing inflamatory bowel disease. Obviously, much still needs to be learned here.

Because ulcers have been experienced throughout history, people have found effective natural therapies. Most physicians are not aware of these therapies, but nutritionally oriented physicians have been using them with promising results. Some recommend a combination of antibiotic therapy and bismuth, with DGL licorice, citrus seed extract, goldenseal, activated charcoal, and aloe vera. Glutamine, gamma oryzanol, SanoGastril, cabbage juice, comfrey, and calendula have also been shown to heal ulcers.

Other natural substances that have been shown to be effective against this bacterium include oil of oregano, turmeric, cumin, ginger, chili, borage, and licorice root. Several of these, turmeric, borage, and parsley, also inhibited the ability of H. pylori to adhere to the stomach.

Dietary recommendations for people with ulcers may be useful. Low-fiber diets may contribute significantly to ulcers. A South African physician, G. Borok, studied more than a thousand patients with ulcers and concluded that elimination of refined sugars, white-flour products, milled maize, chocolate, fries, soft drinks, and desserts will reduce gastric irritation. He also suggests avoiding tea and coffee. Another plug for a whole-foods diet!

A recent study on the diet of people with duodenal ulcers found that people who had good vitamin-A intake, followed a high-fiber diet, or ate seven or more servings of fruits and vegetables per day rather than three servings or fewer reduced risks of developing ulcers by 54 percent, 45 percent, and 33 percent, respectively. Again, this shows that a great diet can reduce your risk of all sorts of health problems.

One new therapy uses lactoferrin, which is found in colostrum and transfer factor, to eradicate H. pylori. Research has shown that use of triple therapy with added lactoferrin improves the success rate. Alone, it probably won't do the job. People with high levels of gastritis and helicobacter also have concurrent high levels of lactoferrin in their stomach. Is the lactoferrin helping the H. pylori gain a foothold and helping it gain necessary iron for its metabolism? Or is the lactoferrin called in by the body's immune system to help rid us of the bacteria? At this point, no one really knows.

Research for ulcer healing has shown good results for a wide variety of natural products. You can also find relief from combination products that contain bismuth, licorice root, grapefruit seed extract, goldenseal root, aloe vera, zinc carnosine, mastic gum, quercetin, sea buckthorn, water hissop, Bolivian medicinal, traditional Chinese formulations, and other herbs. Cranberry juice, ginger juice, broccoli sprouts, Brussels sprouts, plantain (banana type), propolis, evening primrose oil and other polyunsaturated fatty acids, reishi mushrooms, green tea, turmeric or curcumin, and yogurt can also heal ulcers. One study of 1,785 people found that moderate drinking of alcohol killed H. pylori infection. Details on many of these follow.

Functional Laboratory Testing
- **H. pylori test.** This can be done through stool, breath, or blood testing. It is widely available.

Healing Options
- **Drink water.** One very simple remedy for ulcers and gastritis is to drink huge amounts of water. Drink four to six glasses of water during the pain, and it may magically disappear. A fascinating book on this subject is *Your Body's Many Cries for Water*, by Fereydoon Batmanghelidj, M.D. Drink eight to ten glasses of water or more each day.

- **Try licorice.** DGL licorice helps heal the stomach's mucous lining by increasing healing prostaglandins that promote mucus secretion and cell proliferation. It also makes an environment that is inhospitable to H. pylori and has some weak antibiotic effects. Licorice enhances the blood flow and health of intestinal tract cells. It's considered to have the same healing effect as cimetidine (Tagamet). It's important to use DGL licorice to avoid side effects caused by whole licorice. Take 760 to 1,520 mg chewed before each meal. Daily total dosage is 4.5 grams.
- **Use aloe vera.** Aloe vera is a folk remedy for ulcers and has been approved by the FDA for use in oral ulcers. It is soothing, reduces inflammation, and helps to heal gastric ulcers. Take 1 teaspoon of fresh gel after meals. Use gel that doesn't have skin; otherwise it can give you diarrhea. If you buy an aloe vera product, use as directed.
- **Try gamma oryzanol.** Gamma oryzanol, a compound found in rice bran oil, is a useful therapeutic tool in gastritis, ulcers, and irritable bowel syndrome. It acts on the autonomic nervous system to normalize production of gastric juice and has also been shown to be effective in normalizing serum triglycerides and cholesterol, symptoms of menopause, and depressive disorders. Studies involving 375 hospitals in Japan indicate that gamma oryzanol was effective in reducing symptoms in 80 to 90 percent of participants, with more than half of the participants experiencing total or marked improvement. Typical dosage was 100 mg three times daily for three weeks. Occasionally, the dosage was doubled, and often the therapy was used longer. Minimal side effects were experienced by 0.4 percent of the people. Take 100 mg of gamma oryzanol three times daily for a trial period of three to six weeks to determine if it relieves the problem.
- **Drink cabbage juice.** Cabbage juice is a long-standing folk remedy for heartburn. Drink 1 quart of cabbage juice daily for a trial period of two weeks.
- **Drink cranberry juice.** Cranberry juice has been well studied for helping to resolve H. pylori. It appears to block H. pylori from adhering to the stomach tissue, in the same way that it does in the bladder. While it doesn't work for everyone, a Chinese study reports that 11.3 percent of people were H. pylori free after drinking two 9-ounce juice boxes of cranberry juice daily for 90 days. Another report states that when cranberry was used along with oregano, results improved because of the synergy. In another study, when cranberry juice was given to people along with triple therapy, results improved; 82.5 percent of people who drank 9 ounces (250 ml) of cranberry juice twice daily had normal H. pylori breath tests. In women results were even better; 95.2 percent had normal test results.

- **Use mastic gum.** Several studies tout the anti-ulcer benefit of mastic gum. Take 1 gram (1,000 mg) daily in divided doses.
- **Eat yogurt.** Eating 12 to 24 ounces of yogurt containing bifidobacteria lowered H. pylori in breath testing after six weeks of daily consumption.
- **Drink a lot of green tea.** H. pylori was inhibited in gerbils when given green tea extract. The human dosage would be 4 to 8 cups of green tea daily using about ½ teaspoon of dried green tea per cup.
- **Try glutamine.** Glutamine is the most popular antiulcer drug in Asia today. The digestive tract uses glutamine as a fuel source and for healing. It is effective for healing stomach ulcers, irritable bowel syndrome, and ulcerative bowel diseases. Begin with 8 grams daily for a trial period of four weeks.
- **Try grapefruit or citrus seed extract.** Citrus seed extract has widely effective antiparasitic, antiviral, and antibiotic properties. Take 75 to 250 mg three times daily.
- **Use goldenseal.** Goldenseal is soothing to mucous membranes, enhances immune function, and has antibiotic and antifungal properties. Take 200 mg three to four times daily.
- **Try SanoGastril.** SanoGastril is a fermented soy product that contains a specific strain of Lactobacillus bulgaricus (LB-15). It's a chewable tablet that buffers the acidity of the stomach. (SanoGastril is marketed in the United States by Nutri-Cology/Allergy Research Group.) A study using two tablets three times daily involved 93 people with ulcers and gastritis. After one month, each participant was x-rayed to see progress. At that time, 12 out of 22 people with gastric ulcer, 25 out of 58 people with duodenal ulcer, and 4 out of 12 people with gastritis were completely healed. Two tablets of SanoGastril three times daily before meals relieved heartburn completely immediately in 76 percent of 158 people. Take two tablets chewed or sucked three times daily between meals.
- **Try catsclaw/Una de Gato.** The inner bark and stems of Uncaria tomentosa and Uncaria guianesis decrease inflammation. Take 1,000 mg capsules three to five times daily. *Caution: Do not take with Coumadin (warfarin).*
- **Use evening primrose, borage, or flaxseed oils.** These oils increase the levels of prostaglandin E2 series, which promotes healing and repair. Take 4,000 to 8,000 mg of one of these oils or a combination oil three times a day for a trial period of four weeks.

Low dietary intake of linoleic acid, an essential fatty acid, has been associated with duodenal ulcers. Flaxseeds are excellent sources of linoleic acid. A benefit to using ground flaxseeds rather than the oil is that the mucous portion of the flaxseed buffers excess acid, which makes it ideal for inflammation in the stomach and throughout the gastrointestinal tract. Grind them fresh daily or buy products with enhanced shelf life, and store in the refrigerator. Linoleic acid is also found in pumpkin seeds, tofu, walnuts, safflower oil, sunflower seeds and oil, and sesame seeds and oil. Use 2 to 3 teaspoons in smoothies or protein drinks, or on salads and vegetables.

- **Take zinc carnosine.** Studies report 100 percent symptom relief and 80 percent healing of ulcers after taking zinc carnosine for eight weeks. Take 75 mg twice daily.

- **Try Turkish herbs.** Six Turkish plant medicines were studied for their effectiveness against H. pylori in a laboratory setting. Five were found to be highly effective, with Cistus laurifolius (laurel rockrose) being the most effective. The effective herbs were the flowers of Cistus laurifolius, cones of Cedrus libani (cedar of Lebanon), herbs and flowers of Centaurea solstitialis (yellow starthistle), fruits of Momordica charantia (bitter melon), herbaceous parts of Sambucus ebulus (danewort or dwarf elder), and flowering herbs of Hypericum perforatum (Saint-John's-wort). We may begin to see research on some or all of these plant medicines. We may also begin to see them in supplements. There have been no human studies.

- **Try melatonin.** Several studies have looked at the effect of melatonin on GERD. Melatonin is a hormone that helps us fall asleep and is a powerful antioxidant. It's also found in the hormone-producing cells in the GI wall. It works best when given along with Tagamet (cimetidine). Dosages between 3 and 6 mg before bed for four to eight weeks have been found to be an effective treatment for GERD.

- **Try comfrey and calendula.** A Bulgarian study used comfrey and calendula either with antacid medications or alone in patients with peptic ulcers. Eighty-five percent of both groups felt better, but people who also used antacids felt better a few days earlier. Gastric scoping showed equal healing of ulcers in both groups. Comfrey, one of my favorite herbs, has come under fire lately. It contains small amounts of pyrrolizidine alkaloids, which have liver-damaging and possible carcinogenic effects. Although there have been no known cases of toxicity in humans from comfrey, rat testing has caused it to be removed from many products and banned in several countries. Studies were done using the specific pyrrolizidine alkaloids, but in studies with whole comfrey, no adverse reactions were found.

  While the controversy continues, be cautious about using comfrey internally. Restrict its internal use to two weeks. Comfrey has been used medicinally for hundreds of years to promote wound and bone healing. The combination of comfrey and calendula makes sense in terms of today's triple therapy: comfrey promotes healing and protects the gastric mucosa, while calendula has antibacterial effects. Dosage in the Bulgarian study was unclear, but comfrey leaf and calendula flower tea at 3 to 4 cups daily would be appropriate.

GASTROPARESIS

Gastroparesis is delayed gastric emptying. It occurs when the muscles in your stomach don't open to let the food pass into the duodenum properly. It literally means "paralyzed stomach." This can be a very severe disease because your food doesn't move. Symptoms can vary but may include vomiting, nausea, feeling of fullness after eating just a bit, bloating, heartburn, lack of appetite, weight loss and malnutrition, and fluctuations in blood sugar levels. Causes vary but may include damage or unresponsiveness of the vagus nerve, diabetes, H. pylori infection, viral infection, autoimmune disease, nervous system disorders such as Parkinson's disease, and scleroderma. It's more common in people who have had gastric or other abdominal surgeries and in people with eating disorders, hypothyroid, scleroderma, and Parkinson's disease. Gastroparesis can result in weight loss and malnutrition, bacterial overgrowth in the stomach, or food that sits and hardens in your stomach (called a bezoar). An endoscopic exam can determine whether gastroparesis is your problem. It is diagnosed by an upper endoscopy. Ultrasound is also used to rule out gallbladder disease and pancreatitis. The SmartPill is also used to diagnose gastroparesis.

A lot of the medical treatments may work for a while but then stop working. Some of the integrative physicians I have met use a prescription drug called domperidone. It is used in Mexico, Canada, and many European countries for gastroparesis. Physicians like it because it works well and has few side effects. Domperidone can be purchased on the Internet but is not available in the United States. I could find almost *no* research on the use of natural therapies, but here are some that have worked for others and are worth trying.

Healing Options
- **Try d-limonene.** This was highly recommended to me by Patrick Hanaway, M.D. Dr. Hanaway is the medical director of Genova Diagnostic Labs, a family physician, and a speaker at many medical conferences. Take one capsule of d-limonene every other day for 20 days. Take 30 minutes before a meal or 60

minutes after a meal with water or other beverage. Swallow the capsule whole. Do not break it open. Do not take if you are pregnant, nursing, or suspect you have an ulcer.

- **Try Iberogast.** Iberogast, formulated in Germany in 1961, comprises nine different herbs. These include German chamomile, clown's mustard, angelica, caraway, lemon balm, celandine, licorice, and peppermint. The exact mechanism isn't known but has a dual action in that it relaxes smooth muscle, helping when there is spasm, and also helps where there isn't any muscle tone. It also has anti-inflammatory and strong antioxidant properties.

- **Try tangweikang.** A Chinese study found that the herbal combination tangweikang was effective at helping with gastric emptying and blood sugar control in people with diabetes.

- **Try lipoic acid.** Richard Bernstein, M.D., in his book *Dr. Bernstein's Diabetes Solution*, has an entire chapter on gastroparesis and its relationship to diabetes. Lipoic acid helps liver function and regulation of blood sugar. He recommends 600 mg of lipoic acid daily.

- **Try digestive enzymes.** While these will not change your muscle tone, Dr. Bernstein states that many of his patients find that papaya enzymes have helped with symptoms of belching and bloating and help to keep blood sugar in control.

- **Take betaine HCl with pepsin.** Dr. Bernstein also recommends betaine HCl with pepsin to help more fully digest the food into chyme. The better the food is digested, the more easily it will pass through a narrow sphincter. *Caution: This should not be used in people who have ulcers, gastritis, or esophagitis.*

- **Eat pureed foods.** Pureed meats, fruits, and vegetables; soups; smoothies; baby food; protein drinks; yogurt; cottage cheese; ricotta cheese; and other foods that are primarily in a liquid form are more easily digested.

- **Try biofeedback and other mind-body techniques.** I found one study where 26 people with impaired gastric emptying were given a relaxation technique, called autonomic training, along with directed imagery. The authors concluded that this technique or biofeedback therapy might be useful. We do have good research indicating that mind-body therapies, imagery, and biofeedback are useful for other GI motility issues, such as IBS, so it may also work for gastroparesis.

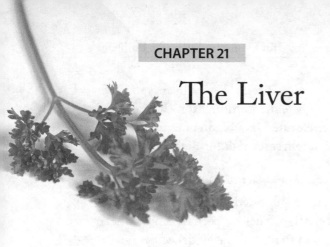

CHAPTER 21

The Liver

The liver is the most complex organ in the body. Unlike the heart, which has one major function—to beat—the liver has a multitude of functions that include regulation of blood sugar levels, making 13,000 different enzymes, humanizing food by acting as a filter, breaking down toxins, manufacturing cholesterol and bile, breaking down hormones, and more. Because of its complexity and the 10,000 pounds of substances it must filter over a lifetime, the liver can easily become overwhelmed. Often the first sign of liver disease is elevated liver enzymes, AST (aspartate aminotransferase) and ALT (alanine aminotransferase).

Common liver conditions include hepatitis, cirrhosis, hemochromatosis, and, more rarely, liver cancer. Jaundice, a yellowing of your skin, is a sign that something is wrong with your liver.

Love your liver once in a while by helping facilitate detoxification. Read Chapter 18 for information on detoxification programs.

FATTY LIVER DISEASE

Fatty liver disease is just that, your liver is accumulating fat. It's not an actual disease but can lead to cirrhosis and liver failure. It's also called nonalcoholic fatty liver disease (NAFLD) and it affects 20 percent of Americans. At this stage, it's completely reversible with changes in diet, exercise, and liver support. You probably will have *no* symptoms. If you do, you may be tired, have pain in your liver area (below your ribs to the right), or be losing weight for no reason. It's detected when your liver enzymes, ALT and AST, are elevated in a blood chemistry panel. It can also lead to metabolic syndrome, which increases risk for diabetes and cardiovascular diseases.

Recently a study of children in San Diego found fatty liver disease in 13 percent of children who died from natural causes and were autopsied. The highest rates were in obese children; 38 percent had fatty liver. High fructose corn syrup has been linked to fatty liver disease in several studies, and there is some evidence that artificially sweetened soft drinks are worse instigators of fatty liver than even the drinks sweetened with high fructose corn syrup. The average American adult consumes 18.6 percent of calories from refined sugars; teens consume on average 20 percent. That's 34 teaspoons (544 calories) for boys and 24 teaspoons (384 calories) for girls. Most of this comes from soft drinks sweetened with high fructose corn syrup. Environmental toxins, junk food, and high-fat diets also contribute to fatty liver. A recent rat study asked the question, will pregnant moms who eat junk food predispose their children to obesity and fatty liver disease? The answer was yes. The alarming part was that much of this was irreversible, even when the baby rats were given a healthy diet to eat.

Healing Options

- **Diet and lifestyle:** Changes in diet and lifestyle are the current medical recommendations for people with fatty liver. Lose weight if you are overweight. Exercise if you aren't exercising. Eat a whole-foods diet, filled with fruits and vegetables. Avoid refined sugars and soft drinks. Stop drinking alcoholic beverages. Take an antioxidant supplement. Take milk thistle and lipoic acid supplements (see Healing Options under Hepatitis for dosages). Check your labs every four to six months. If your ALT and AST levels aren't responding, be more aggressive.

- **Try southern ginseng:** Gynostemma pentaphyllum is known as southern ginseng because it has similar therapeutic properties to ginseng and grows in southern China. A study that combined diet, exercise, and southern ginseng reported additional effects in weight loss, liver enzyme reduction, insulin levels, and HOMA levels. Take 500 mg three times daily.

- **Try keishibukuryogan:** There is a formula used in Japanese medicine called keishibukuryogan (KBG TJ-25). This was found to be of benefit when added to exercise, diet, and weight loss.

HEPATITIS

The eight types of hepatitis are A, B, C, D, E, autoimmune, alcoholic, and nonalcoholic steatohepatitis (NASH). Types A through E are caused by a blood-borne viral infection that causes inflammation in the liver. Autoimmune hepatitis, alcoholic hepatitis, and NASH are not caused by infection.

Hepatitis A

Hepatitis A can occur in isolated cases or spread among large groups of people. You can catch it from close personal contact with a person who has it or from food or water that has been contaminated. It is usually a self-limiting illness with flu-like symptoms. Once you've had hepatitis A, you cannot get it again. It may take several months to recover fully. A vaccine for people over the age of two is available for life-long protection against hepatitis A.

Hepatitis B

Hepatitis B is the most common serious liver infection in the world and is more serious than hepatitis A. It can lead to cirrhosis, liver cancer, or liver failure. In most people, it is a self-limiting illness. However, 90 percent of infected babies, 30 to 50 percent of infected children, and 5 to 10 percent of infected adults will also develop a chronic infection. A vaccine is available to help prevent hepatitis B infection. It is currently recommended by the CDC that all babies be vaccinated.

Each year 100,000 Americans contract hepatitis B and 5,000 to 6,000 Americans will die from it. It is estimated that 1.25 million Americans have chronic hepatitis B. Worldwide, it affects 400 million people and there are 1 million deaths per year. It is passed directly through blood. Since 1992, blood collected for transfusions is carefully screened for hepatitis B (and C). Prior to that time, infection through blood transfusion was common.

You can get hepatitis B from having unprotected sex with someone who has it, by sharing needles for drug use or tattooing, or by an accidental needle poke with an infected needle. During childbirth, a mother could pass it to her child.

Hepatitis C

Hepatitis C accounts for about 15 percent of acute viral hepatitis, 60 to 70 percent of chronic hepatitis, and up to 50 percent of cirrhosis, end-stage liver disease, and liver cancer. In the United States, four million people, or 18 percent of our population, have been diagnosed with antibodies to the disease. This indicates that they currently have an infection or previously were exposed to the virus. There are 10,000 to 12,000 deaths each year because of hepatitis C. Seventy-five percent of people with acute hepatitis C will ultimately develop chronic hepatitis. Millions more of us may be infected but have not been diagnosed.

Many people with hepatitis C are asymptomatic and may not know they have the disease. In those who do have symptoms, they are generally mild and include fatigue, liver discomfort or tenderness, nausea, muscle and joint pains, and a poor appetite.

The course of this disease varies radically. No symptoms might occur for up to 20 years and liver enzymes might not be elevated. If a liver biopsy is performed and the injury is mild, the outcome is usually good. On the other hand, if severe symptoms occur and liver enzymes are elevated, many people will ultimately develop cirrhosis and end-stage liver disease. Or the illness may be characterized by elevated liver enzymes with few symptoms, with an uncertain outcome. It is estimated that 20 percent of those with chronic hepatitis C will develop cirrhosis within 10 to 20 years. After that time, a small group will develop liver cancer. Hepatitis C is the most common reason for liver transplants.

Hepatitis C is passed via blood. The hepatitis C virus was only isolated in 1988, so many people were infected by blood transfusion prior to that time. Since 1992, blood has been routinely screened for hepatitis. You can get hepatitis C from having unprotected sex with someone who has it, by sharing needles for drug use or tattooing, or by an accidental needle poke with an infected needle. During childbirth, a mother could pass it to her child. In 10 percent of cases, the source of the infection is unknown.

Standard treatment for hepatitis C is interferon and antiviral medications. Their success rate is only 30 percent and the side effects can be severe. This is why so many people with chronic hepatitis are looking at alternative therapies. Patients on interferon therapy have found Saint-John's-wort and ginger help with side effects of treatment.

Hepatitis D
You can get hepatitis D only if you already have hepatitis B. It exists as a coinfection. You contract it the same way you contract hepatitis B and C.

Hepatitis E
Hepatitis E spreads by consuming contaminated drinking water and food. At this point in time, the only Americans who contract this form of hepatitis get it outside of the country, probably in a developing nation. For best prevention, drink bottled

water when traveling, and use only ice made with bottled water. Don't eat raw shell-fish, and avoid uncooked fruits and vegetables that are not peeled by you personally.

Autoimmune Hepatitis

Autoimmune hepatitis occurs when your body's immune system attacks your own liver cells, and it is probably due to a genetic defect. About 70 percent of people with this illness are women, and it's usually diagnosed between the ages of 15 and 40. It is a long-term illness and if left untreated can lead to cirrhosis and eventual liver failure. With treatment, about 70 percent of people with autoimmune hepatitis go into remission or experience a decrease in symptoms. It is usually treated with prednisone and azathioprine, both of which have unwanted side effects. About half of the people who are affected also have another autoimmune illness, such as Hashi-moto's thyroiditis, Grave's disease, Sjögren's syndrome, ulcerative colitis, or autoim-mune anemia. The most common symptoms are fatigue, enlarged liver, jaundice, itching, skin rashes, joint pain, lack of menstrual periods in women, and abdominal discomfort.

Alcoholic Hepatitis

Alcoholic hepatitis is a self-inflicted, progressive liver disease caused by the toxic-ity of alcohol. Unlike hepatitis A, B, C, and D, it is not an infectious disease. It is also known as alcoholic steatohepatitis, acute hepatic insufficiency of patients with chronic alcoholism, florid alcoholic cirrhosis, subacute alcoholic cirrhosis, and fatty liver with hepatic failure.

Alcoholic liver disease causes symptoms in more than two million people (1 percent of our population) but affects many more people who remain completely asymptomatic. It is the fourth leading cause of death in urban adult men ages 24 to 65. It is estimated that up to 35 percent of heavy drinkers have alcoholic hepatitis. This is often undetected until the disease has progressed. Women and nonwhite males are more susceptible to alcoholic liver damage with smaller amounts of alco-holic consumption. On average, it is estimated that men develop cirrhosis taking in about two ounces daily of ethanol, and women with less than one ounce daily. This is an illness that can kill you. Overall, the one-year survival rate after hospitalization for alcoholic hepatitis is about 40 percent.

Symptoms, when present, can include abdominal pain, fever, jaundice, and liver failure. It can progress to cirrhosis or liver cancer.

The long-term outcome depends on whether the person stops drinking alcohol and whether the illness has progressed to cirrhosis. If you have this and keep drink-ing alcohol, you will develop cirrhosis. If you stop drinking, it gradually resolves over a period of weeks to months. People may experience a worsening of liver function during the first weeks of abstinence. Because of alcohol excess, many people with alcoholic hepatitis are malnourished and deficient in antioxidant nutrients. They drink instead of eating. Use of Tylenol while drinking alcoholic beverages is well documented to accelerate liver disease. No one should drink booze and take Tylenol.

N-acetyl cysteine (NAC), catechin (from green tea), and milk thistle (silymarin) have been shown to be helpful in recovery.

Nonalcoholic Steatohepatitis (NASH)

NASH is another noninfectious type of hepatitis. It also is called pseudoalcoholic hepatitis, diabetic hepatitis, fatty-liver hepatitis, and alcohol-like hepatitis. It causes few problems in most people who have it but can lead to cirrhosis. Children especially may experience vague discomfort located at the liver. It often goes unrecognized but is common in those with elevated liver enzymes who have no other diagnosis. In a recent study of children with NASH, nearly all were very obese.

NASH was first discovered in 1980. Until recently, it was believed to be primarily a disease that affected obese, diabetic women. However, recent studies have shown that healthy, lean men, women, and children can all be affected. Inflammation of the liver, mitochondrial damage, and free radical pathology are apparent in this disease. Liver enzymes are elevated, and there is an increased need for antioxidant nutrients. Iron, on the other hand, is a pro-oxidant. It has been shown that high iron levels accelerate progression of NASH.

Ultimately, NASH is diagnosed with a liver biopsy. It is believed that a rich diet and lack of exercise can cause this illness. It can also be caused by drugs such as amiodarone, perhexiline maleate, glucocorticoids, synthetic estrogens, and tamoxifen. Surgeries, such as jejunal bypass, gastroplasty (stomach stapling), biliopancreatic diversion, or extensive small bowel resectioning can also trigger NASH. I even had one client who developed NASH from aggressive herbal treatment prescribed by a doctor. This resolved with clean food and some simple recommendations.

If you are overweight and are trying to lose weight, be sure to do so gradually. Quick weight loss can aggravate the disease.

Diagnosis and Treatment of Hepatitis

Many people with hepatitis have no obvious symptoms. But when they do, the most common ones are fatigue, mild fever, headache, muscle aches, tiredness, loss of appetite, nausea, vomiting, and diarrhea. As the illness progresses, sufferers become jaundiced, which is evident by the yellow color of the skin and whites of the eyes.

They may experience stomach pain and have dark-colored urine with pale-colored bowel movements.

Diagnosis of hepatitis is done with a routine blood test for liver enzymes. Further testing needs to be done to determine which type of hepatitis is present. A liver biopsy may be performed.

It is well documented that people with hepatitis have an increased need for antioxidants. While much more research could be done in this area, taking antioxidants offers a simple and effective way to help protect liver function. It is advisable to take several antioxidant nutrients either in combination or separately. Antioxidants include vitamins C and E, selenium, N-acetyl cysteine, S-adenosylmethionine (SAMe), lipoic acid, and flavonoids; many herbs have antioxidant properties as well. In foods, they are found in fruits and vegetables, preferably fresh and organically grown.

Bert Berkson, M.D., is one of the leading experts on lipoic acid. He reports that a combination of lipoic acid, selenium, and milk thistle rapidly dropped viral levels and brought three of his patients with hepatitis C back to normal health. Dosages were 300 mg of lipoic acid twice daily, 300 mg of milk thistle three times daily, and 200 mcg of selenomethionine once daily. He is currently doing a larger study using these three antioxidants. In a German study from 1976, 42 patients with hepatitis were given intravenous lipoic acid. The treatment showed promise for many of the patients and, because of the low toxicity and lack of side effects, was recommended for long-term treatment.

Rest, sleep, and healthful eating help with an easy recovery. It's also critically important not to drink any alcohol because alcohol is a direct liver toxin.

If you are planning on traveling outside of North America, check to see if you are going to a country with known hepatitis problems. You may want to get vaccinated against hepatitis A and B before you go.

There are a huge number of nutrients, antioxidants, herbs, flavonoids, and phytonutrients that may be beneficial in helping reduce symptoms and the long-term effects of hepatitis and cirrhosis. I found information on hepatitis and B-complex vitamins, phyllanthus, shiitake mushrooms, astragalus, fenugreek, schizandra, andrographis, phosphatidylcholine, thymus extract, chlorophyll, and many more natural compounds. If you don't find something here that really helps, keep looking. I could have spent weeks researching this one topic.

Functional Laboratory Testing

Routine medical testing is adequate for diagnosis of hepatitis. People who are infected may also want additional information. Tests to consider include the following:

- Vitamin and mineral status
- Antioxidant status
- Glutathione levels
- Small intestinal bacterial overgrowth testing

Healing Options

Hepatitis is a serious illness. For best results, these healing options are meant to be used in combination. You don't need to use them all, but pick several at least.

- **Avoid alcoholic beverages.** Alcohol is damaging to the liver. Don't drink if you have any type of hepatitis.
- **Eat lots of fruits and vegetables.** They contain antioxidant nutrients, vitamins, and minerals that help support your immune system. Eat at least five servings daily, preferably a lot more. Fresh juicing of organic vegetables is a great way to quickly multiply your nutrients and antioxidants.
- **Take a multivitamin with minerals.** Cover your bases. A good multivitamin will have base amounts of antioxidants, vitamins, and minerals. Look for one with at least 400 IU of vitamin E, 200 mcg of selenium, and 250 mg or more of vitamin C.
- **Take vitamin C.** Studies have shown vitamin C levels to be very low in people with hepatitis. Vitamin C is well known for its antiviral and antioxidant effects. Much research was also done in the 1970s and early 1980s on vitamin C's ability to naturally stimulate interferon production. Interferon is the drug treatment of choice for people with chronic hepatitis (hepatitis C). Interferon is isolated at great expense, it is only 30 percent effective, and the side effects make many people decide not to even try it. Linus Pauling theorized that vitamin C could be used to increase natural production of interferon. Other researchers also reported that this was so.

    Robert Cathcart, M.D., a long-standing advocate of complementary medicine, uses high doses of intravenous vitamin C for hepatitis. He found that with doses of 40 to 100 grams, he was able to greatly improve symptoms in two to four days and clear jaundice within six days. Other people have found similar effects. As little as 2 grams was able to prevent hepatitis B in hospitalized patients. However, there is little published research specifically on vitamin C and hepatitis.

    At a minimum, I recommend taking 2,000 mg of vitamin C daily. Preferably, use dosages up to bowel tolerance and recalibrate your dosage every week. Determine your personalized dosage with a vitamin C flush. (See Chapter 18.)

- **Try milk thistle or Silybum marianum (silymarin).** Milk thistle has been used for liver protection for centuries and has few side effects. There is an ongoing human study sponsored by the National Center for Complementary and Alternative Medicine (NCCAM) at the NIH. They hope the research will show whether silymarin reduces symptoms in people with hepatitis C and/or cirrhosis, whether it prevents the progression of liver disease in people with hepatitis C but who have normal liver enzyme levels, whether it helps clear up the infections, and finally whether it improves people's quality of life. Another study at the NIH is looking at optimal dosages of silymarin. Silymarin has already been shown to be useful in people with cirrhosis caused by alcohol abuse. Look for a product that has been standardized for silymarin content. A company that has done that will clearly label it on the bottle. Take 420 mg daily.
- **Take zinc.** People with hepatitis are commonly zinc deficient. Zinc helps with healing of tissues and is important for prevention of scarring. Take 50 to 75 mg daily.
- **Try whey protein or transfer factor.** There are numerous studies on the use of transfer factor in people with hepatitis. They have been very positive. Transfer factor is isolated from cow colostrum and is loaded with protective antibodies that help us fight infection. A current study also demonstrates that a whey protein product called Immunocal was effective in patients with hepatitis B, but not hepatitis C. Take 12 to 30 grams of whey protein daily and 300 mg transfer factor, once or twice daily.
- **Try N-acetyl cysteine (NAC).** Several research studies have found that glutathione levels are inversely related to the viral loads for hepatitis B and C. German researchers found that when NAC was added to hepatitis cultures, viral load decreased 50-fold. Take 1,000 to 2,000 mcg twice daily.
- **Try lipoic acid.** Lipoic acid, also called thiotic acid, is a strong antioxidant and has been shown to be liver protective in mushroom and chemical poisoning. In studies with chemically induced hepatitis, lipoic acid has been shown to be effective in treatment. Take 200 to 300 mg twice daily.
- **Try S-adenosylmethionine (SAMe).** In one study, 220 patients with liver disease were given 1,600 mg of SAMe daily. Twenty-six percent of the participants had hepatitis. The study found the use of SAMe resulted in a reduction of symptoms of itching and fatigue and an improved sense of well-being. Laboratory testing confirmed these benefits with improvement of conjugated bilirubin and alkaline phosphatase, two laboratory markers that are elevated in people with hepatitis.

- **Take vitamin E.** People with hepatitis have lower levels of vitamin E. A 2001 pilot study published in *Antiviral Research* investigated people with hepatitis B. Thirty-two patients were given either 300 IU of vitamin E twice daily for three months or no treatment. They were followed for one year. In the vitamin E group, 47 percent (seven patients) had normalized ALT, a liver enzyme. Only one of the controls normalized ALT. Hepatitis B DNA was normalized in 53 percent of the vitamin E group and in only 18 percent of the control group. A normalization of both ALT and DNA was seen in 47 percent of the vitamin E group and none of the control group.

  In another study, people with hepatitis B were given 600 IU of vitamin E daily for nine months. All symptoms of hepatitis disappeared in 5 of the 12 people tested.

  In yet another study, looking this time at people with hepatitis C, there was some additional improvement when people were given 544 IU of vitamin E with interferon therapy. And in a different study, in which people with hepatitis C were given 400 IU of vitamin E twice daily for 12 weeks, there was improvement in 11 out of 23 patients (48 percent). ALT levels were decreased by 45 percent, and AST, a liver enzyme, decreased 37 percent after a six-month follow-up. Vitamin E is nontoxic and worth trying in all types of hepatitis. Take 600 to 1,000 IU of vitamin E daily. Look for d-alphatocopherol and mixed tocopherols, rather than dl-alphatocopherol.

- **Try Picrorhiza kurroa.** Picrorhiza, an herb commonly used in Ayurvedic medicine, has been less well studied than milk thistle, but studies indicate that it is equally effective with nearly identical effects. It has anti-inflammatory and liver-protective properties. Indian researchers also used Picrorhiza in acute hepatitis A and showed it to be helpful in a speedy recovery. Take 400 to 1,500 mg in capsules.

- **Try licorice.** Licorice has been shown to reduce elevated liver enzymes in people with hepatitis. It appears to be the glycyrrhizin that tempers NF-kappaB and inflammatory cytokines. It also naturally raises the body's interferon levels. In Japan, it is often used intravenously for hepatitis B and C. Glycyrrhizin can elevate blood pressure levels, so use with caution.

- **Try sho-saiko-to.** Sho-saiko-to is a Chinese remedy that contains bupleurum and other traditional Chinese herbs. Several trials were done in people with hepatitis B infection and one small trial in people with hepatitis C. Sho-saiko-to helps reduce symptoms and normalize blood liver enzymes in people with active viral hepatitis. It has also been found to help reduce the incidence of liver cancer in people with hepatitis. Take 2.5 grams three times daily. *It should not be used in combination with interferon therapy.*

- **Drink or take green tea.** Catechins are a type of flavonoids found in green tea. Study results have been mixed, but favorable results have been seen in dosages of 500 to 750 mg three times daily. A recent Chinese study on ducklings showed significant reduction in liver damage and protected liver function. In two recent studies, catechin was found to reduce liver damage and hepatitis that was chemically induced by halothane, an anesthetic drug used in surgery. Halothane is known to induce hepatitis in people. Regarding dosage, I recommend that you drink green tea as often as you like.

- **Drink Rooibos tea (Aspalathus linearis).** Rooibos tea is also called red tea. It is a relatively new food product and offers a delicious caffeine-free alternative to people who drink tea. Research was done in rats, but I was delighted to see that, at least in this initial report, it showed a regression of liver damage and cirrhosis and a lowering of liver enzymes (ALT and AST). The researchers consider it to be a useful plant for patients with liver disease. Other studies show it to have antioxidant effects. It appears to have the same properties as green tea. I recommend that you drink it as often as you like.

- **Try quercetin with amla.** Another flavonoid with antioxidant effects is quercetin. Although studies need to be done in people, animal research shows that treatment with quercetin dehydrate reduced oxidative damage from hepatitis twofold. Another mouse study found liver-protective effects of quercetin when combined with amla. Bougainvillea spectabilis has been used in Chinese folk medicine for treatment of hepatitis. The active component of Bougainvillea is quercetin. Take 1,000 to 3,000 mg of quercetin daily, plus 900 to 2,700 mg of amla daily.

CIRRHOSIS

Cirrhosis is a disease of the liver. Scar tissue replaces normal tissue and blocks the flow of blood and nutrients. It kills about 26,000 Americans each year and is the 12th leading cause of death. The most common causes of cirrhosis are alcoholism and hepatitis. Some people have diseases that may lead to cirrhosis, such as alpha-1 antitrypsin deficiency, hemochromatosis, Wilson's disease, galactosemia, and glycogen storage diseases. Nonalcoholic steatohepatitis (NASH) can also lead to cirrhosis. NASH is a condition where fat accumulates in the liver and eventually causes scarring. It is usually associated with diabetes, protein malnutrition, obesity, heart disease, and treatment with steroid medications. Blocked bile ducts can also cause cirrhosis, called *biliary cirrhosis*. Because the liver is our body's main filtering system for drugs and toxins, bad reactions to them may also lead to cirrhosis. Overdosing with vitamin A supplements is another cause of cirrhosis. Vitamin A toxicity in the liver is accentuated in an alcoholic.

About one-third of people with cirrhosis have no symptoms during the initial stages of the disease. Loss of liver function may be picked up on routine blood testing. As the scarring progresses, liver function begins to fail. People with cirrhosis may experience some of the following symptoms: exhaustion and fatigue, loss of appetite, nausea, light-colored stools, weakness, weight loss, abdominal pain, or spiderlike blood vessels that break out on the skin. Cirrhosis may also lead to water retention, bruising and bleeding, jaundice, itching, gallstones, increased sensitivity to medication and environmental contaminants, increased insulin resistance, diabetes, liver cancer, osteoporosis, impotence, and infection in other organs.

The scarring caused by cirrhosis cannot be reversed. But treatment can help stop or slow the disease progression. The liver is remarkably able to recuperate when we eliminate the factors that hurt it. Many find that with a nutritious diet, rest, and supplements, they can begin to feel healthy again. It is critical that you stop drinking all alcoholic beverages if you are diagnosed with cirrhosis. Alcohol is a direct liver poison. It is known to cause cirrhosis, liver cancer, and liver failure and generates a large need for antioxidant nutrients, such as vitamin E, selenium, vitamin C, and N-acetyl cysteine. Alcoholics are notoriously deficient in B-complex vitamins.

If possible, stop using hazardous chemicals. If you do need to use them, protect your skin, be in a well-ventilated area, and wear a breathing apparatus. If your work involves use of paint, solvents, cleaning products, or other chemicals, it's probably time to look for a different job. Use greener cleaning supplies, shampoos, and other toiletries.

Research indicates that many people with cirrhosis have increased intestinal permeability, which can lead to infection and problems elsewhere in the body. Nutrients such as glutamine, quercetin, and probiotics can help heal a leaky gut.

Methionine, an amino acid, from our food is metabolized in the liver into S-adenosylmethionine (SAMe). People with cirrhosis have problems metabolizing methionine. SAMe increases glutathione levels, an important antioxidant for detoxification. SAMe is an important methyl donor and is used as a supplement for people with elevated homocysteine levels, heart disease, joint diseases, and depression.

Functional Laboratory Testing
- Functional liver testing
- Intestinal permeability testing
- Vitamin and mineral analysis

Healing Options

- **Avoid alcoholic beverages.** Alcohol is damaging to the liver. Don't drink at all if you have hepatitis or cirrhosis. If you are an alcoholic, you might find Alcoholics Anonymous or a residential program to be of benefit. Support helps ease the way.

- **Eat lots of fruits and vegetables.** They contain antioxidant nutrients, vitamins, and minerals that help support your immune system. Eat at least five servings daily, preferably a lot more. Fresh juicing of organic vegetables is a great way to quickly multiply your nutrients and antioxidants.

- **Take a multivitamin with minerals.** Cover your bases. A good multivitamin will have base amounts of antioxidants, vitamins, and minerals. Look for one with at least 400 IU of vitamin E, 200 mcg of selenium, at least 250 mg of vitamin C, and at least 15 mg of zinc.

- **Take an antioxidant supplement.** In addition to a good multivitamin with minerals, it would be wise to take additional antioxidants. These can be found in a combination supplement and may include mixed carotenoids, selenium, vitamin E, vitamin C, N-acetyl cysteine, lipoic acid, and more. Or you could use what are known as powdered greens or reds. These products typically contain dehydrated green vegetables and grasses or red and orange fruits and vegetables. It's a quick way to get a ton of antioxidants and vegetables in one swoop.

- **Try lipoic acid.** Lipoic acid is a strong antioxidant and has been shown to be liver protective in mushroom and chemical poisoning. In studies with chemically induced hepatitis, lipoic acid has been shown to be effective in treatment. Take 200 to 300 mg twice daily.

- **Try S-adenosylmethionine (SAMe).** In one study, 220 patients with liver disease were given 1,600 mg of SAMe daily. Sixty-eight percent had cirrhosis, 6 percent had biliary cirrhosis, and 26 percent had hepatitis. A reduction of symptoms of itching and fatigue were noted along with an improved sense of well-being.

- **Try sho-saiko-to.** Sho-saiko-to, also called TJ-9, is a Chinese remedy that contains bupleurum and six other herbs. It is being extensively used in Japan for people with hepatitis and cirrhosis and to prevent the development of liver cancer. Take 2.5 grams three times daily. *It should not be used in combination with interferon therapy.*

- **Try milk thistle or Silybum marianum (silymarin).** Milk thistle has long been used for all liver disease. It appears to retard progression of cirrhosis primarily through its antioxidant effects. Animal research has been consistent in its results; human research has been less so. Still, there is little or no risk and the possibility of great benefit. Take 420 mg daily. Look for a product that has been standardized for silymarin content. A company that has done that will clearly label it on the bottle.

- **Take zinc.** People with cirrhosis often have a zinc deficiency. Get your red blood cell zinc level checked. If it's low, take 50 to 75 mg of zinc daily.
- **Drink Rooibos tea (Aspalathus linearis).** Rooibos tea is also called red tea and is a relatively new food product. It offers a delicious caffeine-free alternative for tea drinkers. Research was done in rats, but I was delighted to see that, at least in this initial report, it showed a regression of liver damage and cirrhosis and a lowering of liver enzymes (ALT and AST). The researchers consider it to be a useful plant for patients with liver disease. It contains small amounts of vitamin C, iron, magnesium, phosphorus, sodium, chloride, and potassium. Other studies show it to have antioxidant effects. For dosage, I recommend that you drink as much as you like.
- **Drink green tea.** There isn't much research here, only one rat study. But at least in rats green tea extract protected against liver damage when they were exposed to carbon tetrachloride, a known liver toxin. Green tea catechins are known to be protective and provide antioxidants. Drink green tea or take green tea extract.

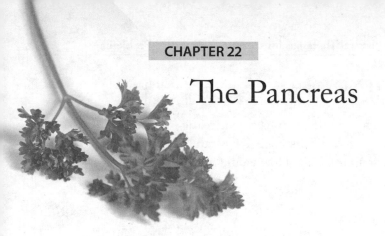

CHAPTER 22

The Pancreas

The pancreas has two main functions in the body. The first is digestive (exocrine function): to produce digestive enzymes to break down fat, carbohydrate, and protein; and bicarbonate to neutralize stomach acid once the food moves from the stomach to the duodenum. The second function of the pancreas (endocrine function) is production of insulin and glucagon to regulate blood sugar levels. Insulin tells your body to store glucose as glycogen; glucagon tells your body to raise blood glucose levels, turning glycogen back into glucose.

The main health problems with the pancreas are insufficiency of enzymes, acute or chronic pancreatitis, pancreatic cancer, diabetes, and cystic fibrosis. In type 1 diabetes, the pancreas is no longer able to produce insulin. Many people with type 2 diabetes have insulin resistance, which can overwhelm the pancreas so that it stops producing enough insulin. Some of the medications used in type 2 diabetes can also affect the beta cells so that they stop producing insulin.

If you have pancreatitis, you will have elevated serum lipase and amylase levels. To assess pancreatic insufficiency, stool testing for pancreatic elastase or chymotrypsin is used. You will often see levels of pancreatic elastase that are less than 400 mcg/g, which indicates pancreatic insufficiency. If pancreatic elastase levels are less than 200, pancreatic insufficiency may be a lifelong issue. For chymotrypsin, the lowest normal value is 100 or 72 mcg, depending on the study. Low chymotrypsin levels were found in people with celiac disease, psoriasis, and gastric surgery. Pancreatic elastase is not affected when you take digestive enzymes; chymotrypsin is.

PANCREATIC INSUFFICIENCY

If your pancreas cannot secrete enough enzymes, you have pancreatic insufficiency. While in conventional medical terms pancreatic insufficiency is rare, for those of us working in integrative health we see it all the time. How would you know?

- Abdominal discomfort
- Bleeding tendency (vitamin K deficiency)
- Bloating
- Can't gain weight
- Failure to thrive in children
- Fatigue for no obvious reason
- Food sensitivities
- Gas
- Hypoglycemia
- Malabsorption
- Steatorrhea—pale, tan colored stools
- Stools that float (fat maldigestion)
- Undigested food in your stools

Pancreatic insufficiency is common in people who have celiac disease, psoriasis, cirrhoses, pancreatitis, and cystic fibrosis. Other triggers are parasites, bacterial overgrowth, dermatitis herpetiformis, inflammatory bowel disease, Zollinger-Ellison syndrome, and AIDS. Stress (mental and physical), getting older, nutritional deficiencies, poor diet, eating only cooked foods, exposure to radiation or toxins, hereditary weaknesses, drugs, and infections also contribute to pancreatic insufficiency.

Functional Laboratory Testing
- Stool pancreatic elastase test
- Stool chymotrypsin test
- Food allergies—IgE test; food sensitivities—IgG or IgG4 test

Healing Options
- **Improve your eating habits.** Eat in a relaxed manner. Chew your food thoroughly. Limit beverage intake with meals. Drinking liquids at meals dilutes the gastric juices in the stomach and pancreatic juice in the small intestines.
- **Take pancreatic enzyme supplements.** Clinical experience shows that pancreatic enzymes work well as a digestive aid. Glandular-based supplements, like

pancreatic enzyme preparations, are directed to specific tissues, helping to initiate repair. Pancreatic enzymes also help restore the balance of GI flora. In studies done on monkeys, it was shown that pancreatic enzymes were able to kill clostridium, bacteroides, pseudomonaceae, enterobacter, E. coli, and klebsiella. Continued use of pancreatic enzymes can help with repair and maintenance of pancreatic tissue.

The United States Pharmacopoeia (USP) regulates the strength of pancreatic enzymes. Take one to two tablets or capsules at the beginning of meals.

- **Try vegetable enzymes.** For people who would rather have a vegetarian alternative to pancreatic enzymes, vegetable enzymes are a suitable option. These enzymes are derived from a fungus called Aspergillus oryzae. Take one to two capsules at the beginning of meals.

PANCREATITIS

Pancreatitis is an inflammation of the pancreas. There are two types of pancreatitis, acute and chronic. Acute pancreatitis is typically caused by gallbladder disease or alcohol abuse. The typical symptoms are abdominal pain, nausea, vomiting, and loss of appetite. Serum amylase and lipase levels are elevated. In acute pancreatitis, it's important to keep electrolytes in balance. People are hospitalized and given IV solutions or medical foods until the inflammation has calmed down.

Chronic pancreatitis is an ongoing inflammation of the pancreas. In 70 percent of people it's alcohol induced. Seven percent of people with pancreatitis have genetic alterations in either the cystic fibrosis gene (CFTR), the serine protease inhibitor gene (SPINK 1/PSTI), or the cationic trypsinogen gene (PRSSI). If it's inherited, it often begins in childhood or adolescence with acute pancreatitis, which eventually becomes chronic. Other causes include tropical pancreatitis (due to unknown nutritional issues), hyperparathyroidism with high calcium levels, extremely high levels of triglycerides, and obstruction of the pancreatic duct.

The main symptom of chronic pancreatitis is a dull pain around the stomach with pain that radiates to the middle of your back. The pain is intermittent and gets worse if you eat. People with pancreatitis gradually lose weight. If the pancreas isn't producing enough lipase, stools will get lighter, float, and have a bad odor. You may need to urinate often and have symptoms of vitamin A, D, E, and K deficiencies. Sometimes people get jaundiced.

It's important to consider the entire DIGIN model in people who have chronic pancreatitis.

Healing Options

- **Stop drinking alcohol.** Easier said than done, but essential. If necessary, join Alcoholics Anonymous or enter treatment.
- **Use a restorative healing diet.** See Chapter 13 for details.
- **Use medical foods.** In some cases, eating predigested foods can provide calories and needed nutrients.
- **Take pancreatic enzymes.** There are many prescription and over-the-counter pancreas enzymes. According to Maurice E. Shils, et al., in *Modern Nutrition in Health and Disease, 10th Edition*, from 4,500 to 20,000 USP will be needed with a minimum of 28,000 IU of lipase. Take one tablet with the first bite of your meal and continue sprinkling your tablets throughout the meal.
- **Take vitamins.** You are likely to be deficient in many nutrients, especially vitamin B_{12} and the fat-soluble vitamins A, D, E, and K. Take an excellent multiple vitamin and have your vitamin and mineral levels assessed.
- **Increase antioxidants to reduce inflammation.** Eat more fruits and vegetables. Make fresh vegetable and green juices. Use wheat grass juice. Use powdered greens or powdered reds, which typically contain dehydrated green vegetables and grasses or red and orange fruits and vegetables, to add antioxidants. Take antioxidant supplements.
- **Alkalize, alkalize, alkalize.** Follow the recommendations in Chapter 17.
- **Try Chinese medicine and acupuncture.** Several studies looked at the combined effect of Chinese herbs with Western treatment for pancreatitis. Patients who received traditional Chinese medicines had better outcomes. Miltiorrhiza, known as red sage, Chinese sage, tan shen, or dan shen, was given to rats and people with pancreatitis with protective effects. There are lots of other studies coming out of China on pancreatitis and herbs. I recommend finding a doctor of oriental medicine to help you with this.

CYSTIC FIBROSIS

Cystic fibrosis is covered well in *Digestive Wellness for Children*.

DIABETES

Diabetes is a worldwide epidemic that's increasing fast. In 1985 30 million people worldwide had diabetes. Today, one billion people have diabetes and a third of the children born each day are expected to have diabetes later in life. In the United

States, 23.6 million people, 7.8 percent of the population, have diabetes. Diabetes rates are highest in Native American populations, where the incidence of childhood diabetes can be up to 45 percent in some communities. Overall, the incidence of diabetes in Native American populations is 17 percent. Blacks, Hispanics, and Asians are also more likely to develop diabetes than whites. Most people with diabetes have never been diagnosed. If you've never had your blood sugar levels looked at, do so.

Diabetes Basics

You may recall that glucose is the main energy source for most of our cells; when blood glucose levels rise, the pancreas normally secretes the hormone insulin, which acts as a transporter, allowing glucose and amino acids to leave the bloodstream and be taken into the cells for use. This process, however, can go awry. Diabetes occurs when the body:

- Doesn't produce insulin
- Or makes insufficient amounts of insulin
- Or is resistant to insulin

Diabetes is a common chronic illness that runs in families, so children with parents or grandparents who have diabetes are more likely to develop diabetes than other children are.

Symptoms of Diabetes

- Blurred vision
- Darkened and velvety areas of skin, most typically in the armpits and neck folds
- Fatigue
- Frequent infections
- Frequent urination
- Increased appetite
- Increased thirst
- Irritability (in children mainly)
- Skin tags
- Slow healing of sores
- Weight loss

Monitoring Diabetes

If you have diabetes, a hemoglobin A1c (HmgA1c; also called glycosylated hemoglobin) test is a simple way to monitor your blood sugar levels. It gives a three-month average of the sugar levels on the outside of red blood cells. Imagine a gum drop.

Recall that it has sugar crystals on the outside of it. Imagine that your red blood cells look like gum drops. The more sugar crystals they have on the outside, the more damaging those crystals are inside a person's blood vessels, heart, eyes, and kidneys and the greater risk of long-term health issues relating to the diabetes. Healthy levels of HmgA1c are less than 7 percent of total hemoglobin. Keeping levels as low as possible helps prevent damage throughout the body.

Uncontrolled diabetes of either type can lead to serious complications later in life. High blood glucose level is the most significant risk factor for developing heart and vascular disease, and diabetes is the leading cause of kidney failure and adult blindness. Careful blood sugar control is essential for preventing these and other complications, including nerve problems and gum disease.

Type 1 Diabetes

Type 1 diabetes is considered to be an autoimmune disorder. It is typically diagnosed in children and young adults. Five to 10 percent of people with diabetes have type 1 diabetes. Type 1 diabetes, which used to be called juvenile diabetes, is more specifically termed insulin-dependent diabetes mellitus (IDDM). Diagnosed in about 13,000 children in the United States each year, its onset is usually sudden and can occur at any time during childhood. People with type 1 diabetes require injections to replace the insulin that their bodies can no longer make. Children with type 1 diabetes are usually thin, and they may complain of thirst. Type 1 diabetes is often triggered by an infection, typically a virus. The body's immune system mounts an attack on the infection and also mistakenly attacks and destroys the insulin-secreting beta cells in the pancreas. Allergy to milk has also been implicated as a possible trigger for diabetes.

New Ideas About Underlying Causes of Type 1 Diabetes. Accumulating research findings suggest that the gut immune system plays an important role in type 1 diabetes. Like all autoimmune diseases, there is a growing consensus in research indicating that people with type 1 diabetes have increased intestinal permeability (leaky gut) and dairy allergy, gluten intolerance, or celiac disease. Alessio Fasano, M.D., medical director at the Center for Celiac Research at University of Maryland School of Medicine, and his research group believe that intestinal permeability is a necessary ingredient for the development of autoimmune conditions, along with genetic and environmental factors. Outi Vaarala and her group report that a disordered gut microbiota contributes to the development of type 1 diabetes. High levels of zonulin have been found in people with type 1 diabetes. Zonulin is a protein that contributes to leaky gut by opening up the tight junctions between cells. Zonulin levels can increase on exposure to specific foods and bacteria. Animal study shows that if zonulin is blocked, destruction of the pancreatic beta cells can be prevented.

There is a small but important crossover in people with type 1 diabetes and celiac disease. A study of 141 children with type 1 diabetes, for example, found elevated antigliaden antibodies in more than 8 percent and found celiac disease in almost 3 percent, which is 10 times the average incidence. Pyira Narula reported a 3.3 percent incidence of celiac disease in children with type 1 diabetes. Another study of 331 children with type 1 diabetes from 1987 through 2004 reported 6.6 percent of the children had celiac disease as well (determined by elevated tTg levels and confirmed with biopsy). Interestingly, the incidence of celiac in these children rose from 3.3 percent in 1994 to 10.6 percent in 2004. One has to ask the question, what specifically has changed in this decade? Two things pop into my mind: increased vaccination requirements and the introduction of large amounts of genetically engineered corn, soy, cottonseed, and canola oil to our food supply.

A considerable amount of research has shown a link between infant allergy to cow's milk and development of type 1 diabetes. In a similar vein, an epidemiological study in 40 countries found that the incidence of type 1 diabetes in children was highest in the countries with the highest consumption of dairy and other animal foods. In children who develop both celiac disease and type 1 diabetes, celiac disease often precedes or develops at the same time as the diabetes. (See sections on autoimmune disease and celiac disease in Chapter 14 for a more complete analysis of the gut-autoimmune connection.)

Children eating a mainly vegetarian diet had a lowered incidence of type 2 diabetes. This needs to be explored more fully to determine what components of a vegetarian diet helped to protect these children. What can be supposed is that vegetarian diets have a higher level of polyphenols and fiber which both have protective properties.

Food Sensitivity and Diabetes. Looking for food sensitivities and allergies may help stabilize the blood sugar levels and reduce the need for medications in people with type 1 diabetes. A recent study done by Russell M. Jaffe, M.D., Ph.D., and colleagues looked at the role of diet and food intolerance in 26 adults with type 1 diabetes. The control group ate their regular diabetic diet and followed their usual lifestyle program. The test group ate a dairy-free diet, removed any additional foods that showed antibody reactions, and were given specific nutritional supplements. After six months, the test group showed significantly greater improvement in blood glucose levels and hemoglobin A1c than the control group. Clinical nutritionist Jayashree Mani reports that by working with an allergen-free and alkalizing diet, she was able to lower blood glucose levels in a type 1 diabetic teenage boy from 350 to 125 mmol/l, while also reducing his insulin needs by more than a third.

Type 2 Diabetes

Type 2 diabetes, which used to be called adult diabetes, is more specifically termed non-insulin-dependent diabetes mellitus (NIDDM). Type 2 diabetes occurs mainly in adults older than 45 and constitutes 90 to 95 percent of all diabetes cases. Type 2 diabetes was virtually unknown in children 30 years ago, but it is on the rise. In some Native American communities, it occurs in 45 percent of children. In children, it is first diagnosed between the ages of 10 and 19 years, and the hormonal changes around puberty seem to be an important trigger. Between 45 percent and 80 percent of children with type 2 diabetes have a parent with diabetes. Children with type 2 diabetes are commonly overweight but typically have no other symptoms until they are diagnosed.

Type 2 Diabetes Is Largely Preventable. Type 2 diabetes at first appears to be a disorder of overly elevated blood glucose (blood sugar) levels. Yet for most people with type 2 diabetes, disordered glucose levels are just the end of a long road that led to diabetes in the first place. Type 2 diabetes is often the result of lifestyle choices. In other words, we "earn" it. It's often termed "a feast in the middle of a famine" because your blood has excessive amounts of glucose (the feast) while your cells starve for the sugar they desperately need to produce energy. If left unchecked, high insulin levels affect our kidneys, eyes, and heart and are linked to fatty liver, nerve damage, brain compromise, gastroparesis or dumping syndrome, maldigestion and malabsorption, sexual dysfunction, and problems with the genitourinary system, such as polycystic ovary disease.

Eating a low-nutrient, highly refined diet; eating a diet low in antioxidants and polyphenols and fiber; obesity; lack of exercise; and lack of sleep all help us build to a point where our metabolism begins showing signs of metabolic syndrome: weight gain around the middle (apple shape or beer belly), low serum HDL cholesterol levels with high LDL cholesterol levels, high insulin levels, rising blood pressure, and/or rising triglycerides. In metabolic syndrome, also called Syndrome X, we don't have the right cellular conditions to properly use glucose. Our pancreas responds by making more insulin to get the glucose into the cells. This is called insulin resistance, which leads to more weight gain and even more insulin resistance in a vicious circle. Eventually we cannot overcome this by just producing more insulin, and our blood sugar levels skyrocket. This condition is diabetes. Often we have decades of warning signs before we are diagnosed with diabetes. We can stop metabolic syndrome by changing our lives, and in most cases we can prevent diabetes.

Eating a low-glycemic diet, getting plenty of exercise, and having the right nutrients can turn type 2 diabetes and metabolic syndrome around.

Gestational Diabetes

A third type of diabetes is called gestational diabetes. It occurs only during pregnancy and typically resolves once the baby is born. This affects about 4 percent of all pregnant women. It's important that these women be closely monitored during pregnancy for the safety of the mom and baby. Babies born of women who developed gestational diabetes are more likely to develop type 2 diabetes later in life.

Other Types of Diabetes

There are three other types of diabetes that have been more recently codified.

- Latent autoimmune diabetes of the adult (LADA) happens in people who are not obese but have antibodies to insulin. They typically have signs of metabolic syndrome, so if monitored they can prevent diabetes decades earlier.
- People with type 1.5 diabetes have anti-insulin antibodies and are typically obese and insulin resistant.
- Type 3 diabetes occurs when people have insulin resistance in the brain. Insulin is probably the most inflammatory molecule in our bodies. When insulin levels increase in the brain, we have accelerated oxidative stress, nerve damage, cell damage, and early death. This can cause memory loss as well. There is a growing body of research that calls Alzheimer's disease "insulin resistance in the brain."

Functional Laboratory Testing

- Certainly do all of the regular medical testing for diabetes, including fasting glucose and hemoglobin A1c levels.
- Blood sugar levels: Buy a glucose monitor and monitor your blood sugars daily or more often.
- One- and two-hour postprandial insulin testing: This is done one or two hours after a high-carbohydrate meal or with a glucose drink.
- Anti-insulin antibodies test.
- Salivary cortisol: Cortisol levels are often high in diabetes.

- Vitamin and mineral assessments, especially B-complex vitamins, RBC zinc, magnesium, and antioxidant status.
- First morning urine pH testing.
- Food sensitivity testing.
- Celiac testing.

Healing Options for All Types of Diabetes

If you are taking medication for your diabetes, it is critical to use it *consistently and exactly as prescribed*. If you need an insulin pump, you'll need specific instructions on its use from your physician or diabetes educator.

Historically, people worldwide have used various natural remedies to control blood sugar levels: glucomannan fiber, young barley shoots, prickly pear cactus juice, fenugreek—the list is long. As we integrate this sort of information, many more options may become available. You can find many of the herbs and nutrients in the following list in products that combine them to help with glucose regulation.

- **Buy a glucose monitor.** Monitoring your glucose levels is essential. Keeping your glucose levels normalized and having a hemoglobin A1c level below 7 will help to prevent much of the damage caused by high insulin levels.
- **If you are overweight, normalize your weight.** Obesity puts an enormous burden on the body. Losing weight can go a long way toward normalizing insulin and glucose levels.
- **Exercise regularly.** Regular exercise helps to lower blood glucose levels, reduce medication needs, and balance mood and behavior. It is essential that you find some type of exercise you enjoy and can do nearly daily. In type 2, exercise can often make oral medications unneeded.
- **Get psychological support.** Seek support to help manage the times when you just can't cope. Managing a chronic disease can be difficult. Having a sick family member puts a strain on everyone in the family; you all may need individual and/or family counseling from time to time.
- **Decrease inflammation.** Eat a diet rich in fruits, vegetables, legumes, nuts, and seeds. These contain anti-inflammatory antioxidants and polyphenols. Monitor first morning pH to ensure that you are getting as much as your body needs. You cannot put out a forest fire with a bucket.
- **Find the diet that works best for you.** Most people with diabetes will find that a low-glycemic diet works best. Vegetarian diets, which are richer in fiber, antioxidants, and minerals than meat-based diets are, can help reduce the incidence of type 2 in children and adults. Yet Loren Cordain, Ph.D., professor at Colorado State University and researcher and author on Paleolithic diets, and James

Anderson, M.D., from the University of Kentucky, have both demonstrated extraordinary benefits from diets that are high in fiber, high in legumes, and rich in complex carbohydrates. If you monitor your glucose levels carefully, you will discover the best type of diet for you.

- **Implement a high-fiber diet.** Use fiber to regulate blood glucose levels. Research shows that eating a high-fiber diet slows the release of glucose into the bloodstream over time. Peas and beans, fruits, vegetables, and whole grains, and especially high-fiber cereals containing 9 or more grams of fiber per serving, can be extremely useful.

- **Add insulin- and glucose-modulating foods to your diet.** Cinnamon, oat bran, fibers, ginger, rosemary, green tea, cranberries, blueberries, lemon balm, fenugreek, holy basil, and bitter melon are all beneficial. So add some cinnamon to that oat bran!

- **Discover your food sensitivities.** Figure out if you have celiac disease, gluten intolerance, or other food sensitivities. I have seen people whose glucose levels spiked with a single bite of carrot or papaya. Monitoring your glucose levels carefully can help you figure this out. Arthur F. Coca also developed the pulse test. Often your resting pulse will rise more than 16 beats per minute 30 minutes after a meal in response to a food that bothers you.

- **Take a multivitamin and mineral supplement.** Take these supplements to counteract inadequacies in basic nutrients.

- **Take an antioxidant supplement.** Use antioxidants to reduce inflammation and help prevent damage throughout the body. An antioxidant supplement will most probably contain carotenoids, vitamin E, selenium, and glutathione or n-acetyl cysteine, and may also contain lipoic acid and additional nutrients. Find a good antioxidant supplement and use as directed. In addition, take lipoic acid, 100 to 600 mg daily.

- **Try magnesium.** Take this to counteract probable deficiency and insulin resistance. Along with supplements, eat magnesium-rich foods such as green leafy vegetables (like kale, broccoli, spinach, chard, and collards) and whole grains. Magnesium glycinate, malate, succinate, orotate, ascorbate, and fumarate are best absorbed. Start with 100 mg daily; increase the dose by 100 to 200 mg until you get diarrhea, and then reduce it 100 to 200 mg until your bowels are normal. *Note:* If the necessary magnesium dosage is higher than 1,000 mg daily, 1 or 2 teaspoons of choline citrate daily can help with absorption and allow the dosage to be reduced.

- **Try chromium.** This nutrient will help reduce insulin resistance, improve blood sugar regulation, decrease visceral fat, and increase lean body mass. Take 800 to 1,000 mcg daily whether from nutritional yeast or a chromium supplement.

Note: Increase dosage slowly, especially if you are taking medication or insulin, because blood sugar levels can drop suddenly.

- **Take vanadium.** Vanadium helps to move glucose into cells without raising insulin levels. Vanadium ascorbate, citrate, fumarate, malate, glutarate, and succinate are much better utilized than vanadyl sulfate. Take 250 mcg daily.
- **Take gymnema sylvestre.** Try this to improve your body's ability to use insulin effectively and stimulate insulin production. In type 1 diabetics it lowered insulin needs and hemoglobin A1c levels. Take 400 to 800 mg daily in divided doses. Look for a product that has been standardized to 25 percent gymnemic acids.
- **Take carnitine.** Low blood levels of carnitine, a nutrient needed for burning fat and proper functioning of heart muscle, have been found in children and teens with type 1 diabetes. Take 500 to 3,000 mg daily. Dosage can also be determined through testing.

Healing Options That Are Specific for People with Type 1 Diabetes and Autoimmune Diabetes

The treatment goal for children with type 1 diabetes is to minimize the amount of insulin needed and prevent long-term complications by prolonging pancreatic islet beta cell functioning for as long as possible, maintaining good glucose control, and maximizing helpful lifestyle changes. It is unlikely that you will need to use every suggested healing option.

- **Consider autoimmunity.** Autoimmune antibodies against the thyroid, parietal cells, adrenal glands, and endomysium have been found in adults with type 1. People with one autoimmune disease are more likely than other people to develop another. Checking for autoantibodies could prevent damage to other organs and glands. If they are high, you'll know to be more aggressive about allergy reduction in your environment and foods.
- **Take digestive enzymes.** Research shows that people with type 1 diabetes often lack pancreatic enzymes. Use of digestive enzymes can enhance digestive function. Take one to two capsules with each meal or snack. Dose depends on the type of enzyme product and the size of the meal.
- **Use nicotinamide.** Nicotinamide has been shown to reduce progression of the disease in newly diagnosed children. It can put some children into remission, improve glucose control, and help preserve some of the beta cell function. Children should take 25 mg per kg body weight daily (1 kg = 2.2 pounds).

- **Take folic acid.** Folic acid can protect against vascular damage. Take 800 mcg daily.
- **Take thiamine.** Thiamine can reduce numbness and tingling, protect beta cells, and help normalize megoblastic anemia. The dosage varies; typically it is between 50 and 200 mg daily.

Healing Options Specific for People with Type 2 Diabetes

The treatment goal in type 2 diabetes is to maximize lifestyle changes and minimize medication use.

- **Use a glucose-control supplement.** These supplements help regulate blood glucose levels with a combination of vitamins, minerals, and herbs. These products commonly contain B-complex vitamins, chromium, vanadium, bitter melon, and gymnema; they may also contain biotin, vitamins E and C, magnesium, CoQ10, lipoic acid, and/or carnitine. Ask at your local health-food store for recommendations. Use as recommended on the bottle.
- **Try holy basil.** Holy basil is used to help regulate blood glucose levels. When I lived in Hawaii, my diabetic clients swore that eating three leaves of holy basil daily helped normalize their blood glucose without medication. Hairy basil seed has been used for the same purpose. Nontoxic and tasty—you can even make pesto out of it.
- **Eat bitter melon.** Bitter melon is a food that helps regulate blood glucose levels. This is a common food in the Philippines. It's pretty bitter and is an acquired taste. It can also be used as a tea, 1 to 2 cups daily. If you purchase this in a supplement, use as directed.

CHAPTER 23

The Gallbladder, Gallstones, and Cholecystectomy

The gallbladder, a pear-shaped organ that lies just below the liver, stores and concentrates bile that is manufactured in the liver. When we eat a meal that contains fat, the liver and gallbladder are stimulated to release bile. Each day, the liver secretes about a quart of bile, which is absorbed into the body from the ileum and colon and returned to the liver to be used again. Between meals, the gallbladder concentrates bile. Gallbladder problems usually indicate poor liver function. Bile emulsifies fats, cholesterol, and fat-soluble vitamins by breaking them into tiny globules. These create a greater surface area for the fat-splitting enzymes (lipase) to act on for digestion. As a result, people who have poor gallbladder function will likely be deficient in fatty acids and fat-soluble vitamins (A, D, E, and K).

Just the other day a young woman came into my office who had had her gallbladder removed. She was concerned that she wouldn't ever be able to digest fats again. She will. What happens is instead of the bile concentrating in the gallbladder, bile is secreted into the common bile duct where it collects. When we eat a fatty meal, bile is released from the liver and through the common bile duct where it mixes with pancreatic juices and moves through the sphincter of Odii into the small intestinal lumen.

The most common digestive problem associated with the gallbladder is gallstones. One in five Americans over the age of 65 has gallstones, and most people who have gallstones are never bothered by them. Medical treatment for gallstones consists of an injection of a drug that dissolves the gallstones, oral medication to dissolve stones, lithotripsy that breaks stones with sound waves, or surgical removal of

261

the gallbladder. Half a million cholecystectomies, that is, gallbladder removal surgeries, are performed each year. Most help to solve the problem. Ten to 15 percent of people complain of persistent symptoms. These typically resolve within six months, although in rare cases the symptoms persist.

Women are two to four times more likely to be affected by gallstones than men. An inflammation of the gallbladder can lead to pain and discomfort. Symptoms can take the form of abdominal discomfort, vomiting, bloating, nausea, belching, or food intolerances. When you have more than one stone, you may experience a sharp pain or a spasm under the ribs on the right side. Occasionally, the pain will be felt under your right shoulder blade. These pains are typically strongest after eating a high-fat meal. If you experience pains like these, see your doctor or, if they are severe, go to the emergency room.

Diet plays an important role in prevention of gallbladder disease. Low-fat, low-meat, and vegetarian diets are recommended, as is a low-sugar, high-fiber intake. In fact, a recent study of more than 1,100 people found that none of the 48 vegetarians in the group had any gallstones at all. There was an increase in gallstones in people who were heavy coffee drinkers. Dennis Burkitt, a British physician who lived and worked in Africa for 20 years, found that he performed only two surgeries for gallbladder removal among Africans eating an indigenous diet.

If you are overweight, losing weight will reduce your risk of developing gallstones. Be careful, because several studies have shown that fasting and extremely low-fat, low-calorie diets increase your risk of developing gallstones. Fasting for more than 14 hours raises the risk of problems due to gallstones. So easy does it while dieting. And always eat breakfast.

Exercise is also important for the prevention of gallstones. In a 1998 study, men who watched fewer than six hours of television per week had a gallstone rate lower than that of men who watched more than 40 hours. The researchers concluded that 34 percent of the cases of symptomatic gallstone disease in men could be prevented by increasing exercise to 30 minutes of endurance-type training five times per week.

Physicians familiar with natural therapies have favorable results treating gallstones without use of drugs or surgery by having their patients detoxify the liver and strengthen liver function. Metabolic cleansing or other detoxification programs are a critical first step in treatment. Food sensitivities also play an important role in the development of gallstones—most patients with gallbladder disease have them and they must be identified.

Functional Laboratory Testing
- Liver function profile
- Home test for bowel transit time

- Test for HCl adequacy
- Food sensitivity testing
- Acid-alkaline home testing

Healing Options

- **Make dietary changes.** Low-fat diets help prevent gallstones and also reduce pain and inflammation associated with gallstones. Saturated fats found in dairy products, meats, coconut oil, palm oil, hydrogenated oils, and vegetable shortening stimulate concentration of bile. While a low-fat diet is optimal, essential fatty acids are vital to gallbladder function and overall health. Make sure you get 1 to 2 tablespoons of uncooked expeller-pressed oils or extra-virgin olive oil each day—the easiest way is in homemade salad dressing. Also, vegetarian diets have been found to be helpful in reducing the incidence of gallbladder disease.

  Several studies have indicated that people who consume a lot of sweets are more likely to develop gallstones.

  Decrease coffee intake and increase water consumption. Coffee may trigger gallbladder attacks in susceptible people. Use of either regular or decaffeinated coffee raises levels of cholecystokinin, a hormone that stimulates the release of bile from the gallbladder and digestive enzymes from the pancreas, and causes gallbladder contractions. Stop drinking coffee and see what effect this produces. Some people get horrible headaches or flu-like symptoms when they withdraw from caffeine. If you do, wean yourself gradually. And don't forget to drink six to eight glasses of water every day.

- **Reduce bowel transit time.** People with gallstones have significantly slower transit times than healthy people. Eat more high-fiber foods and drink more fluids. Get more exercise. Make sure that your magnesium status is good.

- **Investigate food sensitivities.** In 1968, James Breneman, a pioneer in the area of food allergies, reported that food sensitivities play a role in gallbladder disease. He put 69 patients on an elimination diet consisting of beef, rye, soy, rice, cherry, peach, apricot, beet, and spinach. After three to five days, all people were free of symptoms. With a slow reintroduction of foods they were sensitive to, symptoms returned. The most common food offenders were pork (64 percent), onions (52 percent), and eggs (3 percent). Interestingly, beef and soy are often trigger foods for food sensitivity reactions.

- **Rule out deficient levels of hydrochloric acid (HCl).** A study published in *The Lancet* found that about half of the people with gallstones had insufficient levels of hydrochloric acid (HCl). A Heidelberg capsule test or SmartPill test can determine if you have sufficient levels of hydrochloric acid. You can also do a home test. (See Chapter 11.)

- **Try milk thistle (silymarin).** Extracts of the herb milk thistle have been used historically since the 15th century for ailments of the liver and gallbladder. It helps normalize liver function, detoxify the liver, which it does gently and thoroughly, and improve the solubility of bile. Silymarin promotes the flow of bile and helps tone the spleen, gallbladder, and liver. Take three to six 175 mg capsules daily of standardized 80 percent milk thistle extract with water before meals.

- **Try lipotrophic supplements.** Lipotrophic supplements contain substances that help normalize liver and gallbladder functions. They may contain dandelion root, milk thistle, lecithin or phosphatidylcholine, methionine, choline, inositol, vitamin C, black radish, beet greens, artichoke leaves (Cynara scolymus), turmeric, boldo (Peumus boldo), fringe tree (Chionanthus virginicus), greater celandine, and ox bile. Lipotrophics may also contain magnesium and B-complex vitamins (B_6, B_{12}, and folate) to enhance their function. Use lipotrophic supplements as directed on the label. Use 1,000 mg each of methionine and choline daily.

- **Try lecithin or phosphatidylcholine.** Phosphatidylcholine, the most biologically active form of lecithin, and lecithin have been shown to make cholesterol more soluble, which reduces formation of gallstones. Studies have shown that as little as 100 mg of lecithin three times daily will increase lecithin concentration in bile. I recommend 500 mg daily.

- **Take vitamin C.** Vitamin C has been shown to prevent formation of gallstones. Vitamin C is required for the enzymatic conversion of cholesterol to bile salts. People with high risk for developing gallstones have low ascorbic acid levels. Take 1 to 3 grams daily of vitamin C. I prefer mineral ascorbates as the best form.

- **Try black radish.** Lately I've been seeing black radishes at the grocery store. Black radish (Raphanus sativus niger) has long been used as a folk remedy to stimulate bile production and aid in the digestion of fats. Radishes of all types seem to be of benefit. A recent rat study showed that the inflammation and other abnormal parameters that were observed in rats fed a fat-rich diet were reversed with treatment with black radish. Radishes are also high in bioflavonoids and other immune-protective substances. You can eat radishes for the same benefit. Daikon radish, an Asian variety, is a mild-tasting radish for those of us who aren't radish lovers. Or you can take black radish in capsule or tablet form.

- **Try bile salts.** These are useful for people who have already had their gallbladders removed. Take one to two tablets or capsules with fatty meals.

- **Try lipase-loaded digestive enzymes.** Taking digestive enzymes that contain extra fat digestion enzymes, lipase, can be extremely useful in preventing the need for surgery or after you've had a cholecystectomy. Take one with fat-containing meals and snacks.

■ **Do a liver or gallbladder flush.** Anecdotes about people showing up at their doctor's office with a jar full of stones after a gallbladder flush are abundant, but there is little documentation to validate whether what they passed are really gallstones or just congealed olive oil. Nonetheless, many people testify to the benefits of the gallbladder flush. Do this procedure at home only under the supervision of a clinician.

From Monday through Saturday, drink as much natural apple juice as possible. Continue to eat normally and take your usual medications or supplements. On Saturday, eat a normal lunch at noon. Three hours later (3:00 P.M.) dissolve 1 tablespoon of Epsom salts (magnesium sulfate) in 1/4 cup of warm water and drink it. This is a laxative and helps peristalsis move the stones through your digestive system. It doesn't taste great, so you may want to follow it with some orange or grapefruit juice. Two hours later (5:00 P.M.) repeat the Epsom salts and orange or grapefruit juice. For dinner, eat citrus fruits or drink citrus juices. At bedtime, drink 1½ cups of warm extra-virgin olive oil blended with 1½ cups of lemon juice. Go to bed immediately and lie on your right side with your knees pulled up close to your chest for half an hour. On Sunday morning, take 1 tablespoon of Epsom salts in 1½ cup of warm water an hour before breakfast. If you have gallstones, you will find dark green to light green stones in your bowel movement on Sunday morning. They are irregular in shape and size, varying from small, like kiwi seeds, to large, like cherry pits. If you have chronic gallbladder problems, you may want to repeat this therapy in two weeks. The flush can be repeated every three to six months if you continue to form stones.

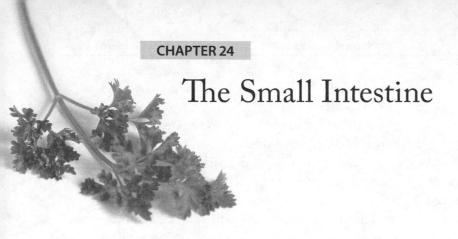

CHAPTER 24

The Small Intestine

G as and bloating are the most common symptoms of small intestinal problems. Other problems that occur in the small intestines are parasites, celiac disease, food sensitivities, and increased intestinal permeability (leaky gut). Use all of the DIGIN approaches to work with these issues.

FLATULENCE OR INTESTINAL GAS

Everyone has gas. It's normal. In fact, we "pass gas" an average of 10 to 15 times a day. Most of our gas comes from swallowed air. Chewing gum, drinking carbonated beverages, and eating whipped foods such as egg whites and whipped cream all contribute to swallowed air. The gas we pass is mainly nitrogen (up to 90 percent), carbon dioxide, and oxygen, which are odorless. Gas and bloating are also a product of the fermentation of small pieces of undigested foods by the bacteria in our intestines. Fermentation produces stinky gases like methane and hydrogen sulfide, which has the odor of rotten eggs. Other substances, like butyric acid, cadaverine, and putrescine are present in tiny amounts, but they are noted for the mighty fragrance they give to gas.

Some of us experience excessive amounts of gas, which can be not only embarrassing but also an uncomfortable sign that something is out of balance. Millions of people have bloating and discomfort associated with gas. If you've ever made wine, you'll recall putting a balloon on the top during the fermentation process that allowed for expansion of the gases produced. Our bellies act like a balloon, expanding to contain the gas produced by fermentation.

Foods from the cabbage family, dried and sulfured fruits, and beans all contain sulfur that gives gas a rotten-egg odor, but sulfur also has critical use throughout our bodies. Cucumbers, celery, apples, carrots, onions, and garlic are all commonly known to cause gas. People with lactose intolerance often experience gas when they eat dairy products. Eating a high-fiber diet is healthful but can cause gas until your intestinal flora adjusts. You may have insufficient levels of hydrochloric acid, intestinal flora, pancreatic enzymes, or a dysbiosis that is causing your problems. Food sensitivities, especially to wheat and grains, can also cause excessive gas.

You will probably find the answers to your gas issues in the DIGIN model. If they're not solved by these simple suggestions, look deeper. I remember one man whose flatulence was causing difficulties at work. His coworkers complained. He had stool testing and discovered he had parasites. Once treated, his gas normalized.

Functional Laboratory Testing
- Small intestinal bacterial overgrowth test
- Organic acid testing
- Comprehensive digestive stool analysis with parasitology
- IgE and IgG allergy testing
- Lactose breath test
- Self-test for lactose intolerance by eliminating all dairy from your diet

Healing Options
- **Chew your food well and eat slowly.** These simple activities can have far-reaching effects on healthy digestive processes and gas reduction.
- **Increase fiber gradually.** Most of us need to dramatically increase the amount of dietary fiber we eat, but raising these levels too quickly can cause a lot of gas and discomfort. Our flora goes wild with sudden increases in dietary fiber, and the fermentation causes gas. Increasing your fiber intake more slowly will solve this problem. High-fiber foods include whole grains, beans, and many fruits and vegetables.
- **Consider possible lactose intolerance.** The inability to digest lactose, the sugar in milk, is a frequent cause of gas. Eliminate all dairy products for at least two weeks and see if there is improvement. Make sure to eliminate all hidden dairy products found in foods. Products such as Lactaid and Digestive Advantage LI really help for the times you do eat dairy products.
- **Supplement with probiotics.** Use of a supplemental probiotic bacteria can make a tremendous difference in your ability to digest foods. Beneficial flora can help

reestablish the normal microbial balance in your intestinal tract. Take one to two capsules or powdered probiotic supplement as directed on label. Products differ in dosage. Mix powdered supplement with a cool or cold beverage; hot drinks kill the flora.

- **Try digestive enzymes.** Many people find that supplementation with digestive enzymes at meals, either vegetable, bromelain, papaya, or pancreatic enzymes, really helps prevent gas. Take one to two digestive enzymes with meals.

- **De-gas your beans.** Beans are an excellent source of vegetarian protein, containing both soluble and insoluble fibers, as well as sitosterols, which help normalize cholesterol levels. However, beans are notorious for their gas-producing effects. They contain substances that are difficult for us to digest. For instance, beans, grains, and seeds hold their nutrients with phytic acid. Soaking or sprouting releases the nutrients so that we can absorb more of them. First, soak the beans for 4 to 12 hours, then drain off the water, replace with new water, and simmer for several hours until they are soft. Some people find that putting a pinch or two of baking soda in the water helps reduce gas. Others add kombu, a Japanese sea vegetable, or ginger. Beano is an enzyme product that contains the enzymes necessary for digestion of beans. Place a drop or two on your food; it helps reduce flatulence for most people. Beano is sold widely in drugstores and health-food stores.

  Also recall that we produce digestive enzymes for foods we commonly eat. If you eat beans rarely, start by eating a tablespoon or two of beans each day. Your body may begin to produce the enzymes necessary for their digestion.

- **Explore food sensitivities.** Although lactose intolerance is the most common food sensitivity, people can be sensitive to nearly any other food. The most likely culprits are sugars and grains. Careful charting of your foods and flatulence levels can help you detect which foods are giving you the most trouble. Food sensitivities don't usually exist by themselves. If you have a number of food sensitivities, check for dysbiosis.

- **Check for dysbiosis.** An imbalance of bacteria, yeast, or parasites often causes excessive gas. These microbes eat sugar and cause fermentation of sugars, fruits, and starches that we feel as gas and bloating. A comprehensive digestive stool analysis, organic acid test, or small intestinal bacterial overgrowth test can determine whether or not you have dysbiosis or other dysbiotic imbalance.

- **Avoid alcohol sugars.** Sorbitol, maltitol, isomalt, and xylitol are indigestible alcohol sugars found in most sugarless candy and gum. They are used by diabetics and dieters because these sugars are sweet but don't affect blood sugar levels. Large amounts of sorbitol and xylitol cause gas, but even small amounts can cause a problem for those who are sensitive.

- **Take chlorophyll.** Chlorophyll liquid or tablets can help prevent gas. Take 1 tablet two to three times daily with meals.
- **Use ginger, fennel, and anise.** Most of us have at least one of these spices in our kitchen, and they are valuable tools for reducing gas. Put a few slices of fresh ginger or ½ teaspoon of dried ginger in a cup of boiling water and steep until cool enough to drink. It will soon begin to dispel your gas from both ends, and you'll be much more comfortable. Fennel and anise can be used in tea or you can simply chew on the seeds to relieve gas. In Indian restaurants, you find small bowls of these seeds. They also cleanse the palate with their sweet pungency.
- **Use herbs and drink herbal teas.** Traditionally herbs and spices were added to foods to aid digestion. Nearly all our common kitchen herbs and spices have a beneficial effect, including basil, oregano, marjoram, parsley, thyme, celery seed, peppermint, spearmint, fennel, bayberries, caraway seed, cardamom seed, catnip, cloves, coriander, lemon balm, and sarsaparilla. You can find many digestive herbal tea blends in health-food stores.
- **Try activated charcoal tablets.** Charcoal absorbs toxins and gases and can be found in nearly any pharmacy or health-food store. Your stools will turn black—that's the charcoal leaving your body. It has been rated "safe and effective" by the FDA for acute poisoning. It's inexpensive and very helpful. Take one to four tablets as needed, with a meal or immediately if you are having gas problems.

CELIAC DISEASE AND GLUTEN INTOLERANCE

Celiac disease, also called gluten-sensitive enteropathy, is a genetic autoimmune disease that affects about 3 million people in the United States. When people with celiac eat gluten-containing grains, there is inflammation and ultimately damage to the lining of the small intestine. It is often discovered in childhood, but it can go on for decades before being recognized. If the disease is left unchecked, people often have other diseases as a result of the undiagnosed celiac. The typical signs of celiac are indigestion, abdominal pain and bloating, diarrhea, inability to gain weight, and anemia. If only a small segment of the intestines is damaged, or the inflammation is mild, symptoms may be different. Celiac disease is like a chameleon: only 1 out of every 8 to 15 people present this way; most people with celiac don't have any GI symptoms at all. Only half of people present with diarrhea at diagnosis. Other common presentations are depression, bone loss, dental erosion, arthritis/joint pain, mouth sores, muscle cramps, skin rashes, irritability, stomach discomfort, and neurological problems. In children the most common symptoms are abdominal pain, bloating, diarrhea, constipation, weight loss, failure to thrive, and vomiting. Malab-

SIGNS AND CONDITIONS ASSOCIATED WITH CELIAC DISEASE

There is an increased incidence of the following conditions in people with celiac disease. Obviously, many of these symptoms and conditions exist in people who do not have celiac disease or gluten intolerance. For example, celiac disease is found in a small percentage of people with type 1 diabetes or schizophrenia. For those few people, knowing that they have celiac is life-changing.

- Abdominal cramps
- Addison's disease
- Allergies/hay fever
- Anemia
- Asthma
- Ataxia
- Autism
- Bloating
- Bowel movements that won't flush
- Bruising easily
- Calcium deficiency
- Carpal tunnel syndrome
- Cerebral vasculitis
- Dairy intolerance
- Dementia
- Depression
- Dermatitis herpetiformis
- Dizziness
- Down's syndrome
- Ear infections
- Epilepsy
- Failure to thrive
- Fatigue/general weakness
- Feeling unwell or tired without other symptoms

- Fibromyalgia
- Fluid retention
- Gas
- Gastroesophageal reflux disease (GERD)
- GI hemorrhage
- Gray or tan-colored stools
- Hives
- Infertility
- Inflammatory bowel disease
- Interstitial cystitis
- Intestinal cancer
- Irritable bowel syndrome
- Juvenile idiopathic arthritis
- Kidney disease (increased risk)
- Liver disease
- Magnesium deficiency
- Migraine headache
- Miscarriages
- Multiple sclerosis
- Muscle wasting
- Muscle weakness
- Myopathy

- Neurological issues
- Nosebleeds
- Obesity
- Oily stools
- Osteoporosis/ osteopenia
- Palor (paleness)
- Panic attacks
- Peripheral neuropathy
- Psoriasis
- Red urine (hematuria)
- Rheumatoid arthritis
- Schizophrenia
- Sjögren's disease
- Small intestinal bacterial overgrowth
- Stomach rumbling
- Stunted growth
- Thyroid disease
- Turner syndrome
- Type 1 diabetes
- Uncoordinated/ clumsy
- Vitamin deficiencies
- Weight loss
- Williams syndrome

Sources: www.celiac.com; www.celiaccentral.com; Alessio Fasano, "Celiac Disease Insights: Clues to Solving Autoimmunity," *Scientific American* (Aug. 2009); Institute of Functional Medicine, GI Module 2010.

sorption of nutrients can cause far-reaching health problems. Often by the time of diagnosis people have other health issues, such osteoporosis, infertility, neurological issues, or other autoimmune conditions, that are a result of this. Dr. Marios Hadjivassiliou and colleagues have estimated that 57 percent of people with neurological dysfunction of unknown cause have gluten sensitivity. Thyroid disorders have been found in 30 to 43 percent of people with celiac disease. There is an eightfold incidence of cirrhosis in people with celiac. With early detection, I wonder how much of the collateral damage we can prevent? The World Health Organization believes that a policy of mass screening for celiac disease is warranted because it is common and because avoiding gluten-containing grains is an effective treatment.

The recognition of celiac disease and gluten intolerance is rising, although it still takes someone with celiac disease an average of 9 to 11 years and at least five doctors to be diagnosed. It affects about 1 in 133 people. Ninety-five percent of people with celiac are thought to be undiagnosed. Ninety-five percent of people with celiac disease have positive HLA-DQ2 and HLA-D3 genes. Yet most people with these genes will never develop celiac disease: 35 percent of us have these gene types, while less than 1 percent have celiac.

As with all of the genetic diseases, three conditions need to be met for it to be expressed: have the right genes, have the right environment to trigger the disease, and have a leaky gut. Changes in the microbiome can predispose us to celiac. This is why some people develop celiac in early childhood and other people are diagnosed well into adulthood. If you have a relative with celiac or other autoimmune diseases (such as type 1 diabetes, rheumatoid arthritis, or lupus) your risk is 8 to 15 times higher than the general population.

Gluten is a protein component of wheat and several other grains. It's what makes bread and pastries elastic and "gluey." Gluten is a complex molecule, and digesting it thoroughly is something that we humans find difficult to do. Gluten is an unusual molecule that is rich in proline and glutamine. Part of the molecule is impervious to our digestion. In healthy people, the molecule stays inside the gut lumen and is passed as waste in stool. In people with leaky gut, the molecule passes through the gut, where it plays havoc. In people with celiac, this molecule provokes immediate and ultimately chronic inflammation and malabsorption. At a couple of the recent Defeat Autism Now conferences, Dr. Alessio Fasano, from the University of Maryland, who is one of the foremost celiac researchers in the world, showed a video of mice, one of which had been exposed to gluten, and the other one who had not been exposed to gluten. In the mouse that was exposed, there was a buildup of intraepithelial lymphocytes (IELs) at the inside of the gut lumen. IELs are white blood cells that immediately release cytokines to get rid of molecules that don't belong there. (At the time of writing, Dr. Fasano's lecture and video can be seen at http://

www.autism.com/pro_categories.asp?con=Baltimore&Year=2010.) Dr. Fasano states that this happens in *all* of us when we eat gluten-containing grains. If we have a leaky gut, then it becomes an issue because every time we eat gluten-containing grains, there is more immune involvement.

The lucky part about celiac is that if you completely stop eating gluten-containing grains, the body heals. You will see big changes almost immediately, and over 3 to 12 months the small intestine will heal. Avoiding all gluten is easier than it used to be, but still it can be daunting. How deeply you have fallen into the celiac rabbit hole will determine how long it will take for you to be renourished and how well some of the coexisting conditions will heal.

About half of all people with celiac disease are also lactose intolerant at the time of their diagnosis. Lactase, the enzyme required to split lactose, is manufactured at the tips of the villi. Because these villi are damaged in people with untreated celiac disease, their bodies can't manufacture the lactase. Once people have gone onto a gluten-free diet and the intestinal lining is repaired, some will be able to tolerate dairy products. Right now the *only* safe treatment for celiac is to avoid gluten 100 percent. Researchers are working hard to find additional approaches for people with celiac. There is some promise with the use of digestive enzymes to break down gluten. Others are trying to inhibit tissue transglutaminase (tTG) so that it doesn't modify undigested gluten particles so that they bind to the HLA-DQ2 and DQ8 proteins. Dr. Fasano is studying a drug, Larazotide, that blocks zonulin (which opens the tight junctions in the intestine, increasing leaky gut). Still others are working on possible vaccines. It's too soon to know for sure what will be discovered, but keep your eyes open.

Gluten Intolerance

Celiac is an advanced disease. Since so many of us have the "right" genes for celiac, many of us are on the road but do not yet have celiac disease. There are two possible theories about gluten intolerance: (1) It's on a continuum and you just haven't developed into celiac disease yet, and (2) there are different genetics involved with gluten intolerance that have yet to be discovered. According to Kristina Harris, Ph.D., a celiac researcher at the University of Maryland, only half of people with gluten sensitivity have the DQ2 type of gene. I see this all the time in my practice—many of my clients have normal celiac tests, yet upon going on an elimination diet they find that many of their health issues resolve. This is why genetic testing alone cannot rule out gluten intolerance.

We are just beginning to see literature in the research that delineates the differences between gluten sensitivity and celiac disease. A 2011 paper by Anna Sapone, Alessio Fasano, and a slew of other researchers has a very interesting report. They did comparisons on 26 people with gluten sensitivity, 42 people with celiac disease, and 39 people used as controls who had neither gluten sensitivity nor celiac disease. Those with gluten sensitivity reported GI symptoms but without any abnormal inflammation when sed rate, C-reactive protein, and mucoprotein were evaluated. Fifty-seven percent of people with gluten sensitivity had genes that predisposed them to celiac disease (DQ2 or DQ8) and 43 percent did not. All three groups were given lactulose/mannitol testing to determine whether they had leaky gut syndrome. Surprisingly, gluten sensitivity was not associated with increased intestinal permeability, and results were even more normal than for people in the control group. People with gluten sensitivity had lower levels of changes in adaptive immunity (IL-6 and IL-21) but had higher markers of innate immunity, like toll-like receptor 2. Also T-regulatory cell marker FOXP3 was reduced in people with gluten sensitivity. T-regulatory cells are like the brakes on the immune system that tell it that the threat is over. Because of these differences, the researchers concluded for the very first time that celiac disease and gluten sensitivity are distinct entities that are both caused by distinct reactions to exposure to gluten-containing grains.

If you have positive food sensitivity testing for gluten, gliaden, and/or gluten-containing grains, think gluten intolerance. You can also test IgG and IgA anti-gliaden and IgG and IgA antigluten antibodies through any physician or medical lab. Positive antibodies are found in about 10 percent of the population. If you test positive for these antibodies, avoid all gluten even in minute amounts for four to six months and take gut-healing herbs, nutrients, enzymes, and probiotics. Then retest with blood testing and by reintroducing gluten into your diet. Gluten intolerance may or may not be permanent. If you can discover underlying causes in the DIGIN model, you may be able to heal your gut and tolerate gluten again. The very best method of testing yourself for gluten sensitivity is to avoid all gluten for three months. Typically, people with celiac disease have additional sensitivites that resolve once the gut is healed. For this reason, I recommend the elimination diet as outlined in Chapter 15.

Testing for Celiac Disease and Gluten Intolerance

Gastroenterologists feel that the most accurate diagnosis of celiac disease is done through jejunal biopsy. I have worked with many people who have negative biopsies yet still get sick on even small bits of gluten. The most specific and accurate blood test for celiac is antibodies to tissue transglutaminase (tTG). If positive, you have celiac disease. There are false negatives, however; tTG testing is negative 31 percent of the time in people with celiac disease. If it's not full-blown, it's not discovered. Genetic testing is useful but limited, since 35 percent of us have the right genetics to develop celiac disease. IgG and IgA antibodies to gluten and gliaden can help to determine whether you have gluten intolerance.

From my viewpoint, an elimination diet and exclusion of wheat from your diet for three months will give you a terrific indicator of whether gluten is your friend or not. I cannot tell you how many times I've worked with clients who feel miraculously better without gluten in their lives who are told by their doctors that in order to diagnose celiac they have to eat gluten-containing grains for three to six months so that the inflammation will show up. Most people seem reluctant to do that. They already know that they feel worse when they eat gluten-containing foods and don't want to feel worse again.

People with celiac disease have malabsorption, so typically they have nutritional deficiencies. It's useful to test for these and/or to take a good multivitamin with minerals.

Functional Laboratory Testing

Celiac panels may contain the following tests:

- IgA and IgG antitransglutaminase Elisa/Act (tTG) (This test is the most accurate, although 31 percent of people with celiac test negative because they do not have enough GI damage.)
- IgA and IgG antigliaden antibodies
- IgA antiendomysial antibodies
- IgA and IgG deaminated gliaden antibodies
- Antiendomysial, antigliadin, and tissue transglutaminase antibodies
- Total IgA (If total IgA is low, then specific IgA antibodies aren't accurate.)

The following tests can help determine if there are additional factors:

- Vitamin and mineral testing
- Organic acid testing
- Comprehensive digestive stool analysis with parasitology
- Intestinal permeability testing
- Lactose breath test
- Food sensitivity testing

Healing Celiac and Gluten Intolerance

- **Avoid all gluten for at least three months.** Avoid all gluten-containing grains and any products that contain them, even in small amounts. Gluten is found in many grains, including wheat (including couscous, semolina, orzo, bulgur, graham, and farina), rye, barley, millet, spelt, kamut, and triticale. Oats don't contain gluten but are often contaminated with gluten from farming practices, transportation, or manufacturing. In addition to obvious sources of gluten, many products have hidden sources. Salad dressings, some hot dogs, ice cream, bouillon cubes, chocolate, and foods containing hydrolyzed vegetable protein may contain gluten. (See Chapters 9 and 10 for more information on gluten and gluten-free grains. Hidden sources of gluten can be found at www .digestivewellness.us.)

Gluten-free grains and grain substitutes include:

Almond meal flour	Potato flour
Amaranth flour	Potato starch
Amaranth grain	Roasted kasha (buckwheat)
Brown rice flour	Quinoa flour
Buckwheat	Quinoa grain
Coconut flour	Sorghum
Cornmeal	Sorghum flour
Cornstarch	Tapioca
Guar gum	Tapioca flour
Millet	Teff
Millet flour	White rice flour
Pecan meal	Xantham gum

Although giving up gluten will be difficult at first, it has become easier over the past few years with the growing number of products, restaurants, and bakeries offering gluten-free options. You'll be able to find delicious breads, pastas, cookies, crackers, and more.

- **Try digestive enzymes.** Either pancreatic or vegetable enzymes can be used to enhance digestive function. Take one to two with each meal. Specific amylase enzymes can be of particular benefit.

- **Supplement with probiotics.** Probiotic flora enhances digestive function. Either eat cultured and fermented foods or take probiotic supplements.

- **Try gut-healing nutrients.** Glutamine, N-acetyl-D-glucosamine, and gamma oryzanol, are all healing to the intestinal lining. While no specific testing has been done on therapeutic use of these nutrients in people with celiac disease, clinical experience with celiac indicates their usefulness.

- **Take a multivitamin with minerals.** Zinc, selenium, folic acid, iron, and vitamins A, B_6, D, E, and K have all been shown to be deficient in people with celiac disease. Get a good-quality multivitamin with minerals. Look for a supplement that is hypoallergenic and contains no grains or dairy.

CHAPTER 25

The Colon or Large Intestine

Common problems in the large intestine, also called the colon, include constipation, diarrhea, diverticular disease, irritable bowel syndrome, inflammatory bowel disease, ulcerative colitis, Crohn's disease, hemorrhoids, polyps, and colon cancer. Proper functioning of the colon requires a high-fiber diet. The colon is home to tens of trillions of beneficial bifidobacteria and other flora that ferment dietary fiber that, in turn, produce short-chain fatty acids, butyric acid, valerate acid, propionic acid, and acetic acid. These short-chain fatty acids are the primary fuel of the colonic cells. They're needed to maintain, fuel, and build new colonic cells. Without adequate fiber, we starve the colonic cells and weaken the integrity of the colon. Butyric acid has been shown to stop the growth of colon cancer cells in vitro and is used clinically to heal inflamed bowel tissue.

The colon's main function is to recycle nutrients and water back into our bodies and eliminate waste products. Adequate hydration is essential for good colon health. Water is our best choice, followed by fresh vegetable juices, diluted fruit juices, herbal teas, coconut water, and fruits and vegetables.

CONSTIPATION

Constipation affects up to 28 percent of North Americans. Physicians write more than a million prescriptions for constipation relief annually, and we spend $725 million a year on laxatives. Constipation is defined differently by different people, and it is often subjective: I feel constipated if I have only one bowel movement a day. The Rome III criteria for constipation includes two or more of the following: straining at least 25 percent of bowel movements; lumpy or hard stools at least 25 percent of the time; sensation of incomplete evacuation in at least 25 percent of bowel movements; sensation of obstruction at least 25 percent of the time; manual maneuvers to facilitate evacuation at least 25 percent of the time; fewer than three bowel movements a week. An additional symptom is hard stools unless you use laxatives. The Rome III criteria attempt to differentiate between constipation and constipation-type IBS, but the latest research indicates that these are artificial divisions that aren't really useful. Constipation affects women twice as often as men and is more common in people over age 65.

Fifty percent of people have bowel movements daily; many people do not have a bowel movement every day; most people are irregular and may not have the same number of bowel movements every day or at the same time of day. In integrative circles, it is considered normal to have one to three soft bowel movements each day. Optimal bowel transit time is 12 to 24 hours, so if you are having only three bowel movements each week, you have a transit time of 56 hours, which is way too long. This makes sense in light of current theories about fecal transit time. If you haven't done the transit time self-test, now would be a good time. (See section on bowel transit time in Chapter 2.)

Bowel movements should be painless. If you experience pain, see your physician. You may have a structural abnormality, fissure, hemorrhoid, or more serious problem. Pain during bowel movements can cause a muscle spasm in the sphincter, which can delay a stool. Magnesium helps relieve and prevent muscle spasms.

Causes of Constipation

Although aging is commonly listed as a cause of constipation, it is due more to the results of lifestyle. Elderly people often eat low-fiber foods, rely on packaged and prepared foods, take medications that interfere with normal bowel function, and have decreased mobility. Medications that constipate include opiate medications, antidepressants such as Elevil and Tofranil, anticonvulsants, iron supplements, calcium channel blockers like Cardizem and Procardia, and antacids that contain aluminum, such as Amphojel and Basaljel.

Many other factors can be the underlying cause of constipation. Dysbiosis and lack of gut microbiome balance are often overlooked causes of constipation. Recent research has confirmed that people who are chronically constipated often have positive methane breath testing, which indicates small intestinal bacterial overgrowth (SIBO). In fact, the more severe the constipation, the more likely that SIBO is present. Magnesium deficiency slows peristalsis, causing constipation. Hormones play a role. Women often notice that their bowel habits change at various times in their menstrual cycles. Pregnancy is a common, but temporary, cause of constipation. Constipation can also be caused by an underactive thyroid. Some diseases can affect the body's ability to have bowel movements. Parkinson's disease, scleroderma, lupus, strokes, diabetes, kidney disease, low or high thyroid function, and certain neurological or muscular diseases, such as multiple sclerosis or spinal cord injuries, can cause constipation. Colon cancer can also cause it. Neurological problems, such as injuries to the spinal column, tumors that sit on nerves, nerve disorders of the bowel, and certain brain disorders are other causes.

Dennis Burkitt, M.D., studied bowel habits of Africans living in small towns and large cities. He found that people who ate indigenous, local foods had an average of a pound of feces each day, with 12-hour transit times. Burkitt found that those who lived in cities on Western diets excreted only five and a half ounces of stool each day, with average transit times of 48 to 72 hours. People on native diets had extremely low incidences of diseases common to Western civilization, such as appendicitis, diabetes, diverticulitis, gallstones, coronary heart disease, hiatal hernia, varicose veins, hemorrhoids, colon cancer, and obesity. When these people moved into cities and ate a Westernized diet, they too developed these diseases. Dr. Burkitt attributed much of this disease to poor dietary fiber intake in a modernized diet.

Overuse of laxatives is common and compounds the problem. Chronic use of laxatives, even herbal laxatives, causes the bowels to become lazy, and the muscles become dependent on laxatives to constrict. Some laxatives can cause damage to the nerve cells in the wall of the colon. If you have used laxatives, you need to retrain your body to have bowel movements on its own. Try sitting on the toilet each morning for 20 minutes and relax. Over time your body will remember how to relax and function normally.

Solving the Problem

For most people, eating more of a whole-foods diet, exercising, and drinking plenty of fluids normalizes bowel function.

Pay attention to your body's needs. When your body gives you the signals that it's time to defecate, stop what you are doing and go to the bathroom. When you ignore your body's urges, the rectum gets used to being stretched and fails to respond normally. Feces back up into the colon, causing discomfort. If you dislike having a bowel movement at work, school, or in a public restroom, readjust your attitude and get used to the idea. Everybody's doing it.

Healing Options

- **Look for infection.** Bacterial, fungal, and parasitic infection can cause constipation. SIBO is evident in many people with chronic constipation.

- **Double your fiber intake.** Legumes, such as kidney, navy, pinto, and lima beans, have a large amount of dietary fiber. Make whole grains the rule and processed grains the exception. The addition of high-fiber cereals at breakfast can make a big difference. Brussels sprouts, asparagus, cabbage, cauliflower, corn, peas, kale, parsnips, flaxseeds, and potatoes contain high amounts of fiber. A recent study compared the use of psyllium seeds, a fiber supplement, with the use of docusate sodium, a common stool softener. The psyllium was more effective at relieving constipation than the stool softener. So use psyllium and eat more fiber. Ground hempseed meal, or ground or soaked flaxseeds also work well to soften stools and normalize bowel movements. Make these changes slowly. A quick change to a high-fiber diet can cause gas and bloating. As your body gets used to this new way of eating, it will adapt. Remember that the requirements for most of us are to double our daily fiber intake.

- **Hydrate.** Be sure to drink six to eight glasses of water, juices, or herbal teas and eat at least five servings of fruits and vegetables each day.

- **Exercise if you don't already do so.** Exercise helps relieve constipation by massaging the intestines. Many of my clients have found that regular exercise keeps their bowels regular.

- **Try psyllium seed husks.** Stop using laxatives and enemas and start using psyllium seeds. They add bulk and water to stool, which allows for easy passage. Though not a laxative, psyllium seeds do regulate bowel function, are beneficial for both diarrhea and constipation, and do not cause harmful dependencies. Build up gradually to 1 teaspoon of psyllium with each meal to avoid gas and cramping from sudden introduction of fiber.

- **Try wheat bran, chia seeds, flaxseeds, hempseeds, or corn bran.** These can all be used in the same way as psyllium seeds. They add bulk and moisture to stool, which allow it to pass more easily. Build up to 1 to 2 tablespoons daily.

- **Improve bowel habits.** Ignoring your body's natural urge to defecate can cause constipation. Take time each morning to have a bowel movement. If you go when nature calls, it takes just a minute or two.

- **Improve bowel flora.** Poor bowel flora causes the digestive system to move sluggishly. Eat cultured and fermented foods and/or take a probiotic supplement two to three times daily. If you are able to digest yogurt, it has a normalizing effect on the bowels and can be helpful for either constipation or diarrhea.

- **Add magnesium.** Magnesium helps keep peristalsis—rhythmic muscle relaxation and contraction—working by proper relaxation of muscles. Americans have widespread magnesium deficiency that contributes to constipation. According to recent studies, 75 percent of magnesium is lost during food processing, and 40 percent of Americans fail to meet the RDA levels for daily magnesium intake. Take at least 400 mg daily. I've had clients who initially needed 2,000 mg of magnesium. Eventually, their deficiency lessens and they need less. If you need large amounts of magnesium, you may want to use 1 teaspoon daily of choline citrate to increase absorption. Too much magnesium can cause diarrhea.
- **Take digestive enzymes.** Many people report that they have more regular and easy bowel movements when they take digestive enzyme supplements.
- **Address lactose intolerance**. People with lactose intolerance sometimes become constipated from dairy products.
- **Assess stress.** See Chapter 16 for stress-management ideas.
- **Evaluate medications.** Many medications can cause constipation: pain relievers, antacids that contain aluminum, antispasmodic drugs, antidepressants, tranquilizers, iron supplements, anticonvulsants, diuretics, anesthetics, anticholinergics, blood pressure medication, bismuth salts, and laxatives. If you noticed that constipation occurred suddenly after you began to take a new medication, discuss it with your doctor.
- **Investigate food sensitivities, dysbiosis, and leaky gut syndrome**. People with chronic constipation who do not respond to diet, fiber, liquids, and exercise should have digestive testing to see if dysbiosis, food allergies, or parasites are the underlying problem.
- **Take vitamin C.** Vitamin C can help soften stool. The amount varies depending on individual needs. Use a vitamin C flush to determine your daily needs. (See Chapter 18.)
- **Try biofeedback.** Biofeedback has been used successfully to treat constipation in people who have problems relaxing the pelvic floor muscles.

DIARRHEA

Diarrhea is a symptom, not a disease. Your body is telling you: "Get this out of me and fast!" If you have chronic diarrhea, it's important to find the underlying cause. Chronic diarrhea can be the result of drugs, diverticular disease, foods or beverages that disagree with your system, infections (bacterial, fungal, viral, or parasitic), inflammatory bowel disease, irritable bowel syndrome, malabsorption, lactose intolerance, laxative use and abuse, contaminated water supply, or cancer. People with gallbladder problems often experience diarrhea after a fatty meal. With careful questioning and laboratory testing, your physician will be able to find the cause. Once you have a diagnosis, you can decide how to approach the problem.

Diarrhea occurs when you have a bowel transit time that is too fast. Feces don't sit in the colon long enough for water to be absorbed back into your body, so the stool comes out runny. (It's truly amazing how much water is usually absorbed through the colon—two gallons every day.) If you have chronic diarrhea, you aren't getting the maximum benefit from foods because you aren't absorbing all the nutrients. Loss of fluids and electrolyte minerals can make us disoriented and weak. In infants, small children, and the elderly, dehydration can be dangerous and can happen suddenly. It's important to replace lost fluids to prevent dehydration. Drink eight to ten glasses of water, fruit and vegetable juices, or broths each day. Infants can be given a Fleet enema, which is easily purchased at drugstores. Follow the directions in the package.

Most diarrhea is self-limiting. It is the body's way of getting rid of something disagreeable—food, microbes, or toxins. So for acute diarrhea, just let it flow and keep drinking plenty of water and fluids. If you have severe abdominal or rectal pain, fever of at least 102 degrees Fahrenheit, blood in your stool, signs of dehydration—dry mouth, anxiety, restlessness, excessive thirst, little or no urination, severe weakness, dizziness, or light-headedness—or your diarrhea lasts more than three days, call your doctor. Be more cautious with small children, people who are already ill, and the elderly.

You usually aren't very hungry when you have acute diarrhea. Many foods "feed" the bugs and you instinctively stop eating. The diet recommended for people with diarrhea is called the BRAT diet, which stands for bananas, rice, applesauce, and toast. These foods are bland and binding. You can make a pretty tasty rice pudding with apples, rice, eggs, and cinnamon. Soda crackers, chicken, and eggs can also be eaten.

With chronic diarrhea, think about food sensitivities, celiac disease, or low-grade underlying bacterial, fungal, or parasitic infection.

Many other substances can cause diarrhea, including an excess of vitamin C or magnesium. For instance, antacids that contain magnesium salts can cause diarrhea. Sorbitol, mannitol, and xylitol are sugars found in dietetic candies and sweets that can cause diarrhea. Even in small amounts, they can cause diarrhea in people sensitive to them. Some people have the same reaction to fructose or lactose.

Functional Laboratory Testing

Prolonged diarrhea is a symptom that warrants thorough investigation. These are a few of the tests that may give you information about what's causing your problem.

- Comprehensive digestive stool analysis with parasitology
- Hydrogen breath test for SIBO
- Lactose breath test
- Food allergy and sensitivity testing—IgG and IgE

Healing Options

Healing options depend on the cause of the diarrhea. See the appropriate sections for complete healing options. Do testing to discover if there is a correctable underlying cause.

- **Supplement with probiotics.** These beneficial bacteria help normalize bowel function. They ferment fiber, which produces short-chain fatty acids to fuel the colonic tissue. You can also take probiotic supplements to help prevent traveler's diarrhea. Take two to six capsules daily.
- **Use Saccharomyces boulardii.** This friendly yeast probiotic has been used successfully to prevent and treat diarrhea caused by antibiotics, traveler's diarrhea, and diarrhea associated with AIDS. It boosts levels of secretory IgA, which is a protective part of the immune system. It is safe for all ages. Take two to six capsules daily.
- **Wash your hands frequently.** The simple act of washing your hands with soap can help reduce the incidence of ongoing diarrhea. In a study done with mothers of children with prolonged diarrhea, the mothers were simply asked to wash their own hands with soap and water before preparing food and eating and to wash their children's hands before eating and as soon as possible after a bowel movement. There was an 89 percent reduction in diarrhea in the hand-washing moms' group in comparison with the control group.
- **Investigate food allergies and sensitivities**. Diarrhea is a common symptom of food sensitivities and allergies. Lactose intolerance is a common source of diarrhea. Avoid milk and dairy foods for two or three weeks to see if the diarrhea stops. Try an elimination diet. Test for food sensitivities.
- **Take goldenseal.** This herb is highly effective for treatment of acute diarrhea caused by microbial infection. Be sure to use goldenseal in recommended dosages as it may also cause diarrhea if used in excessive amounts.

- **Eat yogurt.** This can help stop diarrhea. Yogurt contains active bacteria, L. thermophilus and L. bulgaricus, which help prevent and stop diarrhea. There have been several studies showing yogurt's effectiveness.
- **Use olive oil.** One study showed that oleic acid, the main fatty acid in olive oil, slowed down transit time in people with chronic diarrhea. Because it's so non-toxic, it's worth a try. Oleic acid is also found in olives, almonds, and avocados.
- **Increase fiber.** Adding psyllium, flax, hemp, or other fiber as a daily supplement can help solidify stools. Begin with 1 to 2 teaspoons in at least 8 ounces of water.
- **Avoid alcohol sugars.** Sorbitol, mannitol, maltitol, isomalt, and xylitol are indigestible sugars found in sugar-free candy, gums, and snack bars. They can easily cause diarrhea, gas, and bloating.
- **Take zinc.** Much research has been done on zinc and diarrhea in children. It shortens the duration of acute diarrhea by boosting the body's immune system. Children can take 20 mg daily and adults can take 50 mg daily for up to two weeks.

DIVERTICULAR DISEASE

Diverticula are pea-sized pouches that have blown out of the intestinal wall, primarily in the colon. There hasn't been much research on the underlying cause of these diverticula. It's commonly believed that a low-fiber diet, constipation, and getting older predispose us. Soft, bulky stools easily pass through the colon and respond to peristaltic waves; hard, dehydrated stools are more difficult to push along, and the bowel wall has to work harder. As a result, the muscles in the colon thicken to help this abnormal situation, which results in greatly increased pressures within the bowel. Over time, this prolonged pressure can push out portions of the bowel wall, causing diverticular pouches. It's like pushing on a balloon.

Although diverticulitis was unknown until 1917, currently about half of all people over the age of 60 have diverticular disease, and about 10 percent of the population will have it by the age of 40. It occurs more commonly in women than in men and with increasing frequency with age. In three-fourths of us, diverticula will never cause any problem or issue. When these diverticular pockets don't bother us, we call it diverticulosis.

When the diverticula become infected, it's called diverticulitis. Infection of the diverticular pockets can be a very serious illness. The suffix "-itis" means "inflammation." You will experience pain, most commonly around the left side of the lower abdomen (except in Asians, who present most often on the right side) and often a fever with or without nausea, vomiting, chills, cramping, and constipation. It is usually at this point that a physician will order tests to discover diverticulitis and diverticulosis. These infections are treated with antibiotics and a soft-fiber diet or liquid. In most cases taking antibiotics will clear up the diverticulitis. If not, it's important to figure out why. If your diverticulitis doesn't respond, you may be in the small minority of people who require surgery. The possible complications of diverticulitis are bleeding, bowel obstruction, fistulas, abscesses, perforation, and peritonitis. So, if you think you are having a diverticular problem, call your doctor.

Once the inflammation resolves, a high-fiber diet is recommended. Diverticular pouches don't go away, but a high-fiber diet will prevent most future attacks. Repeated episodes of diverticulitis may require surgery. A disease of Western civilization, diverticular disease occurs rarely in people who consume a high-fiber diet. There is no evidence to support the notion that people with diverticular disease need to avoid nuts, seeds, or corn once inflammation has resolved.

I can find no good research on natural therapies or herbal medicines for prevention of diverticulitis.

Healing Options

- **Consume a high-fiber diet.** A high-fiber diet is of first and foremost importance for preventing the development and recurrence of diverticular disease. If you are recovering from a flare-up of diverticulitis, begin with a soft-fiber diet. Cook vegetables until fairly soft, eat cooked fruits, use easy-to-digest grains like oatmeal, and make vegetable soups with tofu. Foods with seeds (such as strawberries, poppy seeds, sesame seeds, pumpkin seeds) can catch in your diverticula and cause irritation. Until healed, avoid seed foods.

  Once you are feeling well, establish a high-fiber diet as a normal part of your life. Focus on fruits, vegetables, whole grains, and legumes. Meat, poultry, fish, and dairy products contain zero fiber and need to be eaten in moderation. Psyllium seeds are a good fiber supplement choice because they are nonirritating. Studies have shown that people eating a high-fiber, low-fat diet lower their risks of diverticular disease significantly. (Men who eat a high-red-meat, low-fiber diet have even higher incidences.) It may take you some time to get accustomed to a high-fiber, low-fat diet, but it will be worth the effort. The benefits reach further than your digestive tract, lowering your risk factors for cancer, heart disease, and diabetes. Be certain to drink plenty of water and other healthy beverages.

- **Supplement with probiotics**. Friendly flora can help fight the infection while it's active and protect you from future infection. Take one capsule two to three times daily for prevention; two capsules three times daily during flare-up.
- **Take gamma oryzanol**. While studies of gamma oryzanol, a compound in rice bran oil, were not directly involved with diverticulitis, gamma oryzanol is known to have a healing effect on the colon. (See discussion of gastric ulcers and gastritis in Chapter 20.) Take 100 mg three times daily for three to six weeks.
- **Take protective omega-3 fatty acids.** I can find no research on this in relation to diverticular disease, but fish oils and protective omega-6 oils such as evening primrose oil and borage oil increase the levels of prostaglandin E2 series, which promote healing and repair. Take 1,000 to 2,000 mg three times a day.
- **Take aloe vera.** Aloe vera, which contains vitamins, minerals, and amino acids, has been used by many cultures to heal the digestive tract. Its anti-inflammatory properties are soothing to mucous membranes, and it has been shown to reduce pain. Again, I cannot find any published research in connection to diverticulitis, but use of aloe makes sense. Aloe reduces bleeding time, which is important with ruptured diverticula. Dosages vary from product to product, so read the label.
- **Take slippery elm bark.** Slippery elm bark has demulcent properties and is gentle, soothing, and nourishing to mucous membranes. Drink as a tea, chew on the bark, or take in capsules. To make a tea, simmer 1 teaspoon of slippery elm bark in 2 cups of water for 20 minutes and strain. Sweeten if you want and drink freely; it can be used in large amounts without harm. Or take two to four capsules three times daily.

IRRITABLE BOWEL SYNDROME

Irritable bowel syndrome (IBS) affects 10 to 15 percent of all American adults and is the most common gastrointestinal complaint. Seventy-five percent of those affected never seek a physician's help—they just learn to live with it. Over the years, IBS has had a variety of names: spastic colon, spastic bowel, mucous colitis, colitis, and functional bowel disease. It accounts for 10 percent of all doctor's visits and 50 percent of referrals to gastroenterologists. It's the second most common reason why people miss work, and the economic burden was $1.35 billion in 2003. It affects women three times as often as men. It runs across all socioeconomic groups.

Associated symptoms are abdominal pain and spasms, bloating, gas, and abnormal bowel movements. Bowel movements usually relieve the discomfort. Diarrhea alternating with constipation is the most common pattern, although some people are diagnosed with IBS for chronic constipation. (See "Constipation" earlier in this chapter; the lines between IBS-type constipation and chronic constipation are blurry.)

Anemia, weight loss, rectal bleeding, and fever are *not* symptoms of irritable bowel syndrome. Bowel changes accompanied by these symptoms need to be checked out by a physician to discover the cause.

The Rome III criteria break IBS into different types: IBS-C for constipation, IBS-D for diarrhea dominant, or mixed. However, naming something gets us no closer to helping people, and still most physicians tell people to eat more fiber and go home and have a good life.

IBS has often been treated as a psychosomatic illness or just a lack of dietary fiber, and many people just learn to live with it. Yet the quality of life for someone with IBS is equal to that of someone undergoing chemotherapy for cancer or living with rheumatoid arthritis.

IBS sufferers often have reason to feel stressed, nervous, and depressed about their condition. Stressful situations can trigger IBS symptoms. IBS can significantly restrict one's lifestyle. Most of my IBS clients know where every public restroom is in town. They can't make morning appointments because of the unpredictability of their bowels, and eating away from home can be tricky. Their social lives are tricky or nonexistent.

Underlying Causes of IBS

There is no single cause for IBS, but hopefully we can find the causes for each person and work with him or her individually in response to the biochemical uniqueness.

The first place to begin is to look for small intestinal bacterial overgrowth (SIBO). If IBS is accompanied by either fibromyalgia, chronic fatigue syndrome, or restless leg syndrome, the diagnosis of SIBO is pretty assured. Recent studies suggest that IBS is actually SIBO. Dr. Mark Pimentel and his group report that 78 percent of people with IBS have SIBO. Forty-eight percent were successfully treated with antibiotics (Rifaxamin). Dr. Sergio Peralta reports that of 97 patients with IBS, 56 percent had SIBO. Three weeks after treatment with Rifaxamin for seven days at 1,200 mg, breath tests for SIBO were done. Half of the people had normal tests, and most people had significantly reduced symptoms. People with the best results were those who had alternating constipation/diarrhea-type IBS.

IBS can also be caused by other infections, food sensitivities, celiac disease, leaky gut, imbalances in serotonin, lactose intolerance, infection, mind-body interaction, malabsorption of nutrients, hormonal imbalances, endometriosis, AIDS, environmental sensitivities, and more.

In about 25 percent of people, IBS is initially triggered by infection. The infection causes inflammation in the mucosal tissues, which stimulates T-cell-mediated and smooth muscle changes. When this inflammatory response continues over time, the bowels learn to be over- or underreactive to stimuli. People with postinfection IBS are more likely to have diarrhea-type, as well as high serotonin levels. There is usually a good response in postinfectious IBS with use of probiotic supplements. Use of COX2 inhibitors helps to normalize bowel motility. Natural COX2 inhibitors include turmeric, boswellia, and Kaprex (a product by Metagenics).

Parasites and candida overgrowth are overlooked causes of irritable bowel syndrome. One study showed that 18 percent of the study participants had treatable parasitic infections, while another found giardia in 9 percent and parasites in 15 percent of the study population. Leo Galland, M.D., has found that giardia was responsible for problems in nearly half of his patients with IBS. Even benign pinworms can cause severe colonic cramping at a certain stage of their life cycle. Ask your doctor to order a comprehensive digestive stool analysis with parasitology to determine if parasites or candida are making you sick. (Read Chapter 7 on dysbiosis.)

Women may experience a flare-up in their symptoms around their menstrual period. The most common symptom associated with IBS and menstruation is pain.

Other people have an insulin rise after meals, causing an increase in serotonin, which can cause diarrhea.

Food and IBS

Dietary recommendations need to be tailored to your personal reactions. It is commonly advised to avoid alcohol and monitor sugar intake, coffee, beans, and cabbage family foods (broccoli, Brussels sprouts, cauliflower) because they can be difficult to digest. You need avoid those foods only if they bother you. I find that an elimination diet gives better results than simply eliminating these specific foods.

Food sensitivities are found in one-half to two-thirds of people with IBS and are more prevalent in those who have allergies or come from allergic families. The most common foods that trigger IBS are wheat, corn, dairy products, coffee, tea, citrus fruits, and chocolate. In a study in which people were put on an elimination diet for a year, bloating and distension were relieved by 88 percent, colic pain was reduced by 90 percent, diarrhea was reduced 85 percent, and constipation improved in 54 percent. Also, 79 percent of people who had other symptoms, such as hay fever, asthma, eczema, and hives, saw these symptoms improve.

Undiagnosed lactose intolerance is often the cause of IBS. In a recent study of 242 people, it was found that 43 percent had total remission of IBS when they excluded dairy products from their diet, and another 41 percent had partial improvement. Taking the lactose hydrogen breath test is a valuable way to discover who would benefit from a lactose-free diet. (See Chapter 11.) You can also discover this by avoiding all dairy foods and any products that contain dairy foods for at least two weeks to see how you feel. If you have only moderate improvement, other foods may also be playing a role in your symptoms.

Lactose is not the only sugar to cause problems. Our cells use single-sugar molecules (monosaccharides), but many foods contain two-molecule sugars (disaccharides) that must be split. New research suggests that many people are unable to split mannitol, sucrose, sorbitol, fructose, and other disaccharides, and a high percentage of IBS sufferers are intolerant of one or more of these sugars. The result is diarrhea, gas, and bloating. These people find that fruit, especially citrus fruit, aggravates their symptoms. For these people the Specific Carbohydrate Diet, Atkins Diet, or a Paleolithic-type diet works best. It's also important to rule out dysbiosis.

Breath tests can diagnose fructose, disaccharide, and lactose intolerance. You can do a self-test by avoiding all fruit and sugar for at least 10 days. Be sure to read labels carefully and avoid any product that contains glucose, sucrose, malt, maltose, corn syrup, fructose, brown sugar, honey, maple syrup, molasses, and lactose. You'll find that sugar is everywhere, but if disaccharides are the cause of your IBS, it is worth the time and trouble. If sugars and fruits make you feel worse, do the self-test and a blood or stool test for candida infection or bacterial infection.

Antibiotics are well-known causes of temporary diarrhea and GI problems. Steroid medications can also affect the balance of flora. The good flora are eliminated, especially in people who are on repeated doses of antibiotics, which allows other microbes to dominate the intestinal tract. Acidophilus, bifidobacteria, and Saccharomyces boulardii supplements can help restore intestinal balance.

Mind-body techniques can help with IBS. There are good studies on yoga, biofeedback, counseling, and more.

Functional Laboratory Testing

- Comprehensive digestive stool analysis with parasitology
- Lactose breath test
- Hydrogen breath test for methane levels
- Food allergy and sensitivity testing
- Intestinal permeability screening
- Organic acid testing

Healing Options

- **Look for infection.** Since most people with IBS have small intestinal bacterial overgrowth, this is a terrific place to begin your quest. It's possible someone with IBS has a fungal infection, C. difficile or another type of bacterial infection, or Blastocystis hominis or other parasitic infection. (See treatment recommendations in Chapter 9 and testing in Chapter 11.)

- **Increase fiber intake.** High-fiber diets are recommended for people with IBS. You can use high-fiber cereals to boost fiber content, but recent research indicates that wheat bran made the problem worse in 55 percent of cases, whereas it improved symptoms in only 10 percent of patients. This is not surprising because a significant number of people with IBS have a hypersensitivity to wheat products. If you want to add a fiber supplement, use psyllium seeds, flaxseed, or hemp seed. In a study in which psyllium was given to people with IBS, it improved several parameters by increasing the number of bowel movements per week, enlarging stool weight, and speeding up transit times. No negative side effects were reported.

- **Evaluate possible lactose intolerance.** Lactose intolerance is often the underlying cause of IBS. Take the hydrogen breath test or eliminate all dairy products and any products containing dairy from your diet for at least two weeks to help you determine whether lactose intolerance is contributing to your problem.

- **Add probiotics**. In numerous studies, probiotic supplements have been shown to help regulate IBS. Products with multiple strains of microbes would be best. Make sure they at least include lactobacilli and bifidobacteria. Studies on E. coli strain Nissle have also shown much promise.

- **Try an elimination diet.** I've seen pretty amazing responses in IBS in about 50 percent of the people I work with on elimination diets.

After you've tried the dietary approaches, consider these additional options.

- **Explore behavioral therapies**. Biofeedback, self-hypnosis, and other relaxation techniques are widely used to help people with IBS. Stress often triggers bowel symptoms, and learning stress-modification techniques can alter our reactions. If we don't react with alarm to a situation, our body doesn't sense it as stressful.

- **Add glutamine.** Glutamine, the most abundant amino acid in the body, is used by the digestive tract as a fuel source and for healing IBS. Take 4 to 8 grams daily for a trial period of four weeks.

- **Take EPA/DHA fish oil.** Fish oils inhibit the formation of inflammatory prostaglandins and leukotrienes. They may be effective in reducing the pain and inflammation associated with IBS. Take 1,000 to 2,000 mg daily in fish oil capsules, or 300 mg daily of Neuromins.

- **Take peppermint oil.** Peppermint oil is a muscle relaxant that is widely used in England for IBS. More recently there was a published case study on using peppermint oil for a patient with SIBO. That makes sense, since these two diagnoses are interwoven. To get the oil into the intestines intact, use enteric-coated peppermint oil. (The coating prevents it from dissolving in the stomach.) Take one to two capsules daily between meals. During a spasm, you can rub a drop or two of the oil inside your anus with a finger. Caution: it stings!

- **Try herbs.** Chamomile, melissa (balm), rosemary, and valerian all have antispasmodic properties. They help relieve and expel gas, strengthen and tone the stomach, and soothe pain. Valerian, hops, skullcap, and passionflower are all calming herbs and can be found in a combination product. Antidepressant medication is often used by physicians for IBS; these gentle, effective calmatives may give you similar results. Use these herbs in capsules, tinctures, and teas.

- **Eat ginger.** Ginger, either fresh or powdered, helps relieve gas pains. It can be added to foods or used in tea. Within 20 to 30 minutes you'll be belching and/or passing gas, which will relieve the discomfort. To make a tea, take two or three slices of fresh ginger or ½ teaspoon dried ginger in 1 cup of boiled water. Combine it with other herbs, such as peppermint or chamomile, to enhance the effect.

- **Take a multivitamin with minerals.** Taking a multivitamin and mineral supplement will give a good foundation to your nutritional program. If you have had diarrhea long-term, you are likely to be deficient in many nutrients.

- **Take calcium-magnesium citrate.** Anecdotally, many people have found that calcium-magnesium supplements prevent or alleviate the muscle spasms associated with IBS. Take 500 to 1,000 mg calcium, and 300 to 750 mg magnesium. Be aware that too much magnesium will cause diarrhea.

INFLAMMATORY BOWEL DISEASE: CROHN'S DISEASE, ULCERATIVE COLITIS, MICROSCOPIC COLITIS, AND ISCHEMIC COLITIS

Inflammatory bowel diseases (IBD) include four distinct illnesses: ulcerative colitis, Crohn's disease, microscopic colitis (lymphoid and collagenous), and ischemic colitis. Each of these diseases has slightly different characteristics, although the treatment for all of them is aimed at reducing inflammation. IBD affects one million to two million Americans; ulcerative colitis rates are about 2 people per 1,000; and Crohn's disease rates are about 1.7 per 1,000. Rates have risen since 1940 and are rising in other parts of the world where Western diets are becoming the norm. Most cases are diagnosed before age 40. IBD tends to run in families and is more prevalent among people of Jewish descent. There is a higher incidence of IBD in women who take oral contraceptives. Women with a history of IBD or with a family history of IBD may want to choose a different form of birth control.

In all types of IBD, looking for underlying causes or triggers is important. Using the DIGIN model can be extremely useful.

IBD shares many of the symptoms of IBS, but they are very different problems. IBD involves inflammation of the digestive tract, which can occur anywhere from the mouth to the rectum. Malnutrition and malabsorption are common in people with active IBD. Symptoms include abdominal pain, bloody diarrhea, and cramping. If you are having these symptoms, go see your physician. These symptoms may also be accompanied by fever, rectal bleeding, abdominal tenderness, abscesses, constipation, weight loss, awakening during the night with diarrhea, and a failure to thrive in children. Symptoms come and go and can go into remission for months or years. About half of the people with IBD have only mild symptoms. People with IBD often develop complications, which include inflammation of the eyes or skin, arthritis, liver disease, kidney stones, and colon cancer.

IBD is considered an autoimmune disease (your body begins attacking itself). The causes are many and have produced much debate. Current theories suggest that Crohn's and ulcerative colitis have a genetic component, which is triggered to a greater or lesser extent by either infection, a hypersensitivity to antigens in the gut wall, an inflammation of the blood vessels that causes ischemia (a lack of blood supply to the tissues), or food sensitivities. The genes known to be associated with Crohn's disease include NOD2 (also known as CARD15), ATG15L1, IL23R, and IRGM, which all have to do with innate immunity. The NOD gene apparently gives the person a rapid response to gut bacteria and/or their toxic by-products, which causes an overstimulation and production of NF-kappaB and cytokine, which stimulate inflammation. The NOD gene is found in only 10 to 15 percent of people with Crohn's. Obviously, much work still needs to be done to explore the genetics of IBD.

IBD is not caused by emotional illness or psychiatric disorder, though the condition may cause emotional problems because of its chronic nature, painful episodes, and lifestyle limitations. Prolonged treatment with steroid medications can cause side effects of depression, mania or euphoria, and bone loss.

Dysbiosis and IBD

There is a lot of research indicating that dysbiosis plays a significant role in IBD. Since the gut microbiome is the center of our immune system, this makes sense. Studies have reported increased levels of gram negative anaerobic bacteria, such as Bacteroides species, and lower levels of Bifidobacteria species in Crohn's disease, ulcerative colitis, and pouchitis (infection of the diverticula). E. coli has also been implicated in Crohn's disease. We need a lot more research on the use of probiotics, prebiotics, treating known infection, and breaking up the biofilms with probiotics, enzymes, and fiber in these conditions.

The most common microbes involved are E. coli, staphylococcus, streptococcus, proteus, Mycoplasma pneumoniae, Chlamydia psittaci, Clostridium difficile toxin, and Coxiella burnetii. Bacterial infections occurred in one-quarter of all recurrence of IBD.

There is even research implicating poor dental hygiene with increased risk of IBD. Apparently bacterial infection in the mouth can lead to IBD. Brush your teeth—it helps prevent heart disease, too. (See Chapter 29 for more on cardiovascular disease.)

At Digestive Disease Week in 2009, Henrick Nielsen, M.D., of Denmark, presented a study where he reviewed citizens' health records. People who had previously had food poisoning (salmonella and campylobacter) had 2.5 times increased risk of developing IBD over the next 15 years. A flare-up of symptoms commonly occurs with infections.

Ulcerative Colitis

Ulcerative colitis is a continuous inflammation of the mucosal lining of the colon and/or rectum. In the descending colon it is sometimes called left-sided disease, and in the rectum it is called distal disease, ulcerative proctitis, or proctosigmoiditis. If sores are present, they are shallow, and it is generally milder and easier to treat in the rectum. The most common symptoms are abdominal pain, diarrhea, and blood in stools that is maroon colored.

Of people with ulcerative colitis, 20 to 25 percent eventually require surgery because of massive bleeding, chronic illness, perforation of the colon, or risk of colon cancer. Five percent of people with ulcerative colitis ultimately develop colon cancer, and the degree of illness correlates with its incidence. For example, cancer levels aren't higher for people who are affected only in the rectum and distal end of the colon.

The current medications for ulcerative colitis have focused on decreasing inflammation and TNF-alpha. Drs. O. Brain and S. P. Travis at Oxford Radcliff Hospital suggest that this may be wrong. They postulate that defects in barrier function (leaky gut) and innate mucosal immunity (such as a poor ability to kill bacteria) may be the primary causes. These issues then lead to inflammation. If they are correct, then building immunity and healing a leaky gut play a leading role.

Crohn's Disease

The most common symptoms of Crohn's disease include abdominal pain, diarrhea, weight loss, and malnutrition. Crohn's disease can occur anywhere along the digestive tract, from mouth to rectum, but is most common in the colon and ileum near the ileocecal valve. It is sometimes called right-sided disease. Frequent symptoms are fevers that last 24 to 48 hours, canker sores in the mouth, clubbed fingernails, and a thickening of the GI lining, which may cause constrictions and blockage. Inflammation develops in a skip pattern, a little here and a little there, and goes more deeply into the tissues than with ulcerative colitis. In later stages, it can form abscesses and fistulas, little canals that lead to other organs or form tiny caves. If they become serious, surgery may be recommended. If you require surgery for Crohn's disease, it is important to know which part of the intestines were removed and which nutrients may have inadequate uptake. (See Figure 2.1 for an absorption chart.)

Research implicates measles as a possible cause of Crohn's disease. British scientists found measles virus in diseased parts of the colon, while Swedish researchers found a high incidence of Crohn's disease in people who were exposed to measles in utero. Another British study showed that people who had received live measles vaccines had a threefold increase of Crohn's disease, while ulcerative colitis rose by two and a half times. This study did not prove that the bowel disease was actually caused by measles, only that there was a correlation.

Some people with Crohn's disease have flare-ups in a seasonal cycle, which suggests an allergy component to the illness. While studies have shown that allergy is a factor in a small number of people, a survey of members of the National Foundation of Ileitis and Colitis showed that 70 percent of people with IBD listed other symptoms that were probably allergy related. This led one researcher to say "inflammatory bowel disease is just another possible facet of allergy." Mold sensitivity and allergies to candida and other types of fungus have also been proven to provoke IBD symptoms.

Microscopic Colitis

Microscopic colitis is a newer diagnosis. It is characterized by diarrhea, cramps, and abdominal pain. The diarrhea may be continuous or can come and go. There can also be fatigue, fever, or joint pain. When a colonoscopy is done, all looks normal, yet when cells are biopsied under a microscope inflammation is seen. Microscopic colitis is often misdiagnosed because a biopsy is needed to make a definitive diagnosis. Microscopic colitis doesn't appear to morph into Crohn's disease, ulcerative colitis, or cancer. There is some genetic component; it often runs in families.

There are two types of microscopic colitis: collagenous colitis and lymphocytic colitis. In collagenous colitis there is a thickening of the collagen layer in the colon and an increase in inflammatory cytokines. There may also be an increase in lymphocytes, a type of white blood cell. Lymphocytic colitis is characterized by increased numbers of intraepithelial lymphocytes (IELs), which are specific types of white blood cells. This results in watery, nonbloody diarrhea. About half of people have a sudden onset and know exactly when it began. A common trigger is dysentery, giardia, or other intestinal infection.

There are several theories about the origins of microscopic colitis. Some believe it is an autoimmune disease; others suggest that it is caused by a virus, bacteria, or bacterial toxin; and another theory is that it is aggravated or triggered by use of NSAIDs. Probably it's a combination of these that triggers the illness. Like Crohn's disease and ulcerative colitis, microscopic colitis can come and go with flare-ups and healing.

Both types are most often seen in middle-aged women, but they can be found in men, women, and children of all ages. Some cases resolve on their own without any treatment. Fiber and fluids are recommended. Sometimes people might be given a medication to stop the diarrhea. Saccharomyces boulardii is a probiotic that is useful for diarrhea from all causes. If the flare-up is severe, anti-inflammatory drugs, steroids, or antibiotics may be used.

Ischemic Colitis

Ischemic colitis typically occurs in people over the age of 60 and is associated with cardiovascular disease. It occurs when blood flow from arteries to a part of your colon is reduced. Most often this is due to atherosclerosis, a buildup of fatty deposits in your artery. This results in inflammation that can cause temporary or permanent damage to your colon. It can occur anywhere but most often happens on the left side of the colon. When this occurs on the right side of the colon, it can be more serious because the same arteries also feed the small intestine. The most common presentation is abdominal pain, rectal bleeding and often urgent bowel movements, nausea, diarrhea, or vomiting. This usually presents as a flare-up and then subsides. Treatment is typically rest, lots of fluids, and possibly IV antibiotics. Once treated, this typically doesn't recur.

Ischemic colitis can also be caused by or related to other conditions, including vasculitis (inflamed blood vessels), diabetes, blood clotting, radiation treatment to the abdomen, infections (such as Clostridium difficile, shigella, or E. coli), and dehydration. In rare cases medications can precipitate ischemic colitis, including use of birth control pills, estrogen replacement, NSAIDs, migraine medications (triptan and ergot types), antipsychotic drugs, pseudoephedrine, alostron (Lotronex for IBS), and cocaine.

Probiotics in IBD

Where this takes us on a practical level is to look at what we can do to have a healthy gut bacterial environment. Numerous studies have shown that use of probiotic supplements is beneficial for people with IBD. They have been shown to help maintain remission of flare-ups in Crohn's disease, ulcerative colitis, and pouchitis. Probiotic bacteria, like L. acidophilus, bifidobacteria, and the Nissle strain of E. coli, provide competition for other microbes and push them out. Commensal bacteria stimulate our immune response, increase beneficial antibodies such as sIgA, IgM, and IgG, balance pH, and enhance tight junction integrity. Probiotic therapy with E. coli strain Nissle has been shown to be effective in treatment for ulcerative colitis and was found to be equivalent to the drug mesalamine for short-term maintenance of the disease and after use of steroid treatment for remission. VSL#3 is a formula with eight different probiotic species that has been used for pouchitis.

Much more research needs to be done on IBD and probiotics. Different combinations will work for different people and to greater or lesser effect. You'll have to experiment with different brands and see which are most helpful. Remember to begin with a small dosage and increase slowly. You are changing your gut ecology and you want to do it gradually. You can think of them as a medicine that you'll probably need to take daily for life.

A 2004 study tested probiotic bacteria in mice. The exciting part of this study showed that sterilized probiotics worked as well as live probiotics in chemically induced ulcerative colitis. (The use of dead probiotics to modulate the immune system is discussed in Chapter 6.)

Although there is not much research on the yeast connection to IBD, clinicians have often found antifungal therapies to be useful. Friendly flora have been found to be dramatically out of balance in people with IBD, so use of probiotic supplements is highly recommended. Use of the comprehensive digestive stool analysis with parasitology screening and intestinal permeability tests will uncover many of these problems.

Treatment

Medical treatment for IBD consists of anti-inflammatory drugs [e.g., sulfasalazine (Asulfadine), mesalamine (Asacol), olsalazine, balasalazide], steroids (e.g., prednisone), immune suppressors (e.g., azathioprine, cyclosporine, methotrexate), and sometimes antibiotics. While these medications can often relieve symptoms of IBD, they carry their own risks. Some specific drug side effects include bone loss and low cortisol levels due to use of steroid medications, and folic acid deficiency from use of sulfasalazine. Azathioprine (Imuran) has been associated with a small rise in the incidence of lymphoma.

Infliximab (Remecade) and Humira are new drugs that are being used for people who have Crohn's disease and the fistulas caused by it. Research is ongoing for its use in ulcerative colitis too. A monoclonal antibody, infliximab has a high specificity for tumor necrosis factor (TNF-alpha). Humira also targets TNF-alpha. This is an entirely new approach that focuses on stimulating the immune system to stop inflammation in people with severe disease. Many people are able to stop taking steroid medications, and quality of life is increased. Yet, by suppressing immune function, you risk opening yourself up to other diseases.

Another drug called ecabet sodium works by helping to heal and soothe the mucosal lining. Most of the research on this medication focuses on its use in GERD and in treatment for H. pylori. Nonetheless, for people with IBD, it's believed to help by targeting cell-signaling pathways to normalize kinas activation.

A very new approach to IBD is with the use of the Bowman-Birk protease inhibitor, called BBI; testing is in initial stages. BBI is derived from soybeans and is naturally found in all legumes. You'd need to eat huge amounts to get the same effects, but you might find them to be helpful. Remember that legumes are loaded with fiber, help lower serum cholesterol levels, and offer a vegetable protein of high quality.

Medications are often necessary, but use of complementary therapies can reduce the need for them, so that when you really need medication during a flare-up it works effectively. For example, repeated use of prednisone can lead to its failure as an available therapy.

The good news is that effective natural therapies address the underlying factors of the disease, reduce the need for prescription medications, and heal the bowel. Among the hundreds of patients with IBD that Drs. Jonathan Wright and Alan Gaby, two nutritionally oriented M.D.s, have seen, most have improved, many dramatically. The key to success appears to be getting people into remission as fast as possible. To do this effectively, a combination of medication and supplements may be necessary. Once a flare-up has died down, natural therapies are highly successful in preventing a recurrence. It's also really important to take care of yourself when you are well and to practice stress-management techniques to help reduce the number and severity of flare-ups.

One of the most promising new therapies is the use of phosphatidylcholine. People with ulcerative colitis have been seen to have low levels of phosphatidylcholine in their colonic mucus. Phospholipids are essential for the mucous barrier to protect us. When these levels are low, we are likely to have leakiness. Some people are able to stop steroid medications when taking sustained-release phosphatidylcholine at levels of 2 to 4 grams daily. There have been three studies on this therapy, all from the same research group, one of which holds a patent on this particular form of phosphatidylcholine. This gives a possible bias. Also, I wonder whether regular phosphatidylcholine might work as well.

Diet and Nutritional Deficiencies Associated with IBD

No one diet will help all people with IBD, although an elemental diet, the Specific Carbohydrate Diet (details of the SCD program are discussed under "Healing Options"), and the Gut and Psychology Syndrome (GAPS) diet work especially well for people with Crohn's disease. An elemental diet, which has resulted in a reduction of intestinal permeability as well as its symptoms, includes synthetic foods you drink or are given through a tube. It has been found to be as good as steroids in reducing inflammation in a flare-up of Crohn's disease.

Up to 90 percent of people will get huge benefits from going on an elemental diet, which relies in part on medical foods. Medical foods are hypoallergenic foods that contain proteins, fats, and carbohydrates that have been broken down into single amino acids, fatty acids, and simple carbohydrates so that no digestion is necessary. This allows for inflammation to diminish and leaky gut to heal. But there are problems with use of an elemental diet. It is unpalatable to many people, and they won't drink it. Newer products that are tastier are coming on the market.

Food sensitivities play a significant role in a subset of people with IBD. Many IBD patients report significant improvement with use of an elimination diet over a three-week period. After this, they gradually add foods back into their diet to see which ones provoke bloating, pain, diarrhea, bleeding, or other symptoms. One study found that 13 percent of children with IBD were allergic to cow's milk during infancy. It is essential to check for food allergies and food sensitivities. Studies have shown reduction in symptoms and inflammation in people who adhere to a hypoallergenic diet because it reduces inflammation. People with bowel disease are especially sensitive to most grains. Chemicals from some foods are irritating to the bowels. Truly, nearly any food can cause irritation and inflammation. In various studies, citrus, pineapple, dairy, coffee, tomatoes, cheese, bananas, sugar, additives, preservatives, spices, beverages other than water, and bread have all been implicated. You'll need to be tested for both IgE and IgG antibodies to determine your food sensitivities. Testing of IgA and IgM antibodies is also useful.

A low-sulfur diet may be of benefit in Crohn's disease. Studies have shown an increase in sulfur-eating bacteria in people with bowel disease in comparison with other people. In a 1998 study by Dr. William Roediger, four people were advised to avoid high-sulfur foods, including eggs, cheese, whole milk, ice cream, mayonnaise, soy milk, mineral water, sulfited drinks (including wine), nuts, and cruciferous vegetables (broccoli, cabbage, cauliflower, Brussels sprouts, and so forth), and to reduce red meats. They were advised to get protein from fish and chicken. Dr. Roediger found significant changes—participants had no relapses or attacks while on the diet, and there were no adverse effects from the diet itself. The expected relapse rate had been 22.6 percent. Of the four people in the study, one was able to stop taking steroid medication and had been attack free for 18 months, compared to the four attacks experienced in the 18 months before the dietary changes. The other three showed microscopic improvement of inflammation. The average number of daily bowel movements in all four was reduced from six to one and one-half.

Diets that are low in fiber and high in animal fat and sugar have been implicated in the development of IBD. Cigarettes and fast foods have also been implicated in IBD. Oddly enough, eating fried potatoes has also been implicated in increased IBD. It's believed that the glycoalkaloids (alpha-solanine and alpha-chaconine), which are concentrated when potatoes are fried, increase gut permeability.

Because of bleeding and continued irritation, malabsorption of nutrients is often found in people with IBD. These same nutrients are often vital for repair, so the cycle worsens. Low serum levels of zinc, an important nutrient for wound repair, are often found in people with IBD. Folic acid helps repair tissue and prevents diarrhea. Prolonged bleeding can cause deficiencies of copper, zinc, iron, folic acid, and vitamin B_{12}.

Studies have shown an increased need for antioxidant nutrients such as vitamins A, B_3 (niacin), C, E, and K, selenium, calcium, phosphorus, copper, iron, zinc, glutathione, and superoxide dismutase (SOD). Many also have anemia, which is related to iron, B_{12}, copper, and/or folic acid deficiencies.

People with IBD have an increased level of inflammatory cytokines. Many natural substances can modulate these effects. Fish oils have been shown to be helpful for dampening this inflammation in Crohn's disease, although the research isn't entirely conclusive.

Several studies have shown bone loss in people with Crohn's disease and ulcerative colitis. While incidence of loss in some studies is correlated with use of steroid medications, in others it appears to be independent. It is advisable to do at least a baseline bone density study to see if you are at risk. Also check vitamin D levels and try to keep them in the higher end of the normal range. If risk of bone loss is determined, increasing all bone nutrients would be advised. A study on low-impact exercise in people with Crohn's disease found that bone density was significantly increased. So get out there and exercise regularly.

Nicotine and IBD

One unusual twist in the story is that nicotine appears to be protective for ulcerative colitis, while it makes Crohn's disease worse. Although normally I wouldn't recommend nicotine patches, the severity of the disease could warrant a try. Nicotene is certainly less toxic than the usual drugs that are used. The studies show positive results, using 15 to 25 mg patches over periods of four to six weeks along with mesalamine. Many people stayed in remission for up to three months after stopping the patch. One study gave people who were in relapse either nicotine or prednisone with mesalamine for five weeks. The relapse rate was much better in the nicotine group— only 20 percent in comparison to a 60 percent relapse rate for those on prednisone. In the long term, nicotine patches appear to help with flare-ups and maintenance when used with mesalamine.

Less Conventional and Highly Effective Approaches to IBD

There are many additional approaches for IBD. There have been several studies on the use of TSO whipworms to modulate the immune system and halt flare-ups in IBD. (See Chapter 9 for more information on this.) One promising approach involves photopheresis, a process that exposes blood to light and many herbal therapies. Natural COX2 inhibitors, such as curcumin, green tea, and boswellia, also show promise.

You won't believe this, but Dr. Thomas Borody, an Australian physician, took three men and three women with ulcerative colitis and gave them colonic enemas with the bowel movements of healthy people for five consecutive days. Four of the six had total remission of their symptoms within four months. One to 13 years later, they were still completely well and without use of any medications. They call this method fecal bacteriotherapy. Nonetheless, nearly all of his research since then has been on people with C. difficile. It's been highly effective in people with C. difficile infection. I have one client who went to Australia to see Dr. Borody for her bowel issues who had great results. She'd love to have fecal bacteriotherapy done again. A

2010 paper by Faith Rohlke, Cristina Surawicz, and Neil Stollman reports that in 19 people with C. difficile, 18 went into remission after a single treatment and the last person after two treatments. All patients remained symptom free for periods spanning six months to four years.

Functional Laboratory Testing

- Comprehensive digestive stool analysis with parasitology
- Lactose breath test
- Food and environmental sensitivity testing
- Calprotectin or lactoferrin (great for diagnosis and monitoring treatment)
- Intestinal permeability screening
- Antioxidant analysis
- Bone density testing and vitamin D levels
- Immunogenetics testing
- Nutritional analysis of blood

Healing Options

- **Make dietary changes.** Eliminate simple sugars, alcohol, and fast foods (one study showed that flare-ups occurred almost four times as frequently in people with ulcerative colitis when fast foods were eaten twice a week). Grains and dairy products often aggravate the condition. Some people find that going on a raw-foods diet with lots of fresh vegetable juices stops IBD in its tracks. I've had several clients who had IBD early in life who cured it this way. Work with a clinician if you decide to try a raw-foods diet. It's not for everyone.

- **Maintain a normal weight.** While dietary changes can be useful, don't limit your food so severely that you lose weight and muscle mass. Especially in people with Crohn's disease, malnutrition is common. Find a diet that works for you and helps you maintain your weight and health. Don't limit wheat, dairy, other grains, nuts, or seeds unless you are pretty sure that they are causing problems.

- **Correct anemia if present. Correct other vitamin and mineral deficiencies if present. Correct vitamin D levels if they are low. Take a multivitamin with minerals and antioxidant nutrients.** Because of general malabsorption and poor dietary habits in people with Crohn's disease and ulcerative colitis, it is wise to closely measure yourself for nutritional status with testing. Also add a good-quality multivitamin with minerals to your daily routine. Deficiencies of many nutrients have been found in people with IBD: calcium/magnesium; folic acid; iron; selenium; vitamins A, B_1, B_2, B_6, C, D, and E; and zinc. Because oxidative damage plays a significant role in IBD, the supplement should contain adequate amounts of antioxidant nutrients: at least 10,000 IU of beta-carotene or other carotenoids, 400 IU of vitamin E, 250 mg of vitamin C, 200 mcg of selenium, 5 mg of zinc, plus other nutrients. It may also contain CoQ10, glutathione, NAC, Pycnogenol, superoxide dismutase (SOD), and other antioxidants. It is best to buy a supplement that is free of foods, herbs, colorings, and common allergens.

- **Explore possible lactose intolerance.** Hydrogen breath testing or elimination of all dairy products and foods containing dairy from your diet for at least two weeks can help determine whether lactose intolerance is contributing to your problem. Definitely eliminate dairy during a flare-up of your illness.

- **Consider food sensitivities.** Food sensitivities play a significant role in ulcerative colitis and Crohn's disease, occurring approximately half the time. Try an elimination diet, SCD, or GAPS diet. The most common offenders are dairy products, grains, and yeast, followed in frequency by egg, potato, rye, coffee, apples, mushrooms, oats, and chocolate.

- **Try the Specific Carbohydrate Diet (SCD).** Many people have found relief from using the Specific Carbohydrate Diet outlined in Elaine Gottschall's book *Breaking the Vicious Cycle*. Unfortunately we don't yet have any clinical research on the SCD. This diet can be beneficial because it eliminates most foods that cause sensitivities—grains and dairy products. Similar to the candida diet (see Chapter 7), it helps restore intestinal balance. While going on the diet alone may be effective, it is most effective after laboratory testing has determined your unique biochemistry.

- **Take glutamine.** Glutamine is the first nutrient I recommend for bowel and intestinal health. It is the most abundant amino acid in our bodies. The digestive tract uses glutamine as the primary nutrient for the intestinal cells, and it is effective for healing stomach ulcers, irritable bowel syndrome, and ulcerative bowel diseases.

Douglas Wilmore, M.D., has done a lot of clinical research giving high doses of glutamine to people who have short bowel syndrome. This occurs when only a short portion of the colon remains after surgery. These people develop chronic diarrhea and often cannot tolerate any real food. With a high-fiber, high-glutamine diet, and short-term use of growth hormones, Dr. Wilmore was able to normalize bowel function. Glutamine is also great for building muscle mass. Begin with 8 to 20 grams daily for a trial period of four weeks. In clinical settings, up to 40 grams daily have been used.

A study of Nigerian rabbits reported that when honey was added to glutamine supplementation after bowel resectioning, rabbits who got honey had better healing. The researchers report that this might also have benefits in people who have had bowel-resectioning surgery.

- **Try bromelain.** Bromelain, a protein-splitting enzyme derived from the green stems of pineapple, was studied and shown to reduce the incidence and severity of ulcerative colitis with no negative effects even in large doses. Dosages were not listed in this study. Typical doses of bromelain range from 1,000 mg to 3,000 mg daily.

- **Try tormentil.** Tormentil (Potentilla tormentilla), an herb and member of the rose family, is being studied for its effect in ulcerative colitis. According to Grieve's *A Modern Herbal*, it nourishes and supports the bowels and stops diarrhea. It's been reported to have high antioxidant properties and polyphenols. While in early clinical testing, one study with 16 people reported improvements in those treated with 2,400 mg daily. Although the study was done on ulcerative colitis, the benefits could certainly extend to other inflammatory bowel conditions.

- **Take sustained-release phosphatidylcholine.** Recent research on the use of sustained-release phosphatidylcholine in people with ulcerative colitis looks quite promising. Effective doses appear to be 2 to 4 grams daily.

- **Take folic acid.** One of folic acid's main functions is to help with the repair and maintenance of epithelial cells, such as those in the bowel. The drug Asulfadine, commonly prescribed for bowel inflammation, causes a 30 percent loss of folic acid. Even those who don't take Asulfadine may benefit greatly from folic acid supplementation. In one study, 24 people with bowel disease were given either a placebo or 15 mg of folic acid daily. Beneficial changes to the cells were observed in those receiving the folic acid. In my own clinical experience, I have found that a combination of glutamine and folic acid can often rapidly reduce inflammation and irritation in bowel disease. While I used to use high-dose folic acid (5 to 10 mg daily), I've become more cautious because it appears that in susceptible people who already have colon cancer, it may promote cancer growth. Monitor folic acid levels with blood testing and/or organic acid testing.

- **Try wheatgrass juice.** People with ulcerative colitis have had great results reducing flare-ups of the disease by drinking wheatgrass juice. In 2002 Israeli researchers finally put it to the test. Twenty-three people with active distal ulcerative colitis were given either 3½ ounces (100 cc) of wheatgrass juice daily or a green placebo daily for one month. People who received the wheatgrass juice had less severe flare-ups of the disease and less blood loss. Wheatgrass juice is high in glutathione. Low glutathione levels have been found in people with inflammatory bowel disease. There was also improvement in sigmoidoscopy. This is certainly a nontoxic and easy remedy to try.

- **Increase glutathione naturally.** Inflammatory bowel disease is one of increased free radicals. One of the most important reducers of inflammation due to toxicity is glutathione. Two of the simplest ways to increase your glutathione levels are to use a good quality whey protein powder daily and take N-acetyl cysteine (NAC). Dosages of NAC range from 500 to 2,000 mg daily.

- **Increase consumption of omega-3 fatty acids.** Salmon, mackerel, herring, tuna, sardines, and halibut are all excellent sources of EPA/DHA oils. Eating these fish several times a week can supply your body with these essential fats. Seaweeds also provide generous amounts of omega-3 oils, but carrageenan, an extract from seaweed, may increase the inflammation in the colon. While carrageenan is used in animals to produce IBD, in humans the research is not yet clear. To be on the safe side, avoid red and brown seaweeds.

  You can also take capsules of EPA/DHA oils daily. In a recent study, it was found that use of Max/EPA decreased disease activity by 58 percent over a period of eight months. No patient worsened, and eight out of eleven were able to reduce or discontinue use of medication. The dosage was 15 capsules of Max/EPA, which contained 2.7 grams of EPA and 1.8 grams of DHA, per day. Many other studies also show the benefit of fish oils with dosages between 3.5 and 5.5 grams daily.

- **Take probiotics and prebiotic fibers.** E. coli strain Nissle 1917 was found in three studies to be equal to use of 5-ASA medication. VSL#3 has also been studied to keep people in remission and prevent pouchitis. There is much that is unknown, yet probiotics and prebiotics play an important role in modulation of inflammation and immune response. The dose ought to be in proportion to the level of inflammation. (See Chapter 6 for more on probiotics.)

- **Consider TSO whipworm therapy.** Use of benign whipworm eggs can modulate your immune system to calm down and prevent flare-ups. There is a growing body of research on this in IBD. (See Chapter 6 for more information.)

- **Take gamma oryzanol.** Gamma oryzanol, a compound found in rice bran oil, is a useful therapeutic tool for gastritis, ulcers, and irritable bowel syndrome. Try taking 100 mg three times daily for a period of three to six weeks. (See Chapter 20 for more on gamma oryzanol.)

- **Take boswellia.** Boswellia has been used in Ayurvedic medicine as an anti-inflammatory for ulcerative colitis. Only one study has been done so far, but in comparison with sulfasalazine it was equivalent. Take 350 mg three times daily.

- **Try butyrate enemas.** Butyrate is the preferred fuel of the colonic cells. It is produced when fiber in the colon is fermented by intestinal flora, predominantly bifidobacteria. A few studies have shown that butyrate enemas, taken twice daily, helped heal active distal ulcerative colitis.

- **Explore herbal remedies.** Demulcent herbs—marshmallow, slippery elm, acacia, chickweed, comfrey, mullein, and plantain—are beneficial and soothing to the intestinal membranes and help stimulate mucus production. All are gentle enough to be used at will; try them in capsule or tea form. Other herbs used by people with bowel disease include wild indigo, purple cornflower, echinacea, American cranesbill, goldenseal, cabbage powder, wild yam, bayberry, agrimony, neem, aloe vera, chamomile, feverfew, ginger, ginkgo biloba, Saint-John's-wort, milk thistle, valerian, peppermint, hawthorn, and Lapacho.

- **Drink aloe vera juice.** Aloe vera juice has been used as a traditional remedy for digestive disorders of all types. A randomized, double-blind, placebo-controlled trial was done using oral aloe vera gel in people with active colitis. Forty-four people were given 3 ounces daily of either aloe vera gel or a placebo for four weeks. People who received the aloe vera had a significant reduction of all disease symptoms in comparison with people who received the placebo.

- **Try bovine cartilage.** Bovine cartilage is shown to have anti-inflammatory and wound-healing properties. Its benefit has been documented in many illnesses, including ulcerative colitis, hemorrhoids and fissures, rheumatoid arthritis, and osteoarthritis.

HEMORRHOIDS

About half of Americans over the age of 50 have hemorrhoids. They are not life-threatening or dangerous, but they can be painful and might bleed. They occur when blood vessels in and around the anus get swollen and stretch under pressure, similar to varicose veins in the legs. They are found either inside the anus (internal hemorrhoids) or under the skin around the anus (external hemorrhoids). Internal hemorrhoids may become so swollen that they push through the anus. When they become irritated, inflamed, and painful, they are called protruding hemorrhoids.

Straining during bowel movements is a common cause of hemorrhoids. The most common symptom is bright red blood with a bowel movement. Hemorrhoids are also common but temporary during pregnancy. Hormonal changes cause the blood vessels to expand. During childbirth, extreme pressure is put on the anus.

Hemorrhoids also occur in people with chronic constipation or diarrhea. Sitting for long periods, heavy lifting, and genetics are other influential factors. In most cases, hemorrhoids go away in a few days. If you have bleeding that lasts longer, have your doctor examine you to rule out a more serious problem.

Fiber and Hemorrhoids

A high-fiber diet with plenty of fluids—water, fruit juices, and herbal teas—helps prevent hemorrhoids because fiber and fluids soften stool so they pass through easily. No straining with bowel movements means less pressure on the blood vessels near your anus. So, increase your intake of fruits, whole grains, legumes, and vegetables, especially those containing the most fiber: asparagus, Brussels sprouts, cabbage, carrots, cauliflower, corn, peas, kale, and parsnips. Eating a high-fiber breakfast cereal significantly increases your fiber intake.

Could It Be Pinworms?

Hemorrhoids generally don't itch. If your anus itches mainly at night, you might have pinworms. The best time to check for them is at night while you itch. Place a piece of tape around your finger, sticky side out. Put the tape on your anus, pull it off, and check for worms, which look like moving white threads. If you are checking one of your children, you can use the tape method or just look. Another cause of rectal itching is called pruritus ani, which can be caused by food sensitivities, contact with irritating substances (laundry detergent or toilet paper), fungi, bacterial infection, parasites, antibiotics, poor hygiene, or tight clothing. If you have hemorrhoids, you might find relief from the following suggestions.

Prevention

Explore all of the recommendations for constipation (earlier in this chapter).

Healing Options

- **Change your bathroom habits.** In many countries, people squat to relieve themselves. A squatting position on the toilet takes pressure off the rectum and can help during a flare-up of hemorrhoids. (You may feel a little silly, but who's watching!) Also, wipe gently with soft toilet paper. It may help to wash your anal area with warm water after each bowel movement, or if you have a bidet, now is the time to use it.
- **Use salves.** Salves can soothe inflamed tissues. Spread vitamin E oil, comfrey, calendula ointment, or goldenseal salve gently on the anus with your fingers.

Witch hazel is also soothing to hemorrhoidal tissue. Put some on a cotton ball and press gently. Repeat treatments several times daily.

■ **Take sitz baths.** Sitz baths are an old-fashioned remedy for hemorrhoids that are still in favor with the medical profession. Place three to four inches of warm water in the bathtub, and sit in it for 10 minutes several times daily. You can improve the results by adding 1/4 cup Epsom salts or healing herbs. Chamomile, chickweed, comfrey, mullein, plantain, witch hazel, and yarrow are all healing and soothing to mucous membranes. Most of these are weeds and may even be growing in your yard. (Comfrey is a very easy herb to grow; just put it in a place where it can spread. It helps with wound healing of any sort and is also soothing for colds and lung problems.) Bring a large pot of water to a boil. Steep 1 to 2 cups of fresh herbs or 1½ cups of dried herbs until cool; strain and add to bathwater.

■ **Use horse chestnuts.** Horse chestnuts, also called buckeyes, help tone blood vessels, improve their elasticity, and reduce inflammation. They can also be used in a sitz bath. Chop up 2 cups of horse chestnuts, add to boiled water, strain, and add infusion to bathwater. Sit in the bath twice daily for 10 to 15 minutes. You can also take 500 mg of the bark orally three times daily. Horse chestnut salves are also available.

■ **Use butcher's broom.** Butcher's broom helps strengthen blood vessels and improves circulation. Take 100 mg extract three times daily.

■ **Take vitamin E.** Vitamin E helps bring oxygen to the tissues and promotes healing. You can use it topically or take it internally. Take 400 to 800 IU of d-alpha tocopherol and mixed tocopherols daily.

■ **Take vitamin C and bioflavonoids.** Vitamin C and bioflavonoids increase capillary and blood vessel strength so that they don't rupture easily. Bioflavonoids are also essential to collagen formation and elasticity of blood vessels. Berries of all types and cherries have high amounts of protective bioflavonoids. Take 500 to 2,000 mg vitamin C daily plus 100 to 1,000 mg bioflavonoids, which can usually be purchased in a single supplement.

■ **Use dimethylsulfoxide (DMSO).** In the literature, there is one anecdotal study in which a physician used DMSO topically for hemorrhoids. By his report, a 70 percent solution of DMSO will dissolve blood-engorged hemorrhoids almost overnight. It may be worth trying.

Natural Therapies for the Diverse Consequences of Faulty Digestion

"Disease bias means that we take health for granted, waiting to act when health is gone and disease emerges. Once we make this assumption, we can soon become so preoccupied that our horizon is filled with diseases to combat. Because disease looms so large, our sight is obscured to the possibilities of health."

—Russell Jaffe, M.D.

Part V discusses how digestion is linked to issues you would never imagine, including arthritis of all types; autoimmune diseases such as multiple sclerosis, scleroderma, and Behcet's disease; chronic fatigue syndrome; eczema; fibromyalgia; migraine headaches; obesity; psoriasis; schizophrenia; and women's health issues. When looked at through the lens of the DIGIN model and balanced pH, there can be significant improvements in these conditions. (Asthma, autism, ADD, ADHD, and many other conditions have been included in *Digestive Wellness for Children*.)

For each health condition, I have provided general information about the disease, recommendations for functional laboratory testing, and healing options, with the most important ones discussed first. With careful investigation and patience, you may find the underlying conditions that influence how you feel. Many of the supplements and herbs can be found in combination products. You will note that although these health conditions are different, many of the healing options are the same. This goes back to the basic digestive principles presented in the DIGIN model and lifestyle changes from the first half of the book.

Of course, if at first you don't find major improvement, keep working at it. You may not have found the best remedy or combination of therapies on the first try. Patience and perseverance bring the best results. It takes time to resolve chronic illnesses.

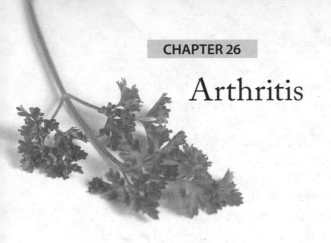

CHAPTER 26

Arthritis

Arthritis refers to more than a hundred diseases that cause inflammation of the joints. The old-fashioned term for arthritis is rheumatism, and today physicians who specialize in arthritis are called rheumatologists. Arthritis affects 40 million Americans and accounts for 46 million medical visits per year. It affects about 15 percent of our population and 3 percent of those severely, but it is severe in 11 percent of people ages 65 and older.

The two most common types of arthritis are osteoarthritis and rheumatoid arthritis. Other common types include psoriatic arthritis, ankylosing spondylitis, gout, Lyme disease, Reiter's syndrome, lupus, and Sjögren's syndrome. Each of these diseases has its own characteristics, but they all share the symptoms of pain and inflammation in joints.

There are many causes for arthritis: genetics, infections, physical injury, nutritional deficiencies, allergies, metabolic and immune disorders, stress, and environmental pollutants and toxins. Several types of arthritis have well-documented associations with faulty digestive function. Osteoarthritis responds well to dietary changes. Rheumatoid arthritis, ankylosing spondylitis, lupus, Sjögren's syndrome, and Reiter's syndrome are all autoimmune conditions. As such, leaky gut probably plays a role, along with environment and genetics.

The current drugs of choice for mild to moderate arthritis pain are nonsteroidal anti-inflammatory drugs (NSAIDs). Although they may help with the pain, many NSAIDs also have a negative effect on the ability of cartilage to repair itself. They block our body's ability to regenerate cartilage tissue by lowering the amounts of healing prostaglandins, glycosaminoglycans, and hyaluronan, and by raising leukotriene levels. NSAIDs block the production of healing prostaglandins, which stimulate repair of the digestive lining. This causes increased intestinal permeability. (See Chapter 4 for more information on NSAIDS and leaky gut.) Use of NSAIDs in children with rheumatoid arthritis showed that 75 percent had gastrointestinal problems caused by the drugs. And the more NSAIDs people take, the leakier the gut wall becomes; the leakier the gut, the more pain and inflammation follows, which sets up a continuously escalating problem. For rheumatoid arthritis and other autoimmune types of arthritis, disease-modifying anti-arthritic drugs, also called DMARDS, are used. There is a wide variety of these, and they all have significant long-term unwanted effects.

Use of natural therapies and dietary change for arthritis can reduce the need for such medications and their accompanying side effects. Natural therapies can be used to help relieve pain, reduce inflammation, help regenerate cartilage, and slow the disease process. These natural therapies can be astonishingly effective. Look to all aspects of the DIGIN model if you have arthritis of any type. Balancing these can be the key to resolving your pain.

FOOD SENSITIVITIES, LEAKY GUT, AND ARTHRITIS

The dietary connection between rheumatoid arthritis and food sensitivities was first noted by Michael Zeller in 1949 in *Annals of Allergy*. He found a direct cause and effect by adding and eliminating foods from the diet. He joined forces with Drs. Herbert Rinkel and Theron Randolph to publish a book called *Food Allergy* in 1951.

Theron Randolph, M.D., is the father of a field of medicine called clinical ecology, which studies how our environment affects health. He found that people with rheumatoid arthritis who were not reacting to foods had at least one sensitivity to an environmental chemical. Randolph sent questionnaires to more than 200 of his patients with osteoarthritis and rheumatoid arthritis to assess how well treatments were working. Their responses showed that when they avoided food and environmental allergens, there was a significant reduction in arthritic symptoms. Randolph also felt that other types of arthritis, including Reiter's syndrome, ankylosing spondylitis, and psoriatic arthritis, have an ecological basis.

Since then, other studies have been done on the relationship between food sensitivities and arthritis. In a study of 43 people with arthritis of the hands, a water fast of three days brought improvement in tenderness, swelling, strength of grip, pain, joint circumference, function, and SED rate (a simple blood test that determines a breakdown of tissue somewhere in the body). When some of these people were tested with single foods, symptoms recurred in 22 out of 27 people. In other studies, the foods most likely to provoke symptoms after an elimination diet were, in order of most to least, corn, wheat, bacon or pork, oranges, milk, oats, rye, eggs, beef, coffee, malt, cheese, grapefruit, tomato, peanuts, sugar, butter, lamb, lemon, and soy. Cereals were the most common food, with wheat and corn causing problems in more than 50 percent of the people.

In another study, it was found that 44 out of 93 people with rheumatoid arthritis had elevated levels of IgG to gliadin. Among these 44 people, 86 percent had positive RA factors. In yet another study, 15 out of 24 people had raised levels of IgA, rheumatoid factor, and wheat protein IgG with a biopsy of the jejunum. Six of the wheat-positive people and one of the wheat-negative people had damage to the brush borders of their intestines. The researchers felt that the intestines play an important role in the progression of rheumatoid arthritis. Increased intestinal permeability allows more food particles to cross the intestinal mucosa, which triggers a greater sensitivity response.

Hvatut and colleagues measured IgG, IgA, and IgM antibodies in serum and intestinal fluid in 17 people with rheumatoid arthritis and 20 healthy controls. They concluded that measuring food antibodies in intestinal fluid gives a more "striking" result between rheumatoid arthritis, food sensitivities, and the immune activation of the mucosal lining (MALT).

Kallikorm and Uibo reported that of 74 people admitted to the hospital with arthritic diseases, 12 percent had elevated antigliaden antibodies, indicating gluten intolerance; 1 person had celiac disease. Because people with one autoimmune disease are more susceptible to other autoimmune diseases, it's good to screen for celiac and gluten intolerance.

The concept of food sensitivity and increased intestinal permeability is gaining acceptance as more physicians see the clinical changes in their patients when they use this approach. Testing for food and environmental sensitivities, parasites, toxic metals, candidiasis, and intestinal permeability and performing a comprehensive digestive stool analysis (CDSA) often provide an understanding of an underlying cause of the disease.

DYSBIOSIS AND ARTHRITIS

Candidiasis frequently plays a role in "fungal" arthritis and is a possible aggravator in rheumatoid arthritis. While common in people who are on immunosuppressant drugs, it is beginning to be seen in people who have normal immune health. It has been found in the synovial fluid of knee joints, yet how often do physicians actually test synovial fluid for infection? Fungus in people with arthritis can be the result of using antibiotics, oral contraceptives, or steroid medications; increased use of alcohol or sugar; or a stressed immune system. Treatment of candidiasis in the digestive system has improved rheumatoid symptoms in many cases.

In many types of arthritis, known microbes trigger a molecular mimicry that then activates the disease. Rheumatoid arthritis is associated with Proteus mirabilis infection; ankylosing spondylitis is associated with Klebsiella sp.; reactive arthritis is triggered by a GI infection of salmonella, yersinia, campylobacter, and in the urinary tract chlamydia.

Infection can trigger arthritis and joint inflammation. Why they move to the joints or cause joint pain is unknown at this time. But the phenomenon is well documented. If candida, Lyme disease, chlamydia, klebsiella, salmonella, or another infection is present, your physician can recommend a variety of therapeutics, including both natural and pharmaceutical remedies.

NUTRITIONAL DEFICIENCIES

There is documentation in the literature about arthritis and deficiencies of nearly every known nutrient. When the needed nutrients are supplied, the body can begin to balance itself. Though many nutritional and herbal products help arthritis sufferers, no one thing works for everyone, so persist until you find the therapies that work best for you. Give each one at least a three-month trial before giving up on it. I remember Abram Hoffer, M.D., speaking about a patient at a conference many years ago. He had recommended the man take 1,000 mg of vitamin C daily for his arthritis. The man took the vitamin C faithfully each day without any improvement. After a whole year, he suddenly became pain-free.

pH BALANCE

People with arthritis are often too acidic. To buffer this acidity, the body pulls alkaline minerals out of the bones. These minerals are sometimes deposited in joints throughout the body. (See Chapter 17 for more on pH balance.)

EXERCISE AND ARTHRITIS

Exercise and stretching are useful for all types of arthritic conditions. Yoga has been found to help with range of motion, pain, stiffness, and joint tenderness. Walking, swimming, physical therapy, and massage therapy may all play a role in reduction of symptoms. Movement is not optional. Even small amounts can give great relief.

OSTEOARTHRITIS

Osteoarthritis is the most common type of arthritis and the one we associate with aging, although nutritionally oriented physicians believe it has more to do with poor dietary habits and biochemical imbalances than age. Pain is usually the first symptom. The main characteristics are stiffness, aches, and painful joints that creak and crack. Stiffness may be worse in the morning and after exercise. Osteoarthritis begins gradually and usually affects one or a few joints, most commonly in the knee, hip, fingers, ankles, and feet. As joints enlarge, cartilage degenerates. Eventually, hardening leads to bone spurs. You lose flexibility, strength, and the ability to grasp, accompanied by pain. Risk of osteoarthritis, especially arthritis in the knee, increases if you are overweight; losing weight helps. Acid-alkaline balance is also important in treating this illness.

RHEUMATOID ARTHRITIS (RA)

Rheumatoid arthritis is characterized by inflammation of joints, most often in the hands, feet, wrists, elbows, and ankles, with symmetrical involvement. It can start in virtually any joint. The onset may be sudden, with pain in multiple joints; or it may come on gradually, with more and more joints becoming involved. Joints become swollen, feel tender, and can degenerate and become misshapen. Joints are often stiffest in the mornings and also feel worse after movement. RA is most common in women and in people who smoke. In a blood test, the rheumatoid factor (RF) will be elevated in most cases of rheumatoid arthritis. While it may get better or worse, once established RA is nearly always present to some extent. Treatment is aimed at lowering inflammation and TNF-alpha.

Many drugs are being used to treat rheumatoid arthritis, and all have complicating side effects. Natural therapies are an adjunct or replacement for medical intervention. For example, fish oils and curcumin lower TNF-alpha.

Rheumatoid arthritis has a genetic component, often running in families. It is believed to be triggered by a bacterial infection (Proteus mirabilis), having the "right" genetics (HLA-DR1/4), and autoimmunity caused by a molecular mimicry. When genes meet the environment, the illness is triggered. The gene marker HLA-DR1/4 is present in 50 to 75 percent of people with rheumatoid arthritis.

There are many microbes that have been associated with rheumatoid arthritis. Here are some of the many microbes that have been indicated in RA: proteus mirabilis, Epstein-Barr virus, mycobacteria, mycoplasma, chlamydia, yersinia, salmonella, shigella, campylobacter, staphylococcus, streptococcus, candida, clostridium, borrelia, leptospira, erysiplotrix, klebsiella, and oral bacteria.

Proteus mirabilis is a bacterium commonly found in the urinary tract and can be found in urine. It causes no problems in most people, but in people who have the HLA-DR1/4 genotype, it acts as a genetic mimic that cross-reacts with collagen XI and hyaline cartilage, breaking down the cartilage. Proteus mirabilis antibodies in people with RA have been found in people in 14 countries. Proteus mirabilis has not been found to have an association with any other disease. I was able to find 44 studies on PubMed regarding the role of Proteus mirabilis, and the mechanisms are beginning to be very well understood. It's postulated that incidence of RA is higher in smokers because smoking puts people more at risk of developing urinary tract infections. In one study, a decrease in antibodies to Proteus mirabilis was observed in subjects on a vegetarian diet. Proteus infections can be treated with either natural or pharmaceutical therapy.

Proteus mirabilis is also found in biofilms. Although there are no studies yet on the relationship of this particular bacteria, biofilms, and arthritis, I look forward to seeing those in the future.

Waldemar Rastawicki and colleagues in Poland studied 92 patients with RA. They were tested for bacterial genes in synovial fluid and blood. While bacterial genes weren't discovered, antigens to pathogenic bacteria were found: salmonella (8.6 percent), yersinia (20.7 percent), and enterobacterial common antigen (34.9 percent).

A 1973 study by Mardh and colleagues reported mycobacteria in synovial fluid. Just recently, a friend with chronic knee issues had her synovial fluid tested and discovered that she had Lyme disease.

Vegetarian, vegan, and raw-food diets have been shown in numerous studies to be successful at reducing the symptoms of rheumatoid arthritis. Vegetable-based diets help balance pH levels. They also provide an abundance of antioxidants, natural anti-inflammatory factors, vitamins, minerals, and phytonutrients. This diet also tends to be more hypoallergenic. Add fish oil to increase the benefits. Short-term fasting prior to beginning the vegetarian diet has also been shown to provide long-term benefits. Please work with a good nutritionist.

It's hard to generalize or predict which of these factors will be found in each person, but usually one or more is present. Each of them needs to be investigated. Leaky gut is probably not a primary cause of rheumatoid arthritis, but long-term use of medications used for the arthritis often makes it a factor.

PSORIATIC ARTHRITIS

Psoriatic arthritis affects 30 percent of people with psoriasis (the incidence used to be 3 to 7 percent), about 1.4 million Americans. People with severe psoriasis are more likely to develop psoriatic arthritis. In addition to the usual symptoms of psoriasis, they also have joint pain, tenderness, or swelling in the fingers, toes, or spine. Other symptoms include reduced range of motion, morning stiffness, redness and pain of the eye that is similar to conjunctivitis, and nail changes with pitting or lifting of the nail. Psoriatic arthritis is rarely found in people who do not also have psoriasis. Psoriatic arthritis is associated with bone erosion and deformities that affect half of the people with this disease. Skin and joint symptoms may flare up or improve simultaneously. Psoriatic arthritis closely resembles rheumatoid arthritis, although people with psoriatic arthritis usually have a negative rheumatoid factor. This disease can be mild, but it can also be severely deforming and disabling.

Like other types of autoimmune disease, psoriatic arthritis has genetic, environmental, and immunologic origins. The gene marker HLA-B27 is present in most people with this disease.

Inflammation of psoriatic arthritis is involved with arachidonic acid pathways and TNF-alpha. New drug therapies, such as injectable infliximab and etanercept, aim at lower TNF-alpha levels. A healthful diet plus essential fatty acids help reduce and prevent further inflammation. Evening primrose, borage, and fish oils; turmeric; curcumin; bromelain; and quercetin all work on these pathways.

Li and Wang used traditional Chinese medicine (TCM) and integrative medicine in working with 47 people with psoriatic arthritis. Seventeen people were given TCM only. Thirty were given a combination of TCM and integrative medicine. Dosages of medications were reduced as symptoms were relieved, cured, or improved. They conclude that TCM and integrative medicine are effective for people with psoriatic arthritis with fewer negative effects than current medical treatment.

ANKYLOSING SPONDYLITIS (AS)

Ankylosing spondylitis is characterized by a progressive fusion of joints in and around the spine. Caucasian men constitute 90 percent of those with the illness, and it typically becomes evident between the ages of 10 and 30. It starts off as a low backache, which is often worse in the mornings. Symptoms get progressively worse and spread from the lower back to the midback and up to the neck. The spine gradually becomes fused. Later, shoulders, hips, and knees may be affected. Symptoms flare and subside.

The role of dysbiosis in ankylosing spondylitis is the most researched and best understood of all the arthritic diseases. Most researchers believe that AS is triggered by an inherited gene and interactions with the environment. Much research has been done on the role of infection as a primary trigger of AS. The gene implicated is HLA-B27, although others may still be found. HLA-B27 is present in 96 percent of people with ankylosing spondylitis. This marker is also present in 8 percent of the general population. Research shows 70 to 80 percent of people with ankylosing spondylitis have klebsiella bacteria in their stools. Yersinia, shigella, and salmonella bacteria are also associated with this process and may contribute to the disease in people who are not infected with klebsiella. These bacteria may not normally cause disease, but in people with the HLA-B27 gene marker, antibodies produced to kill the bacteria cross-react, causing pain and inflammation. This concept of autoimmune disease may explain why some people get certain illnesses and others don't. It's the presence not only of a specific gene but also of a microbe or other environmental trigger that activates the disease process.

What begins as a local infection triggers an autoimmune disease. In the paper "Enteropathic arthritis, Whipple's disease, juvenile spondyloarthropathy, and uveitis," published in *Current Opinions in Rheumatology* 1994, Finnish rheumatology researcher Marjatta Leirisalo-Repo states, "An association between inflammatory bowel disease and enteroarthritis and the spondyloarthropathies has been known for awhile . . . and it now seems evident that chronic gut inflammation is either associated with or is even the cause of chronicity of peripheral arthritis and the development of ankylosing spondylitis."

It is important to make an early diagnosis of ankylosing spondylitis so that progression of the disease can be slowed or halted. Because it usually appears as a low backache, many people will tend to seek chiropractic help or massage therapy or take anti-inflammatory medications. But such remedies can't correct dysbiosis in the intestinal tract. Because many men commonly have low-back pain, they often have irreversible damage before a correct diagnosis is made.

In people with ankylosing spondylitis, also think about gluten intolerance. In one study of 30 people by Togrol, 36.7 percent were found to have antigliaden antibodies. Three of these people (10 percent) also had positive anti-endomysial antibodies. I personally know two men with AS who have experienced positive benefit from being on a gluten-free diet. Other studies have failed to show any significant difference in gluten intolerance in people with AS in comparison with control groups.

Leaky gut syndrome is present in people with ankylosing spondylitis. Unfortunately, NSAIDs are commonly used to treat ankylosing spondylitis, causing even greater intestinal permeability. This, in turn, causes more sensitivity to foods and environmental substances.

About half the people with ankylosing spondylitis experience dramatic improvement when they eliminate dairy products. Thirteen out of 25 people who were studied had good results, and another 4 had moderate improvements. Of the respondents whose results were good, 8 were able to discontinue NSAID medication. Six patients from this study remained dairy-free for more than two years because they were so satisfied with the results. The elimination of dairy products is a simple and effective treatment to try. Although the mechanism for this improvement is unclear, it is suggested that a dairy-free diet modifies the bacterial ecosystem of the gut, which may have benefits. Another hypothesis is that milk allergy causes chronic irritation to the gut as well as gut permeability.

Klebsiella and other disease-producing microbes that can contribute to ankylosing spondylitis use sugars as their main food source. Some physicians are experimenting with a low-starch diet and are getting good results. Eliminate all breads, grains, pasta, cookies, candy, root vegetables, and legumes. Be patient: you may get amazing results, but you will need to stay on the diet for at least six months before you really reap the benefits.

I recently queried two friends with AS about what has been most helpful. They both responded that exercise and stretching have given the best response.

Functional Laboratory Testing

The letters following each list item indicate the illness that that test can be used to detect. Note that O = osteoarthritis, RA = rheumatoid arthritis, PA = psoriatic arthritis, and AS = ankylosing spondylitis.

- Elisa/Act allergy testing for foods, molds, medications, and chemicals (O, RA, PA, AS)
- Organic acid testing (O, RA, PA, AS)
- Comprehensive digestive stool analysis (O, RA, PA, AS)

- Intestinal permeability screening; stop use of NSAIDs for three weeks prior to test (O, RA, PA, AS)
- Candida testing, either separately or in CDSA (O, RA, PA, AS)
- Heidelberg capsule testing for HCl status (RA)
- Small intestinal bacterial overgrowth breath test (RA)
- Liver function testing; people with rheumatoid arthritis are also shown to have reduced function in the detoxification pathways (RA)

Healing Options

Some of these suggestions will significantly help your arthritis; others may not help at all. You can look for products that combine these nutrients and herbs. Be patient and give whatever you try time to work. Try one or two at a time until you find a program that suits your body's unique needs and your lifestyle. Recommendations work for all types of arthritis, unless I've specifically noted a type after the suggestion.

To Reduce Pain and Inflammation

- **Try an alkalizing diet.** Bring your body into acid-alkaline balance. See Chapter 17 for a discussion.
- **Exercise.** It's important to use your body as much as you can without aggravating the condition. Yoga, walking, swimming, stretching, water exercises, physical therapy, massage, and acupressure massage may all be of help. Do something nearly every day.
- **Try an elimination-provocation diet.** Follow the directions outlined in Chapter 15. For best results, work with a nutritionist or physician who is familiar with food sensitivity protocols.
- **Try the Nightshade Diet.** In the 1970s, Norman Childers, a horticulturist, popularized the Nightshade Diet. Elimination of nightshade foods helps only about 15 percent of people with arthritis, but the people who respond are usually helped a great deal. The nightshade foods are potatoes, tomatoes, eggplant, and peppers (red, green, yellow, and chili). An elimination diet of two weeks followed by a reintroduction of these foods provides a good test. Blood testing also picks up these sensitivities.
- **Try yucca.** Yucca has been used by Native Americans of the Southwest to alleviate symptoms of arthritis and improve digestion. It's a rich source of saponins with anti-inflammatory effects. Studies have been done with both rheumatoid and osteoarthritis with significant improvement in 56 to 66 percent of the people who tried it. People taking yucca for more than one and a half years had the additional advantage of improved triglyceride and cholesterol levels and reduc-

tion in high blood pressure, with no negative side effects. Take two to eight tablets daily.

- **Take cetyl myristoleate (CM).** Harry Diehl, a researcher at the National Institutes of Health, found that mice did not develop arthritis when CM was given. When he himself developed arthritis, Diehl took CM and his arthritis resolved. Jonathan Wright, M.D., has found CM to be clinically valuable in about half of his patients. CM appears to actually cure arthritis in many instances. I was able to find two studies on CM that had astounding results. CM was found to be best used in combination with glucosamine sulfate, sea cucumber, and methylsulfonylmethane (MSM). Recommended duration of use is two to four weeks. Carbonated beverages, caffeine, chocolate, and cigarettes are not allowed while taking CM and its associated supplements.

- **Take vitamin C ascorbate.** Vitamin C is an essential nutrient for every antiarthritis program. It is vital for formation of cartilage and collagen, a fibrous protein that forms strong connective tissue necessary for bone strength. Vitamin C also plays a role in immune response, helping protect us from disease-producing microbes. Many types of arthritis are caused by microbes, which vitamin C helps combat. It also inhibits formation of inflammatory prostaglandins, helping to reduce pain, inflammation, and swelling. Vitamin C is also an antioxidant and free radical scavenger; free radical formation has been noted in arthritic conditions. Take 1 to 3 grams daily in an ascorbate or ester form. For best results, try a vitamin C flush weekly for four weeks. (See Chapter 10.)

- **Increase omega-3 fatty acids and fish oils.** Fish oils come from cold-water fish and contain eicosapentaenoic acid (EPA) and docosahexaenoic acid (DHA). The fish with the highest levels are salmon, mackerel, halibut, sardines, tuna, and herring. These omega-3 fatty acids are essential because we cannot synthesize them and must obtain them from our foods. Fish oils inhibit production of inflammatory prostaglandin E2 series, cyclooxygenase, and thromboxane A2, all of which come from arachidonic acid. Fish oils shift the production to thromboxane A3, which causes less constriction of blood vessels and platelet stickiness than thromboxane A2. Research has shown fish oils are really helpful for some people with arthritis, reducing morning stiffness and joint tenderness. Fish oil capsules produce moderate but definite improvement in arthritic diseases at dosages from 8 to 20 capsules daily. Similar results can be obtained by eating fish with high EPA/DHA two to four times a week. Because fish oils increase blood clotting time, they should not be used by people who have hemophilia or who take anticoagulant medicines or aspirin regularly. High dosages in capsule form should be monitored by a physician.

- **Take gamma-linolenic acid (GLA) (RA).** In one study, patients with rheumatoid arthritis were given 1.4 grams of GLA from borage oil daily. It significantly reduced their symptoms: swollen joints by 36 percent, tenderness by 45 percent, swollen joint count by 28 percent, and swollen joint score by 41 percent. (Some people responded in more than one area.) Use of evening primrose oil in the study group and olive oil for the control group showed that both oils helped reduce pain and morning stiffness. Several people were able to reduce use of NSAIDs, but none were able to stop the medication. The modest results in this study were probably due to the use of NSAIDs with the evening primrose oil. The same results could be obtained by use of evening primrose or borage oil alone. Take 1,400 mg.
- **Take and/or eat ginger.** Ginger is an old Ayurvedic remedy that was given to people with RA and OA. In one study it reduced pain and swelling in various amounts in 75 percent of the people tested, with no reported side effects over three months to two and a half years. Ginger can be used as an ingredient in food and tea or taken as a supplement. Take 2 ounces fresh ginger or 3,000 to 7,000 mg powdered ginger daily.
- **Take niacinamide.** Most of the B-complex vitamins have been shown to reduce inflammation and swelling associated with arthritis. Dr. Kaufman, M.D., Ph.D., an expert on arthritis, recommends using niacinamide at a rather high dosage with excellent results. It doesn't cure the arthritis, but it really helps while you take it. If you are going to try this, do so with your physician's supervision. High levels of niacinamide can be liver toxic. Take 250 to 500 mg daily. Soft gel capsules are recommended. Make sure to get a brand without colors, preservatives, or solvents.
- **Take folic acid plus vitamin B_{12}.** In a recent study, those with osteoarthritis in their hands were given 20 mcg vitamin B_{12} plus 6,400 mcg folic acid daily. They reported a significant reduction in symptoms. This is a tiny amount of vitamin B_{12} and a large amount of folic acid, which is nontoxic even at these high levels.
- **Take superoxide dismutase (SOD).** SOD plays an important role in reducing inflammation and has been used alone, with copper, manganese or copper, and zinc for various arthritic conditions. Some physicians are using SOD in injections. Oral SOD doesn't seem to work as well, except when used in a copper-zinc preparation. Wheatgrass extracts of SOD can be purchased at health-food stores. Most people who try them experience benefits, but there is little scientific research to date. Some veterinarians are using wheatgrass SOD with arthritic animals with excellent results.

- **Take S-adenosylmethionine (SAMe).** A recent player on the scene is SAMe, a chemical that is found naturally in every living cell. Research in 10 studies that included more than 22,000 people has shown SAMe to have powerful antidepressant effects without the side effects of pharmaceutical antidepressant medications. SAMe has also been shown to be as potent an anti-inflammatory drug as indomethacin and other NSAIDs, with fewer negative effects. This product is expensive because it is difficult to stabilize. Use it with a good multivitamin that contains B-complex vitamins. Take 400 mg twice daily. Adjust up or down as needed.

- **Take methylsulfonylmethane (MSM) or dimethylsulfoxide (DMSO).** DMSO is highly effective for reducing arthritis pain when used on skin. It has a distinct odor that prevents many people from using it, but MSM is odorless. MSM, a naturally occurring derivative of dimethylsulfoxide, is now being used as a supplement. MSM has been found to be an antioxidant and anti-inflammatory in animal studies, probably because of its high sulfur content. It helps reduce pain and inflammation and gives the body the sulfur compounds necessary to build cartilage and collagen. It is also useful in allergies, blood sugar control, and asthma. Take 1,000 to 5,000 mg daily. It is best when taken with 1,000 to 5,000 mg of vitamin C for absorption. Or use DMSO topically on skin.

- **Take bromelain.** Bromelain is an enzyme derived from pineapple that acts as an anti-inflammatory in much the same way that evening primrose, fish, and borage oils do. It interferes with production of arachidonic acid, shifting to prostaglandin production of the less inflammatory type. It also prevents platelet aggregation and interferes with the growth of malignant cells. It appears to be as effective as NSAID medications at reducing inflammation. Bromelain can be taken with meals as a digestive aid, but as an anti-inflammatory, it must be taken between meals. Take 500 to 1,000 mg two to three times daily between meals.

- **Take quercetin.** Quercetin is the most effective bioflavonoid in its anti-inflammatory effects; others include bromelain, curcumin, and rutin. Bioflavonoids help maintain collagen tissue by decreasing membrane permeability and cross-linking collagen fibers, making them stronger. Quercetin can be used to reduce pain and inflammatory responses and for control of allergies. Take 500 to 2,000 mg daily. It appears to reduce inflammatory cytokines.

- **Take boswellia.** Boswellia is taken over the long term as a treatment for rheumatoid arthritis, not specifically for immediate pain. Boswellia serrata, an Ayurvedic remedy that has been traditionally used for arthritis, pain, and inflammation, has been shown to moderate inflammatory markers such as nitric oxide and 5-lipoxygenase. In a study, a specific preparation of boswellia called H-15 was given to 260 people and found to be effective in treating rheumatoid arthritis. Fifty to 60 percent of the subjects had good results. Take 1,200 mg two or three times daily.

- **Take turmeric or curcumin.** Turmeric has been shown to have powerful anti-inflammatory properties. Some of the mechanisms involved include its ability to block leukotrienes and arachidonic acid, both of which cause inflammation and pain. An effective dosage of turmeric is 10 to 60 grams daily. Curcumin, the active pain-relieving ingredient, can be taken in much smaller doses, 500 mg three times daily. For those lucky enough to live in warm areas where turmeric can be grown and used fresh, it can be juiced, grated, used in stir-fry, and eaten freely. Turmeric is also a lovely flowering garden plant.

- **Take devil's claw.** Devil's claw (Harpagophytum procumbens) is a South African root that is commonly used as an arthritis remedy. It reduces pain and inflammation. Several studies have shown it to work as well as phenylbutazone, a common NSAID medication. It is commonly used in low-potency homeopathic dilutions of 2X in Germany. This is a dilution of one part per hundred of devil's claw in a homeopathically potentized form.

- **Use black cohosh.** Black cohosh (Cimicifuga racemosa) has long been used by European and American herbalists to reduce muscle spasm, pain, and inflammation. It can be used as either a tincture or in capsules.

- **Use capsicum (cayenne pepper).** Cayenne has been well studied for its temporary relief of arthritis pain. Creams with capsicum are used topically to relieve pain. (These creams may burn when first applied.) In various studies, typically more than half of topical-cream users experience pain relief. These are available over the counter and by prescription.

- **Try DL-phenylalanine (DLPA) (RA).** DLPA is an amino acid that is used therapeutically for pain and depression. It is effective for treating rheumatoid arthritis, osteoarthritis, low-back pain, and migraines. "D" is the naturally found form, and "L" is its synthetic mirror. The combination of DL slows down the release of the phenylalanine. It appears to inhibit the breakdown of endorphins, our body's natural pain relievers. Take 400 to 500 mg three times daily.

To Nourish and Regenerate the Joints and Connective Tissue

- **Take a multivitamin with minerals.** People with arthritis are often deficient in many nutrients. Aging, poor diet, medications, malabsorption, and illness all contribute to poor nutritional status. At least 21 nutrients are essential for formation of bone and cartilage, so it's important to find a supplement that supports these needs. Look for a supplement that contains 500 to 1,000 mg calcium, 400 to 500 mg magnesium, 15 to 45 mg zinc, 1 to 2 mg copper, 10,000 IU vitamin A, 200 mcg selenium, 50 mg vitamin B_6, and 5 to 10 mg manganese in addition to other nutrients. Follow dosage on bottle to get nutrients in the appropriate amounts.

■ **Take glucosamine and chondroitin.** Glucosamine sulfate and chondroitin sulfate are nutrients used therapeutically to help repair cartilage, reduce inflammation, and increase mobility. Studies have consistently shown benefits of both glucosamine and chondroitin supplementation. Green-lipped mussels are a rich source of glycosaminoglycans. Use of glucosamine sulfate has no associated side effects, although anecdotally it may raise serum cholesterol levels. It either works or it doesn't. Give it a three-month trial. It's important to buy a product that has been broken down into a molecular size that your body can use. It's worth it to spend more on this product.

■ **Take vitamin E.** Twenty-nine study participants with osteoarthritis were given 600 IU of vitamin E or a placebo daily. Out of 15 who received vitamin E, 52 percent reported improvement. Another study showed no improvement in those with osteoarthritis who were given vitamin E supplementation of 1,200 IU daily. Try 800 IU for two to three months. It is very safe and may help some people. Best is the "d-alpha" form of mixed tocopherols. Look for high levels of gamma-tocopherol.

■ **Use copper to treat RA symptoms.** Copper is involved in collagen formation, tissue repair, and anti-inflammatory processes. Rheumatoid arthritis sufferers often have marginal copper levels. Traditionally, copper bracelets have been worn to help reduce arthritic symptoms. W. Ray Walker, Ph.D., tested those who had benefited from copper bracelets by having them wear copper-colored aluminum bracelets for two months. Fourteen out of 40 participants deteriorated so much they couldn't finish the two months. More than half reported that their arthritis had worsened. Dr. Walker found that 13 mg of copper per month was dissolved by sweat, and presumably much of that was absorbed through the skin. Supplementation with copper increases levels of superoxide dismutase (SOD). Wear a copper bracelet or supplement with 1 to 2 mg daily in a multivitamin preparation. If you are working with a physician, you may temporarily add a supplement of copper salicylate or copper sebacate until copper levels return to normal.

■ **Eat or take alfalfa.** Alfalfa is a tried-and-true folk remedy for arthritis. Many people attest to its benefits, but more research is needed on it. Alfalfa is an abundantly nutritious food, high in minerals, vitamins, antioxidants, and protein. Alfalfa may help because of its saponin content or its high nutrient and trace mineral content. It is widely used as a nutritional supplement in animal feed. Take 14 to 24 tablets in two or three doses daily, or grind up alfalfa seeds and take 3 tablespoons of ground seeds each day. You can mix them with applesauce, cottage cheese, or oatmeal or sprinkle them on salads. Another method is to cook 1 ounce of alfalfa seeds in 3 cups of water. Do not boil them, but cook gently in a glass or enamel pan for 30 minutes and strain. Toss away the seeds and keep the tea. Dilute the tea with an equal amount of water. Add honey if you like. Use it all within 24 hours. Yet another method is to soak 1 ounce of alfalfa seeds in 3 cups of water for 12 to 24 hours. Strain and drink the liquid throughout the day.

Diagnose and Treat Dysbiosis

- **Address hypochlorhydria and small intestinal bacterial overgrowth (RA).** Low levels of hydrochloric acid (HCl) were found in 32 percent of people tested with rheumatoid arthritis. Half of these people had small intestinal bacterial overgrowth. Thirty-five percent of patients with normal levels of HCl had SIBO compared with none of the control group. SIBO was found most in people with active arthritic symptoms. (See Chapter 2 for information on HCl and Chapter 8 on small intestinal bacterial overgrowth.)

Look for Environmental Triggers

- **Examine side effects of breast implants.** Silicone breast implants may cause rheumatoid-like symptoms in some women, although research is divided. If you have rheumatoid arthritis and silicone or saline breast implants, it would be smart to be tested for silicone antibodies or allergies on an annual basis. Many women feel remarkably better once breast implants have been removed.

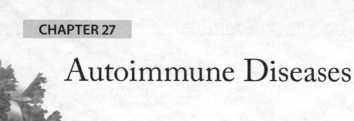

Autoimmune Diseases

There are many autoimmune diseases discussed in the previous chapters and throughout this one. They include type 1 diabetes, celiac disease, autoimmune hepatitis, primary biliary cirrhosis, inflammatory bowel diseases, rheumatoid arthritis, psoriatic arthritis, ankylosing spondylitis, Behcet's disease, fibromyalgia, scleroderma, psoriasis, and Parkinson's disease.

This chapter gives you a general overview of autoimmune diseases. The definition of an autoimmune illness is one in which your body mistakes healthy cells for harmful ones and attacks them. The function of the immune system is to distinguish self from nonself. In these diseases, this goes awry. There are about 80 known autoimmune diseases, and they can affect virtually every body tissue; many of these have overlapping symptoms, which makes them hard to diagnose. Typically these conditions flare up and then go into remission so that you may feel better for a while.

The most common autoimmune diseases include:

Addison's disease	Diabetes type 1
Alopecia areata	Glomerulonephritis
Ankylosing spondylitis	Grave's disease
Antiphospholipid antibody syndrome	Guillain-Barré syndrome
Autoimmune hepatitis	Hashimoto's disease
Celiac disease	Hemolytic anemia
Crohn's disease	Multiple sclerosis
Dermatomyocitis	Myasthenia gravis

Myositis	Raynaud's disease
Parkinson's disease	Rheumatoid arthritis
Pernicious anemia	Scleroderma
Polymyalgia rheumatica	Systemic lupus erythematosus
Primary biliary cirrhosis	Ulcerative colitis
Psoriasis	Vitiligo

These illnesses affect 23.5 million Americans. You are most likely to get an auto-immune disease if you are female, have a family history of autoimmune conditions, work around solvents or other chemicals, and/or are African, Native American, or Latin in descent. Rheumatoid arthritis is two to three times more common in women. Women have 90 percent of lupus; lupus is also three times more common in African American women than in Caucasian women. Ankylosing spondylitis is one of the rare autoimmune diseases that are more common in men.

In autoimmune diseases the immune system overreacts. There is increased inflammation and oxidative damage from free radicals. Your job is to dampen it down so that it doesn't see the world as unsafe. (Read Chapter 9 on inflammation and immunity to get a deeper understanding.)

For an autoimmune illness to thrive it needs the following conditions:

1. The right genetics
2. An environmental trigger (could be stress, sunlight, solvents, other chemicals, a virus, bacteria or parasite, heavy metal, pesticide, or some other exposure)
3. And in some autoimmune conditions, a leaky gut

Alessio Fasano states that for celiac disease to develop, increased intestinal permeability is needed. The relationship between leaky gut and other autoimmune illnesses has also been demonstrated in autoimmune types of arthritis, multiple sclerosis, inflammatory bowel diseases, fibromyalgia, chronic fatigue syndrome, autism, primary biliary cirrhosis, psoriasis, Behcet's disease, and Parkinson's disease. (See Table 27.1.) It has not been studied in many other autoimmune conditions yet, so we don't know if it always plays a role. (For a larger list of diseases associated with leaky gut, see Chapter 4.)

These diseases can develop quickly or over many years. You can typically find autoantibodies in your blood many years prior to the onset of the disease. Arbuckle reported that 88 percent of 130 patients who ultimately developed systemic lupus erythematosus (SLE) had elevated antibodies 9.4 years prior to the diagnosis. Ask your doctor to look for antinuclear antibodies (ANA) antibodies or other more spe-

Table 27.1   **Association Between Viruses and Autoimmune Disease**

EBV = Epstein-Barr virus CMV = cytomegalovirus VZV = Varicella zoster virus RA = rheumatoid arthritis ITP = idiopathic thrombocytopenic purpura (The double plus sign indicates that there is stronger research.)

	EBV	CMV	herpes-1	herpes-2	herpes-6	VZV	measles
autism	+	+	+	+	++		++
RA	++	++					
thyroiditis	++						
Sjögrens	++				++		
myocarditis	+	+					
multiple sclerosis	+				++		++
type 1 diabetes	+	+					
Guillain-Barré syndrome	+	+					
uveitis		++	++	++			
keratitis			+				
autoimmune hepatitis			+			++	
Reiter's syndrome	+	-	+			+	
polymyositis	+						
pemphigus	+					+	
scleroderma		+					
psoriasis		+					
ITP	+	+					
IgA nephritis	++	+-					
glomerulonephritis	++						

Adapted from and used with permission from Aristo Vojdjani, Ph.D., MT.

cific antibodies if you suspect you may have an autoimmune condition. Some of the regular tests that may tip you off include sedimentation rate, complete blood count, elevated C-reactive protein, 25-OH vitamin D testing, and looking for oxidative damage. Functional tests include organic acid testing, food allergy and sensitivity testing, lactulose/mannitol testing for leaky gut, looking at methylation pathways through homocysteine or liver detoxification profiles, and looking at 2:16 ratios of hydroxyestrone. People with one autoimmune illness are more likely to develop additional autoimmune conditions. In 2009 Bardella and colleagues in Milan, Italy, reviewed 297 consecutive patients to determine the prevalence of autoimmune conditions in people with celiac and inflammatory bowel disease. They report that 25.6 percent of people with celiac had another autoimmune condition; 21.1 percent of people with Crohn's disease also had a second autoimmune condition; and 10 percent of people with ulcerative colitis had a second autoimmune condition. Various studies have reported the incidence of people with celiac disease who also have type 1 diabetes to be between 3 and 6 percent. Togrol reports that of 30 people with ankylosing spondylitis, 11 (36.7 percent) also had positive antigliaden antibodies; 3 of the 11 also had positive antiendomysial antibodies (10 percent). People with autoimmune conditions can also display systemic inflammation. It has been reported that people with lupus have increased risk of developing atherosclerosis and osteoporosis.

In my own practice I have seen people with lupus, scleroderma, and multiple sclerosis (MS) improve significantly when on an elimination diet. Fasting has proven to be effective at reducing inflammation in people with lupus and rheumatoid arthritis; an elimination diet is something that can offer similar results, since fasting cannot be sustained. Although research doesn't indicate that people with MS have celiac more often than other people, anecdotally there are certainly many people who respond to a gluten-free diet. Hopefully more research will be done in this area.

People with autoimmune conditions can also have problems with GI motility, causing constipation or IBS-like symptoms. Elderly people with Parkinson's disease were found to have lengthened stool transit time and some malabsorption, which was indicated by decreased mannitol absorption on intestinal permeability testing.

Conventional treatments for autoimmune diseases include medications to reduce inflammation and symptoms, eating well, getting as much exercise as you can without overdoing, getting rest, and using stress-management techniques. Rather than focusing on a single organ or system, using a broader view of the body will get you better results. Try chiropractic treatments, acupuncture, hypnotherapy, and chi gong. Meditate, listen to music, and cultivate methods of training your mind to feel safe and relaxed.

Whatever autoimmune condition affects you, look at the DIGIN model (discussed in Part II, Chapters 3 through 10) to discover whether you can reduce the severity of the illness and/or reduce the incidence of flare-ups. Reducing inflammation is key, so looking for what triggers your inflammation can be critical. While many people may need prescription medications to reduce inflammation, remember that food is typically our most inflammatory contact. So, trying elimination diets and discovering your specific dietary triggers is important. Healing a leaky gut, caused by your medications or other triggers, is another important step to keeping you healthy. Looking for dysbiosis and the competency of your digestive function can also give you significant information. Think about using probiotics to help modulate your immune system and to reduce inflammation. Consider using natural anti-inflammatory supplements and diet to enable you to reduce your reliance on prescription medications.

Selenium, magnesium, and zinc deficiencies have been associated with autoimmune diseases; low vitamin D levels are also seen in autoimmune conditions with frequency, so have these tested. The incidence of autoimmune conditions rises as you move away from the equator; less sunlight, more autoimmune disease. Vitamin D modulates immune function and inflammation when it is at normal or optimal levels.

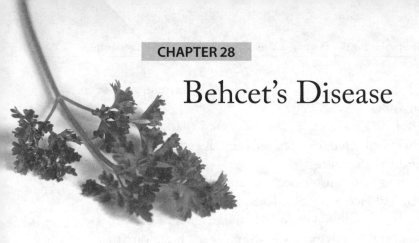

CHAPTER 28

Behcet's Disease

Behcet's disease (BD) is an inflammatory autoimmune disease that affects blood vessels throughout the body, causing vasculitis, an inflammation of the blood or lymph vessel. It was first recognized in 1937 by a Turkish doctor, Hulusi Behcet. It is also known as Silk Road disease because the incidence is greatest in the Mediterranean, the Middle East, and the Far East, although there have been cases in people of all nationalities and descent. In the United States, it is more common in women than in men. In Middle Eastern countries, it is more common in men than women. Symptoms most commonly appear in one's 20s or 30s but can begin anytime. Fifteen thousand to 20,000 Americans have been diagnosed, and many more are undiagnosed.

Symptoms vary depending on where the inflammation is in your body and are due to an overactive immune system. It is chronic and the course is unpredictable. Some people are debilitated by the disease, while a lucky few may go into complete remission. The most common symptoms are recurrent sores in the mouth and genitals and eye inflammation. The sores often have a white or yellow center with redness at the edges and are very painful. There may be additional symptoms, including skin lesions, painful joints, bowel inflammation, and meningitis. Symptoms may involve the nervous system, causing Parkinson-like symptoms; memory loss; impaired speech; hearing loss; loss of balance; blindness; headaches; stroke; and digestive complications, such as bloating, gas, bloody stools, and diarrhea. About 15 percent of people with BD also have heart disease complications. Sufferers sometimes experience a profound sense of fatigue. BD usually presents itself in a rhythm of remissions and flare-ups of disease activity. It may be worsened by extremes of hot and cold climates or menstrual cycles.

There is no known cause for Behcet's disease. It is suspected that an environmental exposure, such as a viral or bacterial infection, can trigger the illness in people who are already genetically susceptible.

A large body of research focuses on the insufficiency of antioxidant nutrients and enzymes in people with BD. Glutathione peroxidase levels are lower in people with BD. Glutathione is an enzyme that depends on vitamin E and selenium for optimal function. Superoxide dismutase (SOD) activity is also diminished. It appears that production of nitric oxide is excessive in people with BD. Use of antioxidant nutrients can bring nitric oxide under control.

One recent study examined levels of vitamin C and malondialdehyde in people with BD. Malondialdehyde is a metabolite that is produced when there is lipid peroxidation, which is a chain reaction requiring antioxidant nutrients. Vitamin C levels were lower in people with BD than in controls, and malondialdehyde levels were higher than in controls. Vitamin C levels were low in people with BD even when the illness was in remission. Different researchers looked at vascular health and found that one hour after IV vitamin C was given there was improved function in the blood vessels.

Another study looked at vitamin E supplementation in BD. It was found that vitamins A and E, beta-carotene, and glutathione levels were lower in people with BD than in controls. When given vitamin E supplementation for six weeks, levels of blood antioxidants rose in the treatment group and were higher than in the untreated control groups.

BD sufferers have significantly increased intestinal permeability. Leaky gut syndrome can be aggravated by use of certain foods. Use of dairy products, gluten-containing foods (see section on celiac disease in Chapter 24), and other foods may trigger an immune response and symptoms. Testing for food and environmental sensitivities and allergies makes sense. Use of nutrients such as glutamine, quercetin, probiotics, and antioxidants can be helpful.

No specific diagnostic test exists for Behcet's disease. Diagnosis is made by elimination of other possibilities and through symptom analysis and is best done by a physician experienced in the treatment of Behcet's patients. A list of patient-recommended physicians is available at the American Behcet's Disease Association website at http://www.behcets.com. BD may begin gradually at first, with sores that come and go, and may be undiagnosed for a long time; it may also be misdiagnosed as herpes. Like patients with chronic fatigue syndrome, people with BD are often told it's "all in your head" because they look so healthy. Most of the inflammations are internal and not readily apparent to family and friends. To be diagnosed with BD, a person must have had recurrent oral ulcers, at least three times in a year. They must also meet two of four additional criteria: recurrent genital ulcers, eye lesions, skin lesions, or a positive "pathergy test." The pathergy test is simple. The forearm is pricked with a sterile needle, and if a small red bump or pustule occurs, the result is positive. This is very useful in Middle Eastern populations, where 70 percent of people with BD test positive, but less so in Europe and America, where the majority test negative.

Conventional treatments are similar to those for other autoimmune conditions and involve the use of immunosuppressive medications such as steroids, interferon alpha 2A and B, Levamisole, cyclosporine, Cytoxan, colchicine, Trental, and thalidomide. Not a group to be dealt with lightly.

This is a perfect condition in which to use the DIGIN model to try to find underlying imbalances and triggers.

Functional Laboratory Testing
- Intestinal permeability testing
- Organic acid testing
- Lactose intolerance test
- Testing for gluten and antigliadin antibodies
- IgE, IgG, IgM food and environmental sensitivity testing

Healing Options
After testing, you'll have a better idea of any underlying problems. Look up related sections in this book to help you with the specifics. Then detoxify if necessary, clean up your diet, take probiotics, and increase your intake of vitamins, minerals, and other antioxidants.

- **Try metabolic cleansing.** Metabolic cleansing involves going on a hypoallergenic food plan for one to three weeks and taking a nutrient-rich protein powder designed to help restore your liver's detoxification capacities. For a thorough discussion of metabolic cleansing, see Chapter 18.
- **Take and eat antioxidants.** You'll find fruits and vegetables to be great natural sources of antioxidants. Make sure you eat 5 to 12 servings daily, if not more. They probably won't give enough protection by themselves, so add nutritional supplements. Vitamin C, vitamin E, glutathione, trace minerals, and other antioxidants may be helpful in decreasing the incidence and severity of flare-ups. Research shows that BD patients have an increased need for antioxidants.

Therefore, supplementation with trace elements involved in the antioxidative processes may increase scavenger enzyme activities, and consequently, an improvement in clinical symptoms may be expected. While much more research is needed in this area, there is no reason not to add them to your daily routine. Take an antioxidant combination with carotenoids, selenium, glutathione, or N-acetyl cysteine, and that may contain lipoic acid, grape seed extract, Pycnogenol, or other antioxidant nutrients.

- **Take vitamin E.** Take 800 to 1,000 IU d-alpha tocopherol with mixed tocopherols daily. Look for a product with a high gamma-tocopherol or high tocotrienol content.

- **Take vitamin C.** Take a minimum of 2,000 mg of vitamin C daily. To maximize effects see the section on vitamin C flush in Chapter 18.

- **Try BG-104.** This is a Chinese herbal supplement. One study looked at the effectiveness of BG-104 in people with BD and Sjögren's disease. Both BG-104 and vitamin E were found to have an anti-inflammatory effect. They enhance antioxidant activity to reduce sedimentation rates (a measure of tissue breakdown) and number of neutrophils (white blood cells) and lower C-reactive protein levels, which is a measure of inflammation.

- **Balance your pH.** See Chapter 17 for more information.

- **Try acupuncture.** There is limited research in this area, but one study showed a positive effect on improving immune function and trace mineral status; however, a 2002 letter in the *British Journal of Ophthalmology* (Murray and Aboteen, 2002) discussed a BD patient who developed pathergy-like pustules at the sites of acupuncture needle placement, indicating caution in the use of this treatment.

- **Investigate allergies and sensitivities.** Although more research needs to be done in this area, one study indicated an immune response when patients were given cow's milk. Eliminate dairy products for two weeks. See if you have improvement in symptoms. Then add back cultured dairy, such as yogurt, kefir, and cottage cheese. See how you feel. It may be necessary to avoid dairy products altogether. Rule out other food sensitivities with an elimination-provocation diet and/or food-allergy or food-sensitivity blood testing.

Cigarettes, toothpaste, mouthwash, and flavored dental floss can cause irritation. In a conversation I had with Joanne Zeis, the author of several books on Behcet's disease (http://www.behcetsdisease.com), she said, "ironically, according to some research studies people who quit smoking cigarettes sometimes develop excessive oral ulcers, which can be a real problem for BD patients who quit—some go right back to smoking again. This is a paradox but will vary from person to person.

"Toothpastes containing sodium lauryl sulfate may create aphthous ulcers in some BD patients, and should be avoided."

■ **Take probiotics and eat probiotic-rich foods.** Lactobacillus acidophilus is often beneficial in prevention and treatment of canker sores and may be useful in BD. No clinical research has been done in this area, but it makes sense. Take one to two capsules or ⅛ to ¼ teaspoon of the powder three times daily; take between meals.

■ **Practice stress-management skills.** Stress can contribute to a flare-up of the disease. Development of strong support systems is vital. This is a lifelong illness and you can greatly benefit from support groups, many of which are available on the Internet. Exchange of information and dialogue with others who understand what you are going through can expedite recovery. Take time for yourself, rest, and relax.

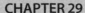

CHAPTER 29

Cardiovascular Disease: The GI Link

Cardiovascular disease certainly has more aspects to it than just the digestive ones. This section covers the GI-cardiovascular links.

PERIODONTAL DISEASE AND BRUSHING TEETH

It's been known for over a decade that people who have periodontal (gum) disease have increased risk for heart disease. There are two mechanisms that are known for this: systemic inflammation and bacterial infection. The bacteria Porphyromonas gingivalis and Streptococcus mutans have been identified as the main oral culprits that increase risk of heart diseases. Different studies have noted increases in atherosis, aneurysms, heart disease, heart valve issues that cause endocarditis, and Buerger's disease.

It has been demonstrated that simply brushing teeth twice daily can reduce risk of heart disease. A Scottish study with 11,000 participants demonstrated a 70 percent increased risk in people who brushed less than twice daily.

PREBIOTICS AND PROBIOTICS

Prebiotics and probiotics are another boon to our cardiovascular system. Their benefits are well documented. They help to normalize high total cholesterol, high LDL cholesterol, and triglycerides and can help boost HDL cholesterol levels. In a 2006 study by E. Fabinan and I. Elmadfa, 17 women were given a probiotic supplement daily for eight weeks, while 16 others ate 3½ ounces of commercial yogurt daily for four weeks, followed by two more weeks of 7 ounces of yogurt daily. Both groups had lowered total cholesterol levels with increases in HDL cholesterol and improved cholesterol ratios.

H. PYLORI INFECTION

People who have H. pylori infection in their stomach have been shown to have increased risk of developing ischemic heart disease. Although it's not completely understood why this happens, it appears that H. pylori helps to initiate an environment that increases heart disease; inflammation increases heart disease risk, and H. pylori increases inflammation. In mice, H. pylori increases platelet clumping and blood coagulation. H. pylori also increases heat shock proteins, which have also been implicated in cardiovascular disease. A recent study looked at people who had previously had H. pylori infections or stomach ulcers. After they were treated for infection, they were followed for five years. With the H. pylori taken care of, HDL cholesterol levels increased, while C-reactive protein and fibrinogen levels decreased. Another study indicated that in men with diabetes, H. pylori infection increased risk of heart disease. Another study showed little association with H. pylori and increased heart disease risk in women.

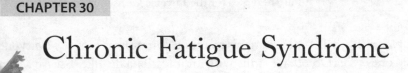

Chronic Fatigue Syndrome

Fatigue is one of the most common complaints that bring people into a physician's office. Fatigue can be caused by nearly every illness and is part of the natural healing process. Excessive fatigue that lasts and lasts may be a sign of illness or of chronic fatigue syndrome. Also called CFIDS (chronic fatigue and immune dysfunction syndrome), CFS, myalgic encephalomyelitis (ME), chronic Epstein-Barr virus (CEBV), and yuppie flu, chronic fatigue syndrome is a long-lasting, debilitating fatigue that is not associated with any particular illness. Although people have been fatigued for millennia, the term *chronic fatigue syndrome* was only coined in 1988. CFIDS affects more than half a million people. Incidence has increased two to four times within the past decade. According to the Centers for Disease Control and Prevention (CDC), 200 people per 100,000 experience CFIDS. About 50 percent return to normal health within five years. The rest may be affected for decades.

By definition, individuals with chronic fatigue syndrome have been extremely tired for at least six months for no obvious reason. The CDC has provided the following criteria for diagnosis of CFIDS. First, the fatigue is not eliminated by rest, and the fatigue substantially reduces the person's ability to function normally. Second, the diagnosis includes at least four of the following symptoms for a period of at least six months: loss in ability to concentrate or short-term memory function; sore throat; swollen and tender lymph nodes; muscle pain; multiple-joint pain without swelling or redness; headaches of a new type, pattern, or severity; sleep disturbances; and exercise-caused fatigue that lasts more than 24 hours.

People with CFIDS share many common symptoms, but not everyone has all the same ones. CFIDS often begins with an infectious flu-like disease accompanied by fevers that come and go. There is often accompanying joint stiffness and pain, sore throat, cough, sleep disturbances, light sensitivity, night sweats, and extreme exhaustion after the slightest exertion. Commonly, a short walk or bit of exercise will wipe out your energy for days afterward. Some people have the Epstein-Barr virus, or cytomegalovirus, but others don't. Sometimes healthy people have high blood antibodies for these viruses and have no symptoms of CFIDS. It's possible that these viruses trigger CFIDS, but it's also possible that the low immune function in people with CFIDS increases their chances of catching a wide variety of infectious illnesses. Although you can chase the virus, it's often just the trigger and not the ultimate cause of the illness. As with many illnesses, there is speculation on the part of researchers that there may be an autoimmune mimicry that gets triggered by a virus.

Many with CFIDS cannot hold down a job and become depressed because the fatigue is so extreme. Those who do work come home exhausted and go immediately to bed so they can generate enough energy for work the next day. Because there isn't any apparent cause and no observable symptoms, people with CFIDS are often confronted by people and doctors who just don't believe it's real.

In 1990, the CDC began to keep records and study people with CFIDS to understand more about possible causes and therapies. We now know that CFIDS is multifactorial and affects many biochemical systems. Cytokine production of interleukin-2 (IL-2) is low and causes poor immune function. Other immune parameters appear to be overstimulated. Although this seems paradoxical, it's probably not. According to Hans Selye, an expert on stress, our systems initially react to stress by overproducing. If working harder doesn't eventually solve the problem, they underproduce. Many people with CFIDS have exhausted adrenal glands and produce low amounts of cortisol and other adrenal hormones. They often have thyroid insufficiencies and may require thyroid hormone replacement. Other hormones, such as estrogen, progesterone, DHEA, and testosterone, may also be out of balance.

To find relief for CFIDS, use the DIGIN approach discussed in Part II. People with CFIDS almost always have dysbiosis, and most have candidiasis. Leaky gut syndrome is usually present, accompanied by a host of food and environmental sensitivities. There is often malabsorption. The liver is overburdened and overworked, so the toxic by-products of life accumulate in tissues, and the cycle deepens.

Eventually, the mitochondria are affected. Mitochondria are the energy factories inside our cells, creating ATP from glucose in a complicated process called the citric acid cycle, or Krebs cycle. Mitochondrial DNA is extremely susceptible to environmental damage from nutritional deficiencies, infection, disrupted sleep, pregnancy, changes in pH balance in the cell, magnesium status, hormonal deficiencies, and stress. Mitochondrial function can be inhibited by magnesium insufficiency, changes in cellular pH, and abnormal products of metabolism. These can be interpreted by the body as toxins. Magnesium is essential for mitochondrial functioning and is part of the matrix. Mitochondria also require vitamins B_1, B_2, B_3, B_6, lipoic acid, manganese, zinc, CoQ10, glucose, fatty acids, and amino acids. Mitochondrial function can be tested with an organic acid test, which has provided evidence that mitochondrial DNA is damaged much more easily and is more susceptible to environmental toxins and other stressors. As chronic fatigue symptoms progress, the mitochondria often need nutritional support of their own.

Jacob Teitelbaum, M.D., a specialist in CFIDS and fibromyalgia, speculates that this is a mitochondrial and hypothalamic disorder. Viral infections can disrupt hypothalamus and mitochondrial function. The hypothalamus controls sleep, autonomic nervous system function, body temperature, and hormone balance. When energy stores in the hypothalamus are depleted, all of these systems become imbalanced.

With the blood pressure test used with a tilt table, researchers have found that many people with CFIDS have low postural blood pressure. Complementary medicine physicians have long used reclining and standing blood pressures to detect poor adrenal function. Individuals with healthy adrenal function experience only a five- to ten-point rise in blood pressure when they move from a reclining to a standing position. In people with poor adrenal function, blood pressure remains the same or drops. So, is the tilt-table hypotension the primary culprit or an indicator of poor adrenal function? In any case, some people with low blood pressure respond to an increase in salt intake to at least 1,000 mg daily or by taking medication to increase blood pressure.

There aren't any panaceas for CFIDS, but there are therapies that can gradually help restore people to health. It's important to address detoxification, viral load, digestive function, dysbiosis (including candida and parasites), mitochondrial function, intestinal flora, environmental contaminants, heavy metals, underlying allergies, and hormone imbalances (especially thyroid and adrenal), as well as to restore functioning of the immune system. If this seems daunting, it can be. The causes and specifics are different for each person. Careful partnership between practitioner and patient will give the very best results. CFIDS is one area in which conventional, mainstream medicine has little to offer. If you've tried everything that your doctor has recommended and still aren't any better, you need to broaden your approach.

Restoration of digestive competency and nutrition go a long way toward normalizing CFIDS. Work with a nutritionally oriented health professional to design a program that meets your specific needs. The first steps are discovering any underlying problems that aggravate and drive the condition using the tests listed. It's important to check carefully for parasites; one study found giardia in 28 percent of subjects with CFIDS. Develop and follow a diet based on foods that are healthful for you and a nutrient-rich program designed to boost immune, brain, and cellular function. When you are ready, add exercise, a little bit at a time. People with CFIDS often feel worse after exercise, so go slowly. Several researchers link elevated cytokines and TNF-alpha and low levels of antioxidants and heat shock proteins in people with chronic fatigue. Increasing anti-inflammatory nutrients and antioxidants could be really beneficial. (See Chapter 9 on inflammation and the immune system.)

Physical therapy, counseling, occupational therapy, acupuncture, chi gong, Emotional Freedom Technique, and mind-body techniques can all be of great benefit.

The biological, rather than medical, approach to chronic fatigue saves money and works better. In one study of cost-effectiveness it was determined that a nutritional approach costs $2,000 compared to $10,000 for a medical approach. The patients on nutritional programs reported greater improvements in function and subjective well-being. They were able to significantly reduce the amount of medication they used.

Functional Laboratory Testing
- Comprehensive digestive stool analysis with parasitology
- Testing for food, environmental, mold, and chemical sensitivities
- Food allergy testing
- Liver function profile
- Intestinal permeability screening
- Organic acid testing
- Blood analysis for nutrients
- Fatty acid analysis

Healing Options
After testing, you'll have a better idea of any underlying problems. Look up related sections in this book to help you with the specifics.

- **Investigate food and environmental sensitivities.** Try an elimination diet. Use shampoos, soaps, and toiletries that are hypoallergenic for your specific needs and natural household cleaning products that are healthier for you, your family, and the environment. Some people are sensitive to their mattresses, gas stoves, carpeting, and upholstery. If you are, you may need to wear 100 percent cotton or other natural fiber clothes and use 100 percent cotton sheets and blankets.

Cotton is one of the largest genetically engineered crops, and some people are so sensitive to manmade substances that they can tolerate only organic cotton. Work with a health professional who can help you thread your way through the details.

- **Try an alkalizing diet.** See Chapter 17 for details.
- **Supplement with probiotics.** Supplemental use of beneficial bacteria can make a tremendous difference in your ability to digest foods. Beneficial flora can help reestablish the normal microbial balance in your intestinal tract. A recent study of people with CFIDS found that 6 of the 15 participants reported cognitive improvements in the four-week study.
- **Try digestive enzymes.** Pancreatic or vegetable enzymes supply the enzymes that your body needs to digest fats, proteins, and carbohydrates. Products differ. See Chapter 3 for more information. Take one to two capsules with meals.
- **Take a multivitamin with minerals.** Because people with CFIDS have difficulty with absorption and utilization of nutrients, a highly absorbable, hypoallergenic nutritional supplement is necessary. Although products that contain herbs, bee pollen, spirulina, and other food factors are good for many people, people with CFIDS often feel worse after taking food-based supplements. Make sure you buy the supplements that are herb and food free. Choose a supplement that contains the following nutrients: 25 to 50 mg zinc, 5,000 to 10,000 IU vitamin A, 10,000 to 25,000 IU carotenes, 200 or more IU vitamin E, at least 200 mcg selenium, 200 mcg chromium, at least 25 mg of most B-complex vitamins, 400 to 800 mcg folic acid, and 5 to 10 mg manganese.
- **Take vitamin C.** Vitamin C boosts immune function, helps detoxification pathways, and has been shown to have antiviral effects. Clinicians, including me, have found it useful in people with CFIDS. Take 3,000 to 5,000 mg daily. Do a vitamin C flush (detailed in Chapter 10).
- **Increase magnesium.** Magnesium is found in the ATP complex. Found in green leafy vegetables and whole grains, magnesium is involved in more than 300 enzymatic reactions in the body. It is essential for energy production, nerve conduction, muscle function, and bone health. People with CFIDS are often deficient in magnesium. Supplemental magnesium can improve energy levels and emotional states, while decreasing pain. Most people improve with use of oral magnesium supplements, but some need intravenous injections. Physicians can give 1,000 mg magnesium sulfate by injection. In one study, magnesium injections improved function in 12 out of 15 people, compared to only 3 receiving the placebo. Magnesium can be hard for many people to use. Adding 1 teaspoon of choline citrate daily for each 200 mg of magnesium taken can sig-

nificantly improve magnesium uptake. Take 500 to 2,000 mg magnesium glycinate, potassium aspartate, malate, or ascorbate. Caution: too much magnesium causes diarrhea.

- **Try coenzyme Q10 (CoQ10).** CoQ10 is necessary for energy production, immune function, and repair and maintenance of tissues. It also enhances cell function. CoQ10 is widely used in Japan for heart disease and has been researched as an antitumor substance. Take 60 to 300 mg daily.

- **Take essential fatty acids.** Several studies have shown people with CFIDS to have fatty acid imbalances. In a recent study, a combination of evening primrose oil (primarily omega-3) and fish oil (primarily omega-6) or a placebo of olive oil was given to 70 people with CFIDS. Of the people taking fish and evening primrose oils, 74 percent showed improvement at 5 weeks, and 85 percent showed improvement at 15 weeks. In comparison, the placebo group showed 23 percent improvement at 5 weeks and 17 percent at 15 weeks. Another study of the use of supplemental fatty acids showed improvement in 27 out of 29 people with CFIDS over 12 to 18 weeks. Twenty people who had previously been unable to work full-time for an average of more than three years were able to go back to work full-time after an average of 16 weeks. Sixteen months later 27 out of 28 remained improved, and 20 were still progressing. Do fatty acid testing, and then adjust doses to match your needs.

- **Add methionine.** Methionine, an essential sulfur-containing amino acid, is commonly deficient in people with CFIDS. It acts as a methyl donor for transmethylation reactions throughout the body, especially in the brain. It also helps sulfoxidation for liver detoxification pathways and is a precursor for other sulfur-containing amino acids such as cysteine and taurine. People with CFIDS probably have an increased need for methionine. Some people find improvement with a general amino acid supplement that supplies methionine, lysine, and carnitine simultaneously. Take 500 to 1,000 mg daily.

- **Try SAMe.** S-adenosylmethionine (SAMe), a compound that is naturally found in every cell in our body, is made from methionine. Research on SAMe shows it to have powerful antidepressant effects without the side effects of pharmaceutical antidepressant medications. SAMe has also been shown to be as potent an anti-inflammatory drug as indomethacin without the negative side effects in people with arthritis.

- **Try acetylcarnitine.** The vast majority of people with CFIDS have low levels of acetylcarnitine, although their levels of free carnitine are normal. Carnitine, vital for the conversion of fats into energy, also plays some role in detoxification and is believed to be essential for heart function. Finally, carnitine helps transport long-chain fatty acids into the mitochondria. Carnitine deficiencies result in muscle weakness, aches, and poor tone. Take 500 mg of carnitine two to four times daily for three months. For those on a budget, L-carnitine will also work.

- **Try D-ribose.** Ribose is a structural sugar that helps provide energy. Dr. Jacob Teitelbaum did a pilot study with 41 people with either fibromyalgia or chronic fatigue syndrome. Overall two-thirds reported benefits, with 45 percent reporting improvements in energy, and 30 percent reporting improvements in overall well-being after about 20 days; several also reported pain reduction. Take 5 grams three times daily, for three weeks, and then reduce to 5 grams twice daily. Mix in a cold, cool, or room temperature beverage.

- **Try lysine.** Often people with CFIDS also have herpes infections. Some people find good results with a general amino acid supplement, which supplies carnitine, lysine, and methionine as well as other amino acids. Take 1 to 2 grams lysine daily at the first sign of an outbreak; 500 mg daily for prevention.

- **Try malic acid.** Malic acid comes from apples and is important in energy production at a cellular level. Several physicians have found malic acid supplementation reduces fatigue and pain of fibromyalgia. Take 6 to 12 tablets daily, decreasing dosage over time. Each tablet contains 300 mg malic acid–magnesium hydroxide.

- **Use immune-modulating herbs and mushrooms.** Echinacea, goldenseal, astragalus, phytolacca (pokeweed), licorice, and lomatium all have immune-stimulating properties. Also eat immune balancing mushrooms, such as maitake, shiitake, or reishi. They can help prevent secondary infections while you are in a susceptible state. Take them preventively or therapeutically as directed.

- **Provide adrenal support.** People with CFIDS often need adrenal support. Think first about rest and nurture. Then also consider supplements, such as adrenal glandular supplements or herbal supplements, such as licorice and Siberian ginseng. Vitamin C and pantothenic acid (vitamin B_5) are also needed for proper adrenal function. If your blood pressure is low, you can use whole licorice; if not, use DGL, which will not affect blood pressure. It's best to take adrenal support in the morning and at lunch. If taken too late in the day, adrenal support can stimulate energy when you want to be winding down.

- **Consider nicotinamide adenine dinucleotide (NAD).** In a study monitoring the effect NAD has on people with CFIDS, 26 subjects were given the reduced form of it for four weeks and a placebo for an additional four weeks. Thirty-one percent showed improvement when on NAD, while only 8 percent improved when taking the placebo. Subjects were less fatigued and had improvement in quality of life. NAD is integral to the citric acid cycle of energy production. Once again, we are reminded that each person has unique needs. While most people did not benefit, NAD may be a useful treatment for some people. More research needs to be done to see if 10 mg daily, the amount given in the study, is the proper dosage; if a longer treatment program would be of additional benefit; and what, if any, the long-term benefits are.

- **Try Meyer's cocktail.** IV nutrients, given by a physician, can quickly help revitalize your nutrient status. Nutrients can be absorbed and used at higher concentrations. Meyer's cocktail is a combination of magnesium, calcium, vitamins B_{12} and B_6, pantothenic acid, and vitamin C. It has been used successfully in people with a variety of ailments.

- **Exercise.** People with CFIDS find exercise to be totally exhausting and draining. It is common for one period of exercise to be followed within 6 to 24 hours by 2 to 14 days of exhaustion and muscle aches. Paradoxically, exercise is helpful for restoring function in people with CFIDS, so it's advisable to begin with simple walking, swimming, or biking for five minutes daily. If you can, increase by one or two minutes a day each week. If you feel that you are at your maximum, maintain your present length of exercise time until your fatigue decreases. Don't push yourself hard. Slow and steady wins the race. Studies have shown that two-thirds of people with CFIDS benefit through exercise, although it is critical to not overdo.

  A new hypothesis suggests that those with CFIDS are functioning in an anaerobic state, so light anaerobic exercise may be most beneficial. Working with light weights, leg lifts, and use of weight machines to your capacity without causing fatigue may be more beneficial than aerobic exercise. As you begin to feel better, incorporate aerobic exercise—walking, biking, swimming, and dancing. Prioritize, so you have energy for what's most important. Be patient, kind, and loving to yourself.

- **Practice stress-management skills.** Development of strong support systems is vital. People with CFIDS often have the illness for a long time and can greatly benefit from support groups. Exchange of information and dialogue with others who understand what you are going through can expedite recovery. Take time for yourself, rest, and relax.

CHAPTER 31

Eczema or Atopic Dermatitis

Eczema, or atopic dermatitis, is a chronic skin condition characterized by redness, itching, and sometimes oozing, crusting, and scaling. The itch makes us scratch, which causes redness and inflammation. It affects 15 million Americans. Approximately 0.5 to 1 percent of the population has eczema, and it affects 10 to 20 percent of all infants. Fifty percent of children outgrow it by age 15; the rest may have mild to severe eczema throughout their lives. It can first appear at any age but most often during the first year of life. Babies can have eczema on their faces, scalp, bottom, hands, and feet. In children and adults, it may be more localized. Eczema is on the rise in industrialized countries. The causes are multifactorial and include imbalanced intestinal flora; leaky gut syndrome; food allergies; environmental contaminants, such as air pollution and tobacco smoke; and genetic predisposition.

The red patches are itchy, scaly, and dry, which encourages people to use lotions and creams to which they are often allergic. This complicates the problem further. Eczema varies over time, flaring up and calming down, at times better and worse. Emotional stress, heat, increase in humidity, bacterial skin infections, sweat, pets, hormone fluctuations, dust, molds, pollens, toiletries, cosmetics, and wool clothing commonly aggravate eczema. As children age, they may continue to have eczema; it may disappear; or they may develop other allergies, including asthma. People with eczema have high levels of IgE, secretory IgA, and eosinophils, all allergy signs.

Strong connections exist between eczema and food, microbial, and inhalant allergies. The word *atopy*, which is often used by physicians synonymously for allergy, refers to inflammations of the skin, nasal passages, and lungs. People with eczema often have allergies to dust, mold, dander, pollens, and foods.

Food allergies diagnosed through IgE and skin testing are apparent in most children with eczema. In a study of 165 children between the ages of 4 months and 22 years, researchers found that 60 percent had at least one positive skin-prick test for food allergies. When they challenged these results with a double-blind, placebo-controlled study, 39 of 64 subjects had a positive test, with milk, egg, peanut, soy, wheat, codfish, catfish, and cashews accounting for 89 percent of the positive food-allergy challenges. Undoubtedly, many more would be borne out by IgG, IgA, and IgM testing. Another study of children with eczema showed that eczema improved in 49 out of 66 children after elimination of the particular foods. Foods that aggravated eczema in this particular study, in descending order, were eggs, cow's milk, food coloring, tomatoes, fish, goat's milk, cheese, chocolate, and wheat.

A study was made of 122 children, aged four months to six years, with food intolerance. Of them, 52 children had eczema; the rest had chronic diarrhea. The allergies caused damage to the intestinal lining, and there was a decrease in the body's ability to defend itself because of lactose intolerance and dysbiosis, which caused leaky gut syndrome, leading to more food antigens and sensitivity. Children with eczema had more intestinal damage than those with chronic diarrhea.

Although the research is mixed, some studies report that eczema can be prevented in about half of children who have allergic family histories when probiotics are given at birth to both mother and nursing babies. When my son, Kyle, was 10 days old he began getting eczema on his bottom. By the time he was three months old, he looked like a burn victim despite my tries to heal him. I took him to Andrea Rentea, an anthroposophic pediatrician in Chicago, who recommended that I give him Bifidus infantus and that I take it myself. After 10 days, his eczema had completely healed. So had his cradle cap, and his fussiness also had ceased.

Breast-feeding dramatically reduces a baby's risk of developing eczema and allergies. Babies with eczema, and probably most babies, should not be given cow's milk, milk products, eggs, or wheat before one year of age. As their digestive system matures, they can better handle these complex foods. Babies with eczema who drink formula should be tested by skin prick to determine which formulas are most suitable for them. Because babies are born without intestinal flora in their digestive tracts, giving supplemental flora to the baby (and the mother, if she's nursing) can quickly alleviate baby eczema. (See more on this in Chapter 6.)

Elimination of foods, stress, and allergens can significantly alter the course of the disease. Even though you cannot control all factors, controlling enough of them will allow you to stay under the symptom threshold.

Jonathan Wright, M.D., had success in 39 out of 40 patients with eczema who followed this combined program: 50 mg zinc three times daily for six weeks, plus 2 mg copper daily, 5 grams omega-6 fatty acids (evening primrose or borage oil) twice a day for three months, and 1 to 2 grams omega-3 fatty acids (EPA/DHA fish oils) three times daily for four weeks.

Many people with eczema have low HCl levels. See Chapter 3 for more information and to take the HCl self-test.

The main treatments for eczema are steroid creams. These are good for symptom relief, but eczema starts from within the body and needs to be addressed systemically. The most common treatment for eczema is cortisone cream, which suppresses your body's normal immune function. It's very effective; however, there is often a rebound effect after you stop using the cream, and your symptoms return worse than before. A new class of medications, called topical immunomodulators, is available by prescription. In test studies, they relieve symptoms in most people and have less side effects than steroid creams. Patients are often told that these steroid and immunomulating creams act only locally. I disagree. When used over large areas of skin for a long time, they can have dramatic systemic effects. This is borne out by lab testing. Natural creams with chamomile, licorice, and comfrey root are also very effective at soothing and healing eczema without negative side effects. It's important to remember that even though eczema shows up on the skin, it is a systemic problem. Use creams to decrease irritation, but look for the underlying irritants.

Exercise may be especially beneficial for people with eczema. A recent study indicated that exercise reduced the inflammation associated with eczema by increasing the body's adaptability to stress.

To cut down on allergens in the home, vacuum fastidiously and use air purifiers in bedrooms and other rooms you are in frequently. One recent study attributed a reduction in eczema severity to a reduction in mattress dust and carpet mites by using a high-filtration vacuum cleaner and mattress covers. Keep your bedroom clean and clutter free.

Functional Laboratory Testing
- Allergy testing for IgE, food, mold, dust, and inhalants
- Elisa/Act testing for food, chemical, mold, and pharmaceutical sensitivities
- Comprehensive digestive stool analysis
- Heidelberg capsule test for adequacy of hydrochloric acid production

Healing Options
- **Investigate food and environmental sensitivities.** For more information see Chapters 14 and 15. An elimination-provocation diet can significantly reduce eczema. Often foods that you are sensitive to will make you itch. The itching may start soon after the meal, but it can be delayed up to 48 hours, which makes tracking down the foods a bit tricky. Food allergy and sensitivity testing

can help you determine which foods to eliminate from your diet. Eliminate all foods and chemicals that you are sensitive to for four to six months. Use natural household cleaning products and shampoos, and select soaps and toiletries that are hypoallergenic. If you are sensitive to mattresses, gas stoves, carpeting, and upholstery, you may need to use cotton and other natural fiber clothing and sheets that allow the skin to breathe naturally. Work with a health professional who knows how to help you meet your needs.

- **Supplement with probiotics**. Restoring the normal balance of flora in your intestinal tract can help reduce eczema. Use of supplemental beneficial bacteria can make a tremendous difference in your ability to thoroughly digest foods.

- **Check for candida infection.** Fungal infections are a common cause of eczema. In a study of 115 men and women with eczema, 85 were sensitive to fungus; after they were treated with fungal creams, oral ketoconazole, or a yeast-free diet, there was much improvement. Take the yeast self-test and do blood testing or CDSA to determine if yeast is contributing to your eczema. (See Chapter 11 for the quiz.)

- **Try black cumin seed oil.** In four human studies, black cumin seed oil (Nigella sativa) has been shown to alleviate the symptoms of eczema and other allergies. It also moderately helps to normalize serum triglycerides and cholesterol. Black cumin seeds are a food, so there is low toxicity. Take 20 to 40 mg daily per pound of body weight. A 150-pound adult could take 3,000 to 6,000 mg. This is about ½ to a bit more than a teaspoon of black cumin oil daily. Take internally or drizzle on food. It can also be mixed with lotion and put on the skin.

- **Use natural eczema creams.** Herbal creams can be as effective as cortisone creams in reducing eczema, and they don't have the negative side effects. Licorice root stimulates production of healing and anti-inflammatory prostaglandins. Use of a 2 percent licorice cream is recommended. Chamomile creams are widely used in Europe. A recent study compared a chamomile product, Kamillosan, against 0.5 percent hydrocortisone cream. After two weeks, the Kamillosan was reported to give slightly better results than the hydrocortisone cream. Look in health-food stores or ask your health professional to find a product that works for you.

- **Try Jonathan Wright's protocol.** This is outlined earlier in the chapter.

- **Take vitamin C.** A study of 10 young people with severe eczema showed that supplementation with vitamin C significantly improved eczema and immune function. They needed only half as many antibiotics for treating skin infections as the control group. Take 1,000 to 3,000 mg mineral ascorbates or Ester-C daily. Do a vitamin C flush once a week. (See Chapter 18.)

- **Try evening primrose, flaxseed, and borage oils.** Studies show that people with eczema generally have low levels of both omega-3 and omega-6 fatty acids. The first step in metabolism of linoleic acid, which allows for the conversion into gamma-linolenic acid (GLA), is often impaired in people with eczema. Taking GLA directly in evening primrose, flaxseed, or borage oil circumvents blockage. GLA has an anti-inflammatory effect and benefits immune function. Take 1 to 2 grams three times daily of any of these oils or a combination.

- **Increase fish oil consumption.** One recent study on people with eczema showed a 30 percent improvement in a four-month trial of eight capsules of fish oil per day. Though the placebo group was given corn oil, which gave an improvement of 24 percent, results suggest that people with eczema have a generalized need for essential fatty acids. Eating cold-water fish—salmon, halibut, sardines, herring, tuna—two to four times each week can provide you with the omega-3 oils you need. If you use fish oil capsules, do so under the supervision of a physician. They cause a significant increase in clotting time and should not be used by people with hemophilia or those on aspirin or anticoagulant drugs.

- **Try quercetin.** Quercetin, the most effective bioflavonoid for anti-inflammation, can be used to reduce pain and inflammatory responses and control allergies. Take 500 to 1,000 mg three to four times daily.

- **Use turmeric.** For eczema, turmeric can be used in combination with neem, an Ayurvedic remedy for parasites and infections.

- **Try a nickel-restricted diet.** The relationship between nickel sensitivity and eczema has appeared recently in scientific literature. Nickel is an essential nutrient that is found in many enzymes. However, excess nickel is an irritant to the GI lining. You can be tested for nickel sensitivity through skin testing or an oral challenge. Nickel is used as an alloy in jewelry, so if jewelry irritates your skin or turns it gray, you may be sensitive to nickel. If you are, a low-nickel diet should be followed for a limited period of time. High-nickel foods are chocolate, nuts, dried beans and peas, and grains.

- **Neutralize reactions.** There are many ways to minimize the effects of food sensitivities. Clinical ecologists can provide neutralization drops to counteract your reaction to particular foods. These drops work like allergy shots—a small amount of what you are sensitive to helps stimulate your body's natural immune response. Malic acid can also curtail sensitivity reactions.

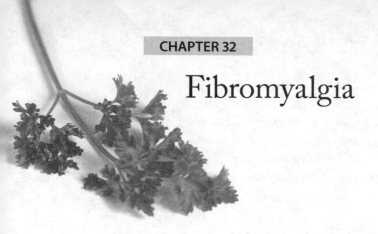

CHAPTER 32

Fibromyalgia

Fibromyalgia is characterized by long-term muscle pain and stiffness. According to the American College of Rheumatology, fibromyalgia affects 3 million to 6 million Americans, 85 to 90 percent of whom are women. It affects about 2 percent of the general population and 20 percent of people with arthritic disease. It used to be called *fibrositis*, which implies an inflammation of fibrous and connective tissues such as muscles, tendons, fascia, and ligaments. Myofascial pain syndrome is similar but is characterized by just a few painful and achy places, most often in the jaw, that are tender when trigger points are touched.

Fibromyalgia is characterized by generalized aching, pain, and tenderness throughout the body. People complain of neck, shoulder, lower back, and hip pain that seems to move around from place to place. People often report fatigue and changes in sleep patterns. They often wake up during the night with a feeling of achiness or stiffness. About 40 to 70 percent of people with fibromyalgia also report irritable bowel symptoms: abdominal pain, constipation, diarrhea, gas, or bloating. Other symptoms that occur with frequency include cognitive decline, extreme sensitivity to touch, fatigue, bladder syndrome, tooth grinding, headaches, jaw pain or temporomandibular joint (TMJ) problems, and depression. Symptoms that occur less often are heightened sensitivity to chemicals; intolerance to cold, heat, or bright lights; bladder problems; Raynaud's phenomenon; difficulty concentrating; mood changes; dry eyes, skin, and mouth; painful menstruation; chest or pelvic pain; dizziness; nasal congestion; and numbness or swelling in the hands or feet.

The American College of Rheumatology bases the diagnosis on just two things: diffuse soft tissue pain for at least three months, and 11 out of 18 paired tender points. "Fibromyalgia" is often a catchall diagnosis for someone with aching muscles and fatigue. It is widely overdiagnosed. One study reported that it was overdiagnosed 66 percent of the time, which means that two-thirds of people didn't get complete enough workups to rule out other medical issues. Symptoms of widespread pain and pain in trigger points can be due to a wide variety of conditions, so looking for an accurate diagnosis is critical.

Fibromyalgia responds well to the DIGIN model presented in this book. Look and look to discover the underlying issues for your fibromyalgia. Find the levers that will help you rebalance. These will be different for each person.

Fibromyalgia can be a physical manifestation of emotional trauma. Statistically people with fibromyalgia have a higher history of chronic stress and emotional, physical, and/or sexual trauma than people without fibromyalgia. People with fibromyalgia often report a traumatic event that triggered initial symptoms: emotional or physical stress, an accident, or a severe infectious illness. This is often accompanied by insomnia due to hypervigilance of the immune system (see Chapter 9). Lack of sleep is associated with a dysfunction of the hippocampus, which can manifest as short-term memory loss and cognitive impairment. These are also classic fibromyalgia symptoms.

Fibromyalgia shares many symptoms with chronic fatigue syndrome, though it is classified as its own disease. People with fibromyalgia, unlike those with chronic fatigue syndrome, usually do not have low acetylcarnitine levels or have a viral infection as a trigger. Recent studies indicate that myofascial pain, fibromyalgia, and CFIDS are on a continuum of the same disease path, with myofascial pain being the mildest, fibromyalgia moderate, and CFIDS the most severe.

Other medical conditions that can masquerade as fibromyalgia include hypothyroidism; anemia; rheumatoid arthritis; Lyme disease; other rheumatic disorders such as ankylosing spondylitis, multiple sclerosis, and Sjögren's disease; and cancers. Dysbiosis, postviral immune suppression, and blood sugar imbalances can also contribute to muscle tenderness. These can all be screened with simple medical testing.

Dr. Mark Pimental reports that 78 percent of people with fibromyalgia have small intestinal bacterial overgrowth (SIBO). When SIBO is treated, fibromyalgia symptoms improve greatly. This is discussed in the sections on IBS and chronic fatigue syndrome.

Nutrient deficiencies play a role in fibromyalgia. Without proper nutrients, energy production in the mitochondria doesn't work correctly. Doing nutritional testing and organic acid testing can help you to optimize your nutritional status.

It's important to be checked for vitamin D status. About half of all people with fibromyalgia are deficient in this nutrient. Vitamin D deficiencies affect about one-third of Caucasians, two-thirds of Hispanics, and 90 percent of people of African descent. Sometimes, just optimizing vitamin D levels can "cure" fibromyalgia. Ask your doctor to check your 25-OH vitamin D level. Normal levels are between 32 and 100 ng/ml. Optimal levels are probably between 60 and 100 ng/ml. People make vitamin D from sunlight, but in northern climates or if people aren't outdoors, they don't make nearly enough. The best food source is cold-water fish, such as salmon, sardines, mackerel, and herring. Vitamin D also helps facilitate magnesium absorption. An increased need for magnesium is found in most people with fibromyalgia.

Use of a single supplement may bring some relief, but a total program is necessary to bring dramatic relief and true healing. Taking coenzyme Q10; vitamins B_1, B_6, and arginine; 5-hydroxytryptophan (5-HTP); S-adenosylmethionine (SAMe); essential fatty acids; antioxidants; niacin; and magnesium malate (magnesium plus malic acid), in addition to a hypoallergenic diet has been shown to have positive effects. Acupuncture has been proven useful in treating fibromyalgia. Chiropractic or osteopathic adjustments and massage treatments may also be of help.

People with fibromyalgia have an increased need for antioxidants. Use of antioxidant supplements and increasing fruits, vegetables, nuts, seeds, and whole foods can reduce inflammation and free radical damage.

People with fibromyalgia are generally put on anti-inflammatory drugs and antidepressants. One study showed that 90 percent of people treated with anti-inflammatory drugs were still symptomatic after three years. Conventional medical therapies for fibromyalgia usually are unsuccessful in the long term because they fail to address possible underlying causes of the illness. Food and environmental sensitivities, candida, toxicity, unresolved emotional issues, and/or parasites can be causal factors in fibromyalgia. A stool test may be useful in diagnosing the cause of fibromyalgia. When the underlying problem has been identified and treated, fibromyalgia resolves.

A small but promising study was done with 32 people who had fibromyalgia for 5 to 10 years. There were 25 active participants and seven controls. The participants were tested for food and environmental sensitivities with the Elisa/Act test and given dietary restrictions. They were put on a detoxification program and personalized nutritional therapies to meet their needs and stimulate repair of cells and tissues. The final component was stress management, with recommendations for relaxation training, exercise, and biofeedback. In 6 to 12 weeks, these people showed a reduction of 80 to 90 percent in their symptoms. They also showed a significant reduction in the number of foods and environmental sensitivities in repeated testing. More research needs to be done in this area.

Nutritional therapies have been successful in the reduction of symptoms. In a study, 50 people with either CFIDS or fibromyalgia were given products made by Mannatech, a multilevel supplement company, including freeze-dried aloe, plant-derived saccharides with freeze-dried fruits and vegetables, and a wild yam product with multivitamins and minerals. Although all subjects in the study had undergone previous unsuccessful medical treatment, a remarkable reduction in symptoms was noted, with continued improvement over the nine-month test period. Although this was a small, preliminary study, it shows promise for the nutritional approach to fibromyalgia and CFIDS.

One approach to fibromyalgia is the use of guaifenesin, a gout medication. Endocrinologist R. Paul St. Amand, M.D., believes that people with fibromyalgia have calcium phosphate deposits on muscles, tendons, and ligaments. St. Amand developed his theory after observing a high level of dental calculus (calcium phosphate deposits) among his fibromyalgia patients. His therapy (which includes a healing crisis, or a period of worsening of symptoms before improvement) begins with a dose of 300 mg of guaifenesin per day. He reports this working in 20 percent of his patients, but if no healing crisis occurs after two weeks, St. Amand increases the dose to 600 mg daily. At this level, another 50 percent of his patients improve, while the remaining 30 percent seem to require higher doses. Typically, if this protocol is going to work, you'll see a change within two months of treatment. The longer you've had the disease, the longer you need to stay on the medication. While doing this therapy, avoid all salicylates, because they negate the treatment. This would include aspirin; herbs such as willow bark and aloe; and some common products such as topical pain-relieving cream, some mouthwashes, eyeliner, and some herbal hairsprays. As guaifenesin is a weak antigout medication with few side effects, the therapy certainly seems worth trying. I know several people who have tried this approach.

Zhang and colleagues report that guaifenesin is a muscle relaxant and is used as an anesthetic to treat the symptoms of fibromyalgia. His group measured specific cytokines in people with fibromyalgia who had taken guaifenesin for at least three months, in people with fibromyalgia who did not take guaifenesin, in family members of people with fibromyalgia, and with controls. People with fibromyalgia had higher levels of inflammatory cytokines, which is to be expected. There were specific differences in which cytokines were elevated in the various groups. More work needs to be done in this area.

Functional Laboratory Testing

- Breath test for SIBO
- Organic acid testing
- Nutritional analysis
- Adrenal stress testing (salivary DHEA and cortisol)
- Elisa/Act food and environmental sensitivity testing
- Oxidative stress evaluation
- Provocation testing for heavy metals
- Hormone testing

Healing Options

- **Look for the underlying cause.** Seventy-eight percent of people with fibromyalgia have small intestinal bacterial overgrowth; others are suffering from post-trauma issues; others have hormone imbalances, food sensitivities, or nutritional deficiencies. Look until you find the clues.
- **Take vitamin D.** Vitamin D deficiency is often diagnosed as fibromyalgia. About half of people with fibromyalgia have low serum vitamin D levels. We make vitamin D in our skin from exposure to sunlight. So, get outdoors more. It's difficult to get enough vitamin D from our foods. Have your vitamin D level tested. Optimal levels in people with fibromyalgia are likely to be between 80 and 100 ng/ml. Dosages range from 2,000 IU daily as a maintenance dose to 10,000 IU daily if vitamin D levels are extremely low.
- **Try an alkalizing diet.** Balancing cellular metabolism by eating an alkalizing diet may be of great help in fibromyalgia. Use pH testing to determine the best diet for you. Include fresh fruits and vegetables, vegetable juices, and sea vegetables. Use baking soda and Epsom salt baths. (See Chapter 9.)
- **Try metabolic cleansing.** Metabolic cleansing involves going on a hypoallergenic food plan and taking a nutrient-rich protein powder designed to help restore your liver's detoxification capacities. Use this protocol for one to three weeks. See Chapter 18 on detoxification and metabolic cleansing.
- **Investigate food and environmental sensitivities.** Eliminate all foods and chemicals that you are sensitive to for four to six months. (See Chapter 15 for an elimination diet.) Get tested to find the specifics. Work with a health professional who can help you with the details.
- **Try ascorbigen and broccoli powder.** A study of 12 patients with fibromyalgia was done with ascorbigen and broccoli powder. Ascorbigen is the most common indole found in cooked cabbage, broccoli, brussels sprouts, and other cabbage

family foods. In one month, symptoms improved by nearly 20 percent. After the supplements were discontinued, symptoms returned to usual levels within two weeks. Take 100 mg ascorbigen plus 400 mg broccoli powder daily.

■ **Take a multivitamin with minerals**. A high-quality, hypoallergenic nutritional supplement is necessary. Although products that contain herbs, bee pollen, spirulina, and other food factors are good for many people, it's best to buy supplements that are herb and food free. Look for the following levels of specific nutrients: 50 to 100 mg vitamin B_1, 50 to 100 mg vitamin B_6, 200 to 400 IU vitamin E, 10,000 IU vitamin A, 10,000 to 25,000 IU carotenes, 200 mcg selenium, 200 mcg chromium, 5 to 10 mg manganese, glutathione, cysteine, or N-acetyl cysteine (NAC), plus additional nutrients. Antioxidant nutrients—carotenes, vitamins C and E, selenium, glutathione, CoQ10, cysteine, and NAC—have been shown to be needed in larger quantities in people with fibromyalgia.

■ **Take vitamin B_1 (thiamin).** People with fibromyalgia have lower levels of red blood cell transketolase, which is a functional test for thiamin status. Researchers found that supplemental thiamin pyrophosphate worked better than other forms. This suggests a metabolic defect rather than a true deficiency. This may also reflect a magnesium deficiency because thiamin-dependent enzymes require magnesium. Take 25 to 100 mg daily.

■ **Take vitamin C.** Vitamin C boosts immune function, helps detoxification pathways, and has antiviral effects. Take 3,000 mg daily. Once a week, do a vitamin C flush (see Chapter 18).

■ **Take magnesium.** It is very common for people with fibromyalgia to be deficient in magnesium. Serum magnesium levels often appear normal, but if more sophisticated tests such as red blood cell magnesium are done, magnesium levels are often low. Supplemental magnesium can improve energy levels and emotional states while decreasing pain. Most people improve by using oral magnesium supplements, but some need an intravenous injection of 1,000 mg magnesium sulfate by a physician (for more on magnesium, see discussion on chronic fatigue syndrome). Choline citrate can greatly enhance oral magnesium utilization (available from Perque, listed in Resources at http://www.digestivewellnessbook.com). Take 500 to 1,000 mg magnesium citrate or magnesium glycinate.

■ **Try arginine.** People with fibromyalgia have been shown to have lower levels of arginine than other people. Take 500 to 1,000 mg or a mixed free amino acid supplement.

■ **Try 5-hydroxytryptophan (5-HTP).** People with fibromyalgia have lower tryptophan levels than controls. Studies have shown 5-HTP to be of benefit in fibromyalgia. Tryptophan is a precursor to serotonin, a neurotransmitter that helps us sleep and prevents depression. Passionflower, an herb with high levels of tryptophan, has been used historically for depression, anxiety, and insomnia, all of which are symptoms of fibromyalgia. Tryptophan is also found in cashews, cheddar cheese, eggs, halibut, peanuts, salmon, sardines, shrimp, turkey, and tuna. Our body produces it when we eat starchy foods. Take 200 to 600 mg daily of 5-HTP. Doses can be divided between morning and bedtime.

- **Try capsaicin (cayenne pepper cream).** The prescription drug capsaicin was used in a study of 45 people with fibromyalgia. It was found to improve grip strength and reduce pain over a two-week period. Capsaicin cream burns temporarily, but this diminishes over time.

- **Try S-adenosylmethionine (SAMe).** A recent study of 47 people with fibromyalgia showed that injections and oral supplementation of SAMe significantly reduced muscle tenderness and the number of tender points, lowered pain severity, and benefited depression and anxiety. SAMe is produced in our bodies from methionine. It is the active methylating agent for many enzyme reactions throughout the body, especially in the brain. It is probably the sulfur that is needed. People with fibromyalgia can probably make this conversion, so oral methionine may be useful clinically (1,000 to 2,000 mg). Other sulfur-containing supplements are dimethylsulfoxide (DMSO), taurine, glucosamine or chondroitin sulfate, and reduced glutathione. In the study, dosages of SAMe were 200 mg given daily as intramuscular injection, plus 400 mg taken orally twice daily.

- **Try Meyer's cocktail.** IV nutrients, given by a physician, can quickly help revitalize your nutrient status. Nutrients can be absorbed and used at higher concentrations. Meyer's cocktail is a combination of magnesium, calcium, vitamins B_{12} and B_6, pantothenic acid, and vitamin C. It has been used successfully in people with a variety of ailments.

- **Try traditional Chinese medicine.** Acupuncture has been established as giving benefit to people with fibromyalgia. A 2010 multicentered study of 186 people with fibromyalgia reported that 65 percent of those who received acupuncture combined with cupping and Western medicine had benefits. This produced better effects than either just acupuncture with cupping or use of Western medicine alone. A 2010 review study of 1,516 people with fibromyalgia (from 25 combined studies) reports that acupuncture reduced the number of tender points and reduced pain scores when compared with conventional medications. When combined with cupping, results improved for pain reduction and improving depression scores. On the other hand, a Cochrane Review in 2009 reported that there was no change in pain intensity when compared to a placebo. Acupuncture and cupping may or may not be of benefit to you but have a low risk and possible benefits that make it worth trying.

- **Try malic acid.** Malic acid, found in apples, is important in energy production at a cellular level. Several physicians have found malic acid supplementation reduces fatigue and the pain of fibromyalgia. It also helps alkalize. Take 6 to 12 tablets of 300 mg malic acid–magnesium hydroxide daily, decreasing dosage over time.

- **Take quercetin.** Quercetin is the most effective bioflavonoid in its anti-inflammatory effects, and it can be used to reduce pain and inflammatory responses and control allergies. Take 500 to 1,000 mg three to four times daily.

- **Take glucosamine sulfate.** Glucosamine sulfate is used therapeutically to help repair cartilage, reduce swelling and inflammation, and restore joint function, with no reported side effects. Take 500 mg two to four times daily.

- **Try digestive enzymes.** Take one to two tablets or capsules with meals.

- **Supplement with probiotics.** Use of supplemental beneficial bacteria can help reestablish the normal microbial balance in your intestinal tract. The supplement you purchase may have additional microbes as well. Take as directed on label as products vary. Mix powdered supplement with a cool beverage.

- **Try coenzyme Q10 (CoQ10).** CoQ10 is necessary for energy production, immune function, repair and maintenance of tissues, and enhanced cell function. Take 60 to 100 mg daily.

- **Try glutamine.** Glutamine, the most abundant amino acid in our bodies, is used in the digestive tract as a fuel source and for healing stomach ulcers, irritable bowel syndrome, ulcerative bowel diseases, and leaky gut syndrome. Begin with 8 grams daily for four weeks.

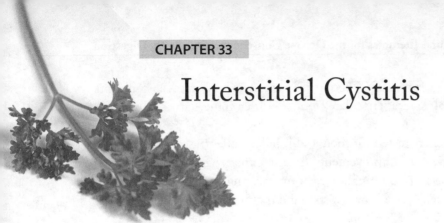

CHAPTER 33

Interstitial Cystitis

Interstitial cystitis (IC) is an illness that results in chronic discomfort or pain in the bladder and pelvic area. The discomfort can be mild to extreme. Common symptoms include urgent need to urinate, pain with urination, frequent urination, pelvic pain, prostitis in men, and pain with love-making. Interstitial cystitis is more commonly diagnosed in women (90 percent) than in men (10 percent). In women, symptoms can get worse during menstruation. The women I have worked with have so much pain after making love that they just don't make love anymore. About half of women spontaneously improve without any medical treatment.

Irritable bowel syndrome and fibromyalgia are common co-diseases. Since in both fibromyalgia and IBS small intestinal bacterial overgrowth (SIBO) plays such a large role, I looked to see if there had been any studies on SIBO in IC. In 2008 Dr. Leonard Weinstock studied 21 women with interstitial cystitis. Seventeen (81 percent) had SIBO as determined by lactulose breath testing. Fifteen women were treated with 1,200 to 1,800 mg Rifaxamin for 10 days. Afterward improvement was sustained with 3 mg of tegaserod nightly. There were moderate to great improvements in 11 (73 percent), and all but one were able to sustain the benefits. Improvements in interstitial cystitis were moderate to great in six of the women (40 percent) and were sustained in seven (47 percent). However, in e-mails with Dr. Weinstock, he said that a placebo-controlled trial had results that were less dramatic. Nonetheless, in an illness where little helps, this is worth exploring.

Entire books have been written about using a low-acid diet and lowering the number of foods containing phenylalanine, tyrosine, tryptophan, asprartate, and tryamine in an effort to control IC. Foods that have been reported as problems include tomatoes, alcohol, spices, chocolate, foods with caffeine, citrus fruits, and artificial sweeteners.

One group of researchers tested for food and inhalant allergies. When specific diets were utilized, there were improvements. In my experience in working with women with interstitial cystitis, elimination diets and testing for food and environmental sensitivities has been useful. I have also found that balancing pH and inflammation is very useful.

Functional Laboratory Testing
- Breath test for SIBO
- Food sensitivity and food allergy testing
- Testing for molds and environmental chemical sensitivities
- Celiac testing
- pH testing

Healing Options
- **Rule out SIBO.** In a 2008 study of 21 women, 81 percent of those tested had SIBO. When treated, most of them improved. Use the SIBO breath test described in Chapter 11.
- **Try an elimination diet.** Bring down the total inflammatory load in your body by trying an elimination diet. This diet eliminates artificial sweeteners and alcohol. You may also want to exclude tomatoes, citrus, and other acidic foods. (See Chapter 15.)
- **Balance pH.** See Chapter 17 for more information.
- **Try quercetin and grape seed extract.** High levels of mast cells have been found in the bladders of women with IC. Quercetin is a mast-cell inhibitor; it reduces inflammation and acts to decrease allergy responses. In one study 22 women were given 500 mg of quercetin twice daily with the protein-splitting enzymes bromelain and papain. In four weeks symptoms improved by 62 percent and the problem index by 55 percent. All but one patient had at least some improvement. Take 1,000 to 3,000 mg of quercetin daily, plus 10 mg grape seed extract daily.
- **Try L-arginine.** Arginine is an amino acid that is needed for synthesis of nitric oxide. One study found high levels of nitric oxide, while another found elevated levels in those with IC. Some women have improved by taking arginine; others haven't. Give it a try and see if it helps you. Take 500 mg three times daily.
- **Try a high-dose probiotic supplement.** Much of the information on interstitial cystitis comes from people who have it. There are many reports from people

who become pain-free after taking high-dose probiotic supplements for several months. There is no published research on use of probiotics in interstitial cystitis as of yet. The main effect of probiotic bacteria is to modulate the immune system, to reduce inflammation, and to protect tissues by making small amounts of antibiotics, anti-cancer substances, and vitamins. Certainly this is a simple remedy to try. Take 100 billion CFU of mixed probiotic cultures once or twice daily.

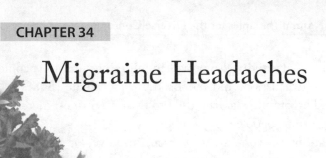

CHAPTER 34

Migraine Headaches

Migraines usually begin with a throbbing pain on one side of the head, which can spread to both sides. About 60 percent of people experience symptoms 24 hours prior to the actual migraine, which include mood changes, food cravings, repetitive yawning, thirst, fluid retention, stiff neck, irritability, fatigue, numbness or tingling on one side of the body, lack of appetite, diarrhea, constipation, a feeling of coldness, lethargy, changes in vision, or seeing bright spots. These symptoms, often called an aura, may let you know a migraine is on the way; they may disappear when the headache appears or remain. Medications and other techniques work best if used at this point. Although symptoms vary from person to person, they have a consistent pattern in each individual. Migraine attacks may last from hours to days and may be accompanied by nausea, vomiting, and extreme sensitivity to light.

Migraine headaches cause periodic disruption in the lives of 28 million Americans, affecting 6 percent of men and more than 18 percent of women every year. It averages just over 10 percent of our population, making it the most prevalent neurological illness. Costs to society are $13 billion annually, which includes 157 million workdays that are lost each year. Migraines have genetic, hormonal, immune, and environmental components.

Migraines usually come on in response to a trigger. Common triggers are foods and beverages, alcohol, stress, emotions, hormone changes, medications such as estrogen therapy, visual stimuli, or changes in routine. A recent study of 494 people with migraines cited the following triggers: stress in 62 percent, weather changes in 43 percent, missing a meal in 40 percent, and bright sunlight in 38 percent. Cigarettes, perfumes, and sexual activity also provoked migraines in some people. Other triggers are red wines, exhaustion, and monosodium glutamate (MSG). Tobacco, birth control pills, and ergotamine (a drug used to treat migraines) increase the frequency of migraines in some people.

Hormone fluctuations in women can worsen, improve, or trigger migraines. Many women experience migraines only at specific times in their menstrual cycle, from ovulation through menstruation. Birth control pills and other estrogen-containing medications are widely recognized to trigger migraines in susceptible women. When women stop taking the medications, their migraines typically disappear. When I was in my teens, I was put on birth control pills for severe menstrual cramps. I developed migraines, but when I asked my doctor if the pills could be triggering migraines he said no because the relationship wasn't yet known. I was put through brain scans and neurological tests. When all was said and done, going off the pill stopped the migraines and I've never had another. Unfortunately this took several years to figure out.

Jean Munro, M.D., an English doctor who specializes in working with people with multiple chemical sensitivities, breaks migraines into four types. The first type is a classic migraine, which begins with a visual disturbance of some sort—flashing lights, blackening, or blurred vision. It usually involves one side of the head, and people often vomit. The migraine usually lasts one to three days and can be quite severe. The second type is called a common migraine and is almost identical to the first except that there is no visual warning. It begins on one side, sometimes progressing to both, and there may be vomiting. The third type is called a basilar migraine, when the blood vessels at the base of the head dilate. It can be quite frightening and often causes a panicky feeling, accompanied by a sense of doom. A generalized headache is accompanied by a pins-and-needles sensation around the mouth, nausea, and tingling hands. The fourth type, called a motor migraine, is a variation on the basilar and may be quite severe. Half the body feels weak, head pain centers around the eye, and vision is distorted.

A 2010 paper in *Headache* looked at comorbid conditions in 1,348 people with migraine: 88 percent were women; 31 percent also had irritable bowel syndrome; 15 percent also had chronic fatigue syndrome; 10 percent had fibromyalgia; 6.5 percent had interstitial cystitis; 25 percent had arthritis; 15 percent had endometriosis; 14 percent had uterine fibroids. Maltreatment in childhood was reported in 58 percent. Interestingly enough, abuse and neglect were associated with different diseases along with migraine. Emotional abuse was associated with irritable bowel syndrome, chronic fatigue syndrome, and arthritis; physical neglect was associated with arthritis in the entire group and with uterine fibroids in women; physical abuse was associated with endometriosis.

Using medications for migraines is the standard medical approach. The main drugs to treat acute migraines are those that increase serotonin (sumatriptan, naratriptan, and zolmitriptan), opiate pain medications, and dihydroergotamine. Drugs that help prevent migraines from occurring include valproic acid, beta blockers, and methysergide. According to Alan Gaby, a prominent nutritionally oriented M.D. and the author of *Nutritional Medicine*, the most effective medications reduce frequency only by half and have significant side effects. In his book, Dr. Gaby writes, "In my experience at least two-thirds of patients who comply with an appropriate regimen of dietary modification and nutritional supplements experience a substantial reduction in, or a complete cessation of, migraine headaches."

PREVENTING MIGRAINES BY CHANGING WHAT YOU EAT

One common trigger of migraine headaches is dysregulated blood sugar levels: hypoglycemia, diabetes, and/or high insulin levels. It's one of the first things that I consider, and why I always ask my clients to keep track of what they have eaten or if they have eaten prior to a migraine. If migraines appear early morning or late afternoon when glucose levels are typically lowest, hypoglycemia is a likely suspect.

Avoiding caffeine or salt can help others. One study reports that people had significant improvement on a low-fat diet. Whether the results were from eating healthier foods or from the low-fat aspect of the diet is unknown to me. Virtually any food can be a migraine trigger. Figuring out which ones can be of great personal benefit.

The relationship between food sensitivities or allergies and migraines was studied during the 1930s. In 400 people, complete or partial relief was achieved 50.8 percent to 78 percent of the time. True IgE food allergies trigger some migraines; IgG sensitivities can also play a role. Since the 1930s, many studies have been done which replicate these results. Here are a few of those studies.

Of 282 patients with migraines whom Dr. Munro studied, 100 percent had food allergies or sensitivities; more than 200 of them were sensitive to wheat and/or dairy products. Other common trigger foods were tea and coffee, oranges, apples, onions, pork, egg, and beef. Dr. Munro found that foods eaten daily provoked more reactions than chocolate, alcohol, and cheese, which are thought to be the most common triggers. Dr. Munro also found that people who eliminated these foods from their diet and cleared their homes of environmental contaminants had the best results in prevention of migraines. Using mild household cleaners, getting rid of gas appliances, removing house plants with molds and fungus, frequent cleaning, and making a bedroom an oasis by removing carpets and curtains resulted in fewer migraines. Although these people were still exposed to smoke, perfume, and other environmental triggers outside, changing the home environment and their diets lowered their total load enough so that they became more tolerant.

In a 1979 issue of *Lancet,* E. C. Grant published a study in which 60 adults were put on a strict elimination diet for five days in an in-patient setting. They then added foods back into their diets. Migraines were triggered by wheat (78 percent of the time), orange (65 percent), eggs (45 percent), tea and coffee (40 percent each), chocolate and milk (37 percent each), beef (35 percent), corn, sugar, and yeast (33 percent each). Headache rates dropped 85 percent. A quarter of people who had high blood pressure had normalization of the hypertension.

Dr. J. Egger and colleagues put 78 children on an elimination diet that included lamb or chicken, rice or potato, banana or apple, one vegetable, water, and vitamin and calcium supplements for three to four weeks. Children who did not improve were given a second elimination diet. On the first or second diet, 88.6 percent recovered completely. Fifty-five foods provoked migraines. The most common were cow's milk (31 percent), egg (27 percent), chocolate (25 percent), orange and wheat (24 percent each), benzoic acid (16 percent), cheese and tomato (15 percent each), tartrazine and rye (14 percent each), pork and fish (10 percent each), beef and corn (9 percent each), soy and tea (8 percent), oats, goat's milk, and coffee (7 percent each), and peanuts (6 percent). Forty of these children participated in blinded food testing; this confirmed that food allergies provoked migraine.

John Diamond, M.D., of the Diamond Headache Clinic in Chicago, reports that foods high in amines also provoke migraines in some people. Dietary amines, which promote constriction of blood vessels, are normally broken down by enzymes, but some people with migraines have lower than normal amounts of the appropriate enzymes. The amines that provoke vasoconstriction are serotonin, tyramine, tryptamine, and dopamine. They are found in the greatest quantities in avocados, bananas, cabbage, eggplant, pineapple, plums, potatoes, tomatoes, cheese, canned fish, wine (especially red), beer, aged meats, and yeast extracts.

Nitrates, phenylethalamine, histamine, phenolic compounds, and monosodium glutamate can be triggers of migraine in certain people. Artificial sweeteners have also been implicated in migraines in some people. Aspartame (NutraSweet) was found to trigger migraine in 8.2 percent of people by Lipton and colleagues. Others speculate about the use of sucralose (Splenda). M. E. Bigal and A. V. Krymchantowski reports one woman whose migraines were consistently triggered by sucralose. Dr. R. M. Patel suggest that it's important for doctors to recognize sucralose as a potential trigger of migraines.

PREVENTING MIGRAINES WITH NUTRIENTS AND HERBS

Taking oral magnesium daily can be excellent for preventing migraines. This has been well studied. Magnesium is used in more than 300 enzymatic reactions in your body. Its main role is to relax muscles, nerves, and in this case, blood vessels. Dr. E. Koseoglu and colleagues found that when given magnesium there was increased blood flow to the cortex, frontal, temporal, and insular regions of the brain. Many women have migraines triggered by menstruation. Others have reported that high levels of estrogen and progesterone decrease cellular magnesium levels and also have direct effects on smooth muscles in the brain. People with migraines often have impaired mitochondrial production; magnesium is needed for energy production. It's also used in neurotransmitter production. Various studies report benefits of 0 to 80 percent reduction in severity and frequency of migraine with magnesium supplementation.

Riboflavin (vitamin B_2) was first studied for prevention of migraines in the 1940s and 1950s. More recently, 19 people with recurrent migraines were given 400 mg of vitamin B_2 daily with breakfast for three months. The number of migraines declined by 67 percent and the severity diminished by 68 percent. Its maximum effect is reached after two or three months, so be patient and give it a good try. In another study, 55 people were given either a placebo or 400 mg of riboflavin daily. Over three months, 59 percent of the people on riboflavin improved by at least 50 percent. There were minor side effects in two people—one had diarrhea and the other had frequent urination. If you experience either of these side effects, decrease the dosage. In some people more modest doses can be effective.

Fish oil supplements contain high levels of DHA and EPA oils. They have been shown in many studies to reduce the severity, duration, and frequency of migraine headaches. Most of us can produce EPA and DHA by using flaxseed oil, borage oil, or evening primrose oil, or by taking alpha-linolenic acid (ALA) and gamma-linolenic acid (GLA) supplements. However, this conversion requires that we have not only the genetic ability to complete the conversion but also adequate vitamin B_6 and magnesium. One study gave subjects 1,800 mg of GLA and ALA in six capsules daily, plus 3 mg of niacin, 20 mg of vitamin C, 25 IU of vitamin E, 20 mg of soy phosphatides, 50 mg of magnesium, 1.3 mg of beta-carotene, and 0.3 mg of vitamin B_6. Of the 128 people who participated in the study, 86 percent had a reduction in the severity, frequency, and duration of their migraine headaches, 22 percent became migraine-free, and 90 percent had reduced nausea and vomiting. Fourteen percent of the subjects were able to reduce their medication to simple pain relievers. Stress reduction and relaxation are also recommended.

Twenty people with a history of migraines for more than one year and with a frequency of two to eight per month were given 1 mg vitamin B_{12} daily for three months in a nasal spray. Half of the people had a 53 percent reduction in migraines. In these people there was a reduction from 5.2 to 1.9 attacks on average per month. In the other half, there was virtually no improvement. Vitamin B_{12} is nontoxic, inexpensive, and widely available in sublingual and nasal sprays. Oral forms are not well absorbed.

Supplementing with vitamin B_6, B_{12}, and folic acid can be useful in people with genetic typing that allows for easy use of folic acid. One study found that in people with the CC and CT MTHFR 677 C to T genotypes, supplementing with 2 mg folic acid, 25 mg of B_6, and 400 mcg of B_{12} significantly lowered severity and frequency of headaches. Severity decreased from 75 percent to 28 percent. People with the TT genotype of MTHFR, in which people have difficulty utilizing folic acid, did not have these improvements. It's possible that taking easily utilized folic acid, such as methyltetrahydrofolate, could have helped even these people.

Melatonin has been tested in several studies for migraines in children and adults. Melatonin levels have been demonstrated to be lower in people who have migraines than in people who don't. Melatonin was given to 32 people with migraines at a dose of 3 mg given 30 minutes before bed, for three months. Headache frequency decreased 60.5 percent, intensity by 51.4 percent, and duration by 55.6 percent. The mechanism is unknown. Many of the medications used for migraines modulate serotonin, and serotonin is converted into melatonin. Perhaps that's why this works. In another study, 22 children were given 3 mg of melatonin before bed. In two-thirds of the children, headaches decreased by half, and four children had no headaches at all. One child dropped out of the study because of daytime sleepiness.

Butterbur (Petasites hybridus) is a European herb that has been used for centuries for such diverse problems as plaque, cough, asthma, and skin wounds. It works by lowering inflammatory markers that cause pain. Most recently it has been shown to be effective for hay fever. In its natural state it contains liver toxins, but a patented product, Petadolex, has removed these substances. In a 2004 study of 60 people with migraines, 33 were given 25 mg Petadolex twice daily and 27 were given a placebo twice daily. After three months, the average incidence of migraines decreased from 3.4 per month to 1.8 per month in the Petadolex group. Forty-five percent of the people responded really well and accounted for most of the results. In another study 108 children demonstrated benefits from butterbur: 77 percent had reduced frequency of headaches by at least 50 percent. Frequency was lessened by 63 percent overall. Ninety-one percent of the children felt substantially or slightly improved after four months of treatment.

Numerous studies have shown the herb feverfew (Tanacetum parthenium) to be effective in preventing and minimizing the severity of migraines. Others show no effectiveness. You can try it for yourself and see if it works for you. In one study by Drs. R. Shrivastava, J. C. Pechadre, and G. W. John, feverfew was given to 12 people with migraine without aura. They were given 300 mg feverfew twice daily, plus 300 mg white willow bark twice daily for 12 weeks. There was a significant reduction in frequency, severity, and duration of migraines.

Dr. Alan Gaby has given Meyers cocktail, an intravenous combination of magnesium, calcium, B-complex vitamins, and vitamin C, during migraine in six or more patients. Gaby reports that when given during a migraine, he has found complete or marked improvement within two minutes, with sustained improvement over 24 hours. One patient was treated more than 70 times in six years and responded well nearly all the time.

CHECK FOR DYSBIOSIS

This is an emerging area of research that is worth exploring. Several studies have explored the link between H. pylori infection and migraine. Dr. K. G. Yiannopoulou and colleagues studied 49 people aged 19 to 47 for migraines without aura. In people who had migraines with menstruation or family members who also had migraines, the incidence of H. pylori from gastric mucosal biopsy was 36 percent and 37 percent, respectively. In people who had no predisposing factors, prevalence of H. pylori was 81 percent in men and 87 percent in women. Dr. I. Ciancarelli et al. report that of 30 people with migraine, 16.7 percent had H. pylori IgA and IgG antibodies. Dr. A. Gasbarrini and colleagues report that of 225 people with migraine with and without aura, 40 percent tested positive for H. pylori with 13-urea breath testing. Another study by the same group reports higher levels of H. pylori in people with aura than without aura. Dr. L. Hong and colleagues report that when H. pylori was treated in people who had both migraine and cirrhosis, incidence, duration, and severity of migraines was reduced significantly.

I haven't seen any studies on small intestinal bacterial overgrowth or fungal overgrowth in people with migraine. There is a large overlap among people who have irritable bowel syndrome, chronic fatigue syndrome, fibromyalgia, allergic rhinitis, and migraine. I look forward to seeing further studies on this.

HYPOTHYROID AND MIGRAINE

Many years ago, I worked with a woman who had severe migraines that decreased her quality of life. We discovered that she was hypothyroid. When her physician regulated her thyroid, her migraines were minimal. In 2007, A. J. Huete and colleagues reported in *Headache* the story of a person whose Hashimoto's thyroiditis resulted in symptoms that looked exactly like a migraine headache with an aura. Her thyroid tests were within a normal range, yet she had elevated antithyroid antibodies. While the incidence of hypothyroidism, subclinical hypothyroidism, or autoimmune thyroid disease and migraines has not been well studied, it seems worth checking.

MOOD AND MIGRAINE

People with migraine often have mood and anxiety problems as well. Using strategies that address these at the same time is warranted: psychological counseling, biofeedback, acupuncture, chiropractic manipulation, emotional freedom technique, meditation, relaxation skills, and other mind-body modalities. Some of these modalities will also help with the neck pain that accompanies migraine so often.

Functional Laboratory Testing
- Intracellular magnesium, either RBC or lymphocytes
- H. pylori testing
- Homocysteine levels (will give an indication about folate, B_6, and B_{12} status)
- Elisa/Act testing for food and environmental allergies or sensitivities—IgG, IgE, and if possible IgA and IgM
- Thyroid testing
- Organic acid testing

Healing Options

Migraines have many triggers that vary from person to person. Finding your triggers and the treatments that work best for you is the key. You certainly won't need all the therapies listed here, but hopefully you'll find relief from some of them.

- **Make dietary changes.** Remove all sugars, alcohol, salty foods, refined carbohydrates, and caffeine. Try to figure out what works best for you personally. Simply avoiding caffeine can dramatically reduce the incidence and severity of migraines. Similarly, Dr. Gaby reported on a 1930 study on the effects of salt in migraine incidence. Twelve people avoided all salted snack foods before meals. At a six-month follow-up, migraines resolved completely in three people, and seven more had fewer attacks. Another study found that a low-fat diet of less than 20 grams daily lowered the incidence of headache from nine each month to three each month. Headache intensity and the need for medications also dropped substantially. This information shows the importance of the diet and the quality of fats. In combination with good-quality omega-3 fatty acids, this could give great results for many people.
- **Examine effects of caffeine.** Caffeine plays a mixed role in migraines. For some people, it significantly reduces the number and severity of headaches; for others it triggers them. Find out what works for you.
- **Be sure to eat often.** Low blood sugar levels often trigger migraines, so don't skip meals. You may find that eating five to six small meals each day works better for you than three main meals.
- **Try an elimination diet.** This may be the most significant thing you can do to discover what is triggering your migraines. Avoid foods you are sensitive to.
- **Make your home environmentally safe.** Use only natural cleaning supplies, remove gas appliances, clean out mold and mildew, use a dehumidifier, and make your bedroom into a safe harbor by removing unnecessary items, such as carpeting and drapery.
- **Avoid monosodium glutamate (MSG).** MSG can provoke migraine headaches, asthma, diarrhea, vomiting, and gastric symptoms. These problems can occur immediately after eating or may be delayed up to 72 hours, which makes their relationship to MSG more difficult to discover. Food product labels may be misleading, with MSG labeled as "natural coloring"; some hydrolyzed vegetable protein contains MSG. You can challenge yourself with MSG to see if it brings on a migraine. The Elisa/Act blood test includes tests for MSG and glutamate sensitivity.

- **Begin with a multivitamin and mineral supplement.** Since so many nutrients have been demonstrated to help with migraine prevention, taking four to nine pills a day of multiple vitamin and mineral supplements may be a simple way to approach this with broad nutritional support.

- **Take magnesium.** Try 400 to 2,000 mg magnesium glycinate, ascorbate, keto-glutarate, malate, or other well-absorbed magnesium daily for at least three months. When you've reached saturation, you'll get diarrhea. I use this with my clients to figure out the correct dose. If you need more than 1,000 mg daily before your stools loosen, add 1 teaspoon choline citrate to facilitate the magnesium absorption.

- **Use riboflavin (vitamin B$_2$).** Studies used 400 mg daily. You may have good results on less. There have been reports of benefit using between 15 and 30 mg daily.

- **Take vitamin B$_{12}$.** Take 1,000 mcg B$_{12}$ nasally or sublingually. Use for at least three months to see the best effect.

- **Try niacin.** David Velling and colleagues report on a woman who began taking niacin to help lower cholesterol. Her migraines stopped for a month at 375 mg of sustained release niacin twice daily. When she reduced the dosage, she had two migraines the following month. There are reports of physicians using niacin intravenously during a migraine to decrease the severity and duration of headaches. The dose contains at least 100 mg niacin, which is infused slowly.

- **Try CoQ10.** You can have your CoQ10 levels tested. In 1,550 children with migraines, nearly 33 percent had low levels of CoQ10. Of those who came back for follow-up, CoQ10 levels increased and incidence and headache disability were reduced. In another study, 42 people with migraines took 100 mg of CoQ10 three times daily; another group took a placebo. In the CoQ10 group, 47.6 percent had their frequency of headaches reduced by half. Two other studies have demonstrated about half of people respond to CoQ10 supplements. Take 100 mg three times daily.

- **Increase consumption of omega-3 fatty acids, olive oil, and polyunsaturated fats.** Take 1,800 mg GLA/ALA and 2,000 to 3,000 mg of fish oil daily.

- **Try feverfew.** Feverfew needs to be taken on a daily basis as a preventive measure rather than as a treatment. There is a difference between fresh and dried feverfew and between various samples. If you don't get relief from one type, try another. Fresh feverfew seems to work best. It is easy to grow, so you could just eat a few leaves each day. Tinctures are available and would best approximate fresh leaves. It also comes in a freeze-dried form that seems to be effective.

Twice daily, take 15 to 20 drops tincture, or take one to three capsules or one to three fresh leaves daily.

- **Try butterbur (Petadolex).** If you are one of the lucky, this could be a great remedy for you. Take 25 mg twice daily.
- **Take antioxidants.** Migraines are often triggered by substances that promote free radicals, such as cigarette smoke, perfume, hair spray, pollution, and household chemicals. One researcher found lower levels of superoxide dismutase (SOD) in platelets of people with migraines than in people with tension headaches. More research needs to be done in this area, but taking adequate antioxidants in a multivitamin with minerals may help prevent migraines.
- **Check for H. pylori.** H. pylori infection has been linked to migraines.
- **Explore possible candida infection.** A recent study of the relationship between candidiasis and migraines found that 13 out of 17 migraine sufferers responded to a three-month program of diet and medication with fewer and less severe headaches. Blood testing showed a lowering of candida antibodies as well. The four people who did not respond well didn't stick to the program. Test for candida. (See Chapter 11.)
- **Try acupuncture.** Acupuncture has been shown to reduce the incidence and severity of migraine headaches in some people. Study results vary. You may find great or no benefit.
- **Explore behavioral techniques.** Many studies have been done and biofeedback, hypnotherapy, and stress-reduction techniques have all proven useful to some migraine sufferers. They may be 35 to 50 percent effective. Plus, you'll have better stress-management skills to use in all areas of life. Behavioral techniques help us better understand stressors and how to cope more effectively.
- **Try chiropractic manipulation and massage.** Chiropractic manipulation and massage can help blood and lymphatic supply and relax muscle tension.

CHAPTER 35

Obesity, Metabolic Syndrome, and the GI Connection

Obesity is a complex issue, and you could fill a small library with what has been written on it. Here I'm going to expose you to the new research on the connection between obesity and your digestive system.

There is a growing consensus in research that obesity has several defining characteristics:

- Alterations in gut bacteria
- Low-grade inflammation
- Subsequent leaky gut
- Elevated levels of lipopolysaccharides (LPS) and endocannabinoids

If obesity is left unchecked it can lead to metabolic syndrome, type II diabetes, high serum lipids, and cardiovascular disease.

ALTERATIONS IN GUT BACTERIA

The gut microbiome is responsible for maintaining our metabolism and determining how much fat we store. People who are obese have a different balance of gut micro-organisms than thin people do. This much is known, yet we don't really know yet exactly which bacteria are involved.

Eighty to 90 percent of the bacteria in our gut are from two main families or phyla: Bacteroidetes and Firmicutes. Original work by Dr. R. E. Ley and colleagues demonstrated that fat mice had more than half as many Bacteroidetes and twice as many Firmicutes bacteria than lean mice. They observed the same thing in 12 people. These people then followed either a low-fat or low-carbohydrate diet for a year, which nearly normalized their balance of Bacteroidetes and Firmicutes bacteria. However, the plot thickens because other researches did not find these differences. Dr. S. H. Duncan and colleagues found no differences in the amount of Bacteroidetes in stool of people who were obese, and levels didn't change when people dieted. Firmicutes levels went down when people dieted, which is the opposite finding from Ley's group.

It appears that research looking at specific species of bacteria will yield better results than just looking at humungous phyla. To that point, there seems to be more of an agreement among researchers about the roles of Bifidobacterium species and Streptococcus aureus in obesity. P. D. Cani and Delzenne found in obese rats that there were reduced amounts of bifidobacteria in both species and number. Kalliomaki and colleagues found a higher number of bifidobacteria in children who were lean at age seven than in children who were overweight. Drs. Marko Kalliomaki, Erika Isolauri, and colleagues also found higher amounts of Staphylococcus aureus in children who became overweight and propose that staph may trigger low-grade inflammation. Other research indicates that increasing B. bifidum and B. breve while decreasing B. catenulatum and S. aureus can also make us leaner.

LOW-GRADE INFLAMMATION

It seems well established that there is a low-grade inflammatory process occurring in people who are obese. This is mediated by our gut microbiome. Patrice Cani, Nathalie Delzenne, and colleagues have a large body of work that looks at the inflammatory pathways in obesity. Mice given antibiotics to simulate imbalances in the microbiota had increased inflammation and toxic by-products in the gut and in stools. The changes in the gut bacteria lessened the mice's ability to handle glucose and provoked increases in body fat, weight gain, inflammation, and oxidative stress, which led to increased intestinal permeability. Cani and Delzenne have also demonstrated that lipopolysaccharides (LPS), components of gram negative bacteria, trigger early, low-grade, chronic inflammation. LPS levels are increased with high-fat diet. High-fat diets also increased gut permeability and lowered bifidobacteria levels.

HIGH ENDOCANNABINOIDS IN GENETIC AND CENTRAL OBESITY

Did you ever get the munchies from smoking pot? Well, marijuana is an external cannabinoid, but we also make our own internal cannabinoids in our brain, muscles, liver, digestive system, and fat cells. When turned on, food tastes amazing. Endocannabinoids help to regulate appetite, regulate our perception of pain, affect our mood, protect our nervous system and neurons, control certain phases of memory processing, act as a feedback loop that signals our neurons to stop secreting neurotransmitters, help regulate heart rate, blood pressure, and bronchial function, and has effects on our fat cells, liver, muscles, and pancreas.

This system, called the endocannabinoid system (eCS), is comprised of lipids (fats) and receptors (CB1 and CB2). Along with the hypothalamus, it stimulates production of ghrelin and we feel hungry. It also regulates energy balance. In people who have central adiposity (are apple shaped) the eCS is overactivated and levels are high.

The endocannabinoids slow gastric emptying, slow intestinal transit, and make food taste great. The eCS also aids in nutrient transport and storage of fat. When we eat more calories than we need at any given time, our body converts those extra calories into fat. When we have eaten enough, cholecystokinin is secreted in our duodenum and leptin is secreted, which lowers our appetite and turns off the eCS. Levels of endocannabinoids drop as leptin is secreted. We no longer feel hungry.

In obese people, levels of endocannabinoids stay chronically high. If we keep the eCS activated continually, it leads to high triglyceride levels, which in turn can lower our protective HDL cholesterol, increase LDL cholesterol, and lead to atherosclerosis (plaque buildup in our arteries). High levels of eCS also decrease adiponectin, which in turn decreases insulin sensitivity. This leads to increased weight gain and ultimately can lead to metabolic syndrome and/or type 2 diabetes.

This constant inflammation contributes to increased gut permeability. The increased permeability leads to more inflammation and food sensitivities. If the inner lining of our duodenum is inflamed, we may not release cholecystokinin and our eCS stays activated. When active, eCS stimulates our liver to make fatty acids.

What is not known is how high endocannabinoid levels are in lean people and what the mechanism is that keeps them lean despite it.

FOOD SENSITIVITY

For a long time clinicians working with food sensitivities have noticed that when people deal directly with their food sensitivities, they begin to lose weight. Although there is little research to support this, it makes sense. Food can be inflammatory and obesity is an inflammatory condition, so going on an anti-inflammatory diet can help lower inflammation and help normalize function. Cell Science Systems, maker of the ALCAT food sensitivity testing process, has sponsored a couple of studies that verify that by avoiding foods you are sensitive to, you can facilitate weight loss. In clinical practice, when working with someone who is obese, I often begin by putting someone on an elimination diet. I'm not the only person who finds this useful: Elson Haas, M.D., wrote a book called *The False Fat Diet* (Ballantine Books, 2001), which utilizes an elimination diet for weight loss, and Mark Hyman, M.D., wrote *The Ultra Simple Diet* (Pocket Books, 2007) to express how an elimination diet plus detoxification could jump-start weight loss as well.

Food sensitivities are tightly linked with leaky gut. So, it makes sense that if leaky gut is associated with obesity, food sensitivities will follow. By avoiding inflammatory foods and following the information in Chapter 4, you may find that it's easier to lose weight.

METABOLIC SYNDROME

Metabolic syndrome affects about 47 million Americans. If you have more than three of these factors, you may be diagnosed with metabolic syndrome: large waist size, triglyceride levels higher than 150 mg/dl, low HDL cholesterol levels, high blood pressure, and fasting blood sugar levels of over 100 mg/dl. It's characterized by insulin resistance and difficulty in handling glucose. Most people with metabolic syndrome are overweight and often apple-shaped, but this also occurs in people who are thin. If left unchecked, metabolic syndrome often leads to type 2 diabetes and increased risk for cardiovascular disease.

Functional Laboratory Testing
- **Comprehensive digestive stool testing:** This test will give an indication of microbial balance and probiotic levels.
- **Hemaglobin A1C:** This test gives a three-month average of glucose levels and is a better indicator of pre-diabetes than fasting glucose levels.

- **Frucosamine:** Frucosamine is similar to Hemaglobin A1C but gives about a two-week average of glucose levels.
- **Food sensitivity testing:** Delayed food sensitivities can predispose to obesity.
- **Insulin testing:** While fasting insulin testing can be useful, doing a one- and/or two-hour test after you've been given a glucose challenge gives a result that is more in line with what happens to your insulin levels after you eat a meal.
- **Vitamin and mineral testing:** There are often micronutrient deficiencies in people with metabolic syndrome.

Healing Options

- **Move more.** Probably the most potent regulator of energy, stress, mood, and weight is exercise. Find an exercise program that you enjoy and do it routinely.
- **Take a probiotic supplement.** Find a supplement that contains bifidobacteria and lactobacilli. (See Chapter 6.)
- **Heal inflammation and leaky gut.** See Chapters 4 and 9 for ways to do this.
- **Reduce inflammation.** Clean up your diet. Get rid of all high-fructose corn syrup, sugars, and most processed foods. Add turmeric and spices to your foods to help reduce inflammation. Eat high omega 3 fish, such as wild salmon, sardines, and herring. Take 1,000 to 3,000 mg fish oil daily.
- **Eat bitter melon.** Bitter melon is available in Asian stores. Research repeatedly reports that it helps to stabilize blood sugar levels.
- **Reduce carbohydrates, increase protein.** Trade some grains, starches, and sugars for protein foods such as legumes, fish, chicken, and bison.
- **Take a blood sugar support supplement.** There are many products on the market that are designed to help reduce blood sugar and increase insulin sensitivity. Look for products that contain magnesium, B-complex vitamins, butter melon, holy basil, cinnamon, fenugreek, green tea, Gymnemna sylvestre, chromium, vanadium, and lipoic acid. There may also be some ginseng, prickly pear, banaba, manganese, biotin, zinc, vitamin C, bilberry, and additional antioxidants. Use as directed.

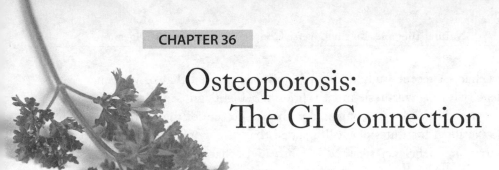

CHAPTER 36

Osteoporosis: The GI Connection

Osteoporosis is a disease where bones are porous and have a tendency to break easily. It affects about 20 percent of women over the age of 50. It also affects men but, due to their higher initial bone mass, less often. Osteoporosis contributes to more than 1.3 million fractures a year. Twenty percent of people who have a hip fracture die within a few weeks, and many others end up needing long-term care.

According to Susan Brown, Ph.D., author of *Better Bones, Better Body,* at least 20 nutrients are needed to build healthy bone. Most of the spotlight falls on calcium, phosphorus, and vitamin D, but an Israeli study reported increases in bone mass from 250 to 750 mg of magnesium taken daily for two years. The group taking magnesium had increases of 1 to 8 percent in bone mass compared to the control group, who lost between 1 and 3 percent of bone mass. Other nutrients needed for proper bone formation include fluoride, silica, zinc, manganese, copper, boron, potassium, strontium, vitamin K, and virtually all other vitamins. Getting enough protein is also essential. You can read about these needs and more at Dr. Brown's website, http://www.betterbones.com/bonenutrition20keybonenutrients.aspx.

BONE LOSS AND CELIAC DISEASE

It has been widely reported that people with celiac disease have a higher prevalence of osteoporosis. A recent study done in Manitoba reports on women with celiac disease who had had bone density testing done within six months before they were diagnosed with celiac. A recent study done in Manitoba reported that of women who had bone density testing within six months prior to being diagnosed with celiac disease, 67.6 percent had osteoporosis compared with 44.8 percent of the controls.

In 2004, the National Institutes of Health stated that osteoporosis was associated with the nutritional deficiencies caused by untreated celiac disease. The NIH consensus statement and subsequent research state that there isn't an increased rate of celiac disease in people with osteoporosis. However, Legroux-Gerot and colleagues report that 8 percent of 140 people with osteoporosis had elevated IgG antigliaden antibodies and 11 percent had elevated IgA antigliaden antibodies. This suggests gluten intolerance.

OUR GUT TALKS TO OUR BONES

It has long been thought that the only mechanism linking osteoporosis and the digestive system was malnutrition due to celiac disease. Now another mechanism has been discovered that seems even more compelling.

Ninety-five percent of the serotonin in the body is produced in the gut in the enterochromaffin cells in the small intestine and duodenum. The other 5 percent is produced in the brain. It's been known for a long time that serotonin modulates peristalsis. Newer research indicates that high levels of serotonin in the gut lower bone density by lowering formation of new bone (osteoblasts) and increasing destruction of old bone (osteoclasts). This is regulated by various genes: Wnt, Lrp5, and Tph1. The Wnt genes regulate how we develop bone, muscle, and nervous system tissues. Genetic research has discovered that there are variations in the Wnt gene that predispose us to having either really strong bones, medium bone density, or bones that are weak from early on in life (causing an early onset of osteoporosis called osteoporosis pseudoglioma).

Inflammation in the gut, such as in Crohn's disease, increases the production of serotonin, which in turn activates the Wnt system. Most people are continually eating foods that cause low-grade inflammation in the gut. The standard American diet is basically an inflammatory diet. Inflammatory cytokines have been shown to increase after eating a high-fat, high-sugar meal. This increases serotonin and activates the Wnt system, reducing bone cell production.

Functional Laboratory Testing
- Vitamin D levels
- Possible celiac and/or food sensitivity testing

- HCl self-test or Heidelberg capsule test
- Nutritional testing for vitamins and minerals

Healing Options

- **Get exercise.** Exercise builds muscle and bone. It's not optional. Find something you like to do and do it regularly.
- **Balance pH.** When cells are in a low level of chronic acidosis, we pull minerals from bone to balance blood pH levels. (See Chapter 17.)
- **Optimize vitamin D levels.** Get your vitamin D level tested. Bringing vitamin D to optimal levels works as effectively to build bone as medications do. Aim for 60 to 100 ng/ml of 25-0H vitamin D. For maintenance, take 2,000 IU daily. For optimizing levels, take 5,000 to 10,000 IU daily.
- **Decrease inflammation.** Eat more fruits, vegetables, nuts, seeds, and beans. Lower your intake of processed foods, salt, low nutrient-density foods, caffeine, and alcohol. Stop smoking. Use herbs and spices in cooking. Eat a rainbow of foods. If this still isn't enough, use anti-inflammatory herbs and nutrients such as fish oil, vitamin D, and curcumin. This is discussed in detail in Chapter 9.
- **Practice stress-management skills.** See Chapter 16 for techniques for lowering stress.
- **Take bone-building supplements.** Take a multivitamin plus a bone-building supplement that contains calcium, magnesium, vitamin D, vitamin K, and other nutrients.
- **Explore HCl adequacy.** Do the self-test in Chapter 11 or get tested for achlorhydria.

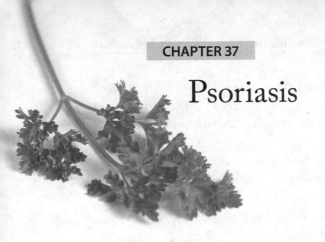

CHAPTER 37

Psoriasis

Psoriasis is a chronic skin rash characterized by scaling, patchy, or silvery-looking skin. It has a cyclic nature, flaring up and simmering down. It can affect just knees, elbows, or scalp or can spread over most of the body. It often occurs at the site of a previous injury. Psoriasis often runs in families and usually develops gradually. It affects about 1 percent of the American population as a whole (4.5 million) but 2 to 4 percent of Caucasians.

Psoriasis occurs when skin cells mature too quickly. Skin cells build up on the surface, causing red, scaly patches that often itch or are uncomfortable. Psoriasis flares up because of stress, severe sunburn, irritation, skin creams, antimalarial therapy, or withdrawal from cortisone, or it can be brought on by other triggers. People with psoriasis have an excess of T-helper cell (Th-1) inflammatory cytokines and relatively few Th-2 cytokines. One of the new theories about psoriasis is that superantigens trigger the disease. These prime the T cells to produce high amounts of inflammatory cytokines. These superantigens also contribute to leaky gut, which allows greater exposure to antigens or toxins, including microbial factors. Subsequently these can be deposited along basement membrane in the skin. Immune complexes develop. It's believed that there is a molecular mimicry between H. pylori antigens and keratin 17, which may cause keratin to proliferate. Keratin is the tough, fibrous protein component of skin, hair, and nails. So when we produce a lot more keratin, the skin gets tough and fibrous. If we look at the DIGIN section of the book, all of these factors play a role: leaky gut, dysbiosis, inflammation, and antigens.

Psoriasis can also occur with joint inflammation as psoriatic arthritis (see Chapter 26), and joint inflammation is found in 3 to 7 percent of people with psoriasis. It isn't clear whether psoriasis and psoriatic arthritis are the same disease or two almost identical diseases.

Thirty-six percent of people with psoriasis have one or more family members with psoriasis, which suggests a genetic component. Psoriasis is also influenced by insulin resistance, impaired glucose tolerance, obesity, liver disease, and high cholesterol and/or triglycerides. It's thought to be an indicator of risk for atherosclerosis and may be an early warning sign.

Digestive issues in psoriasis have been found in many cases. There is a clear relationship between celiac, gluten sensitivity, Crohn's disease, and psoriasis. In psoriasis and these other conditions, researchers found increased intestinal permeability and microscopic bowel lesions. Some people with psoriasis also have gastritis, duodenitis, celiac disease, or inflammatory bowel disease. Disturbances in pancreatic function and even acute pancreatitis have been found to be prevalent in people with psoriasis.

Drs. Michael Murray and Joseph Pizzorno note a number of factors that influence the progression of psoriasis, including incomplete digestion of protein, bowel toxemia, food sensitivities, poor liver function, reaction to alcoholic beverages, and eating high amounts of animal fats.

When protein digestion is incomplete or proteins are poorly absorbed, bacteria can break them down and produce toxic substances. One group of these toxins is called polyamines, which have been found to be higher in people with psoriasis than in the average population. Polyamines contribute to psoriasis by blocking production of cyclic AMP. Vitamin A and goldenseal inhibit the formation of polyamines. Because protein digestion begins in the stomach, low levels of hydrochloric acid there can also cause incomplete protein digestion. Digestive enzymes and/or hydrochloric acid supplementation aid protein digestion. (See Chapter 3.)

Poor liver function may contribute to psoriasis as well. Liver function profile tests and the metabolic screening questionnaire can help you determine liver function, and the metabolic screening questionnaire can also be used to follow your progress. Incorporate a detoxification program with an elimination-provocation diet to determine which foods may trigger your psoriasis. (See Chapters 15 and 18.)

Alcohol consumption contributes to psoriasis because alcohol contains many toxic substances, which stress an overburdened liver. Alcohol also increases intestinal permeability.

DYSBIOSIS AND PSORIASIS

Many studies hypothesize that there is a microbe or pathogen that triggers psoriasis. H. pylori has been found in some people with psoriasis. When treated, some people have had large improvements, while there has been no benefit in others. Studies on dysbiosis in psoriasis are lacking. Dr. Zhan Gao and colleagues extracted DNA from skin lesions of six people with psoriasis. He found increased levels of Firmicutes and low levels of Actinobacteria and Propionibacterium species in people with psoriasis compared to controls. Dr. Luciana C. Paulino and colleagues found no significant differences in yeast levels in healthy skin and psoriasis skin.

In a recent study, 21 out of 34 people with psoriasis were found to have Candida albicans in the spaces between their fingers or toes, and the majority were also affected by fungi from the tinea family. Other research found a 56 percent increase in nail fungus in people with psoriasis. Another study looked at stool samples of people with psoriasis and other skin disorders. Researchers found a high number of disease-producing microbes, predominantly yeasts, in the colon. This may not be the cause of psoriasis but rather an indication of poor gut ecology. Treatment for yeast infection corresponded with a decrease in skin inflammation.

FOOD AND PSORIASIS

Studies on fasting, vegetarian diets, and diets rich in fish oils have all been shown to produce benefit in people with psoriasis. All of these diets reduce inflammation.

Although I have not seen studies on elimination diet, people with psoriasis have high levels of IgE antibodies, which indicates an allergic component. An elimination diet makes sense to try. Allergy and food sensitivity testing could be helpful in figuring out how someone may benefit the most.

Sixteen percent of people with psoriasis have antibodies to gliadin, the protein found in wheat, rye, and barley. However, when tested for gliadin intolerance, their endomysium antibodies were normal. Nonetheless, a gluten-free diet for three months greatly improved the psoriasis. A follow-up study discovered high levels of tissue transglutaminase antibodies in the skin of people with psoriasis. This decreased by half after a three- to six-month gluten-free trial.

The causes and treatments of psoriasis are complex. Successful treatment must encompass several approaches reflecting its complexity. Look for underlying causes and develop a personal program based on your needs.

Functional Laboratory Testing

- Food and environmental sensitivity testing—IgE and IgG4
- Celiac testing
- Candida testing (either blood or stool)
- Organic acid testing
- Liver function profile
- Intestinal permeability testing
- Blood testing for vitamin and mineral status
- Fatty acid testing

Healing Options

- **Try an elimination-provocation diet.** Explore the relationship between your psoriasis and food and environmental sensitivities through laboratory testing and the elimination-provocation diet. For best results work with a nutritionist or physician who is familiar with food sensitivity protocols.
- **Take a multivitamin with minerals.** Take a good-quality multivitamin with minerals every day. Look for a supplement that contains at least 25,000 IU vitamin A, 400 IU vitamin D, 400 IU vitamin E, 800 mcg folic acid, 200 mcg selenium, 200 mcg chromium, and 25 to 50 mg zinc. Each of these nutrients has been shown to be deficient in people with psoriasis. There are several vitamin A topical creams used by dermatologists for psoriasis. Vitamin A is a critical nutrient for healthy skin.
- **Try antioxidant nutrients.** CoQ10, selenium, and vitamin E supplements have shown benefit. One group reported improvement from use of CoQ10 at 50 mg, vitamin E at 50 mg, and selenium at 48 mcg dissolved in soy lecithin for 30 to 35 days.
- **Increase consumption of beneficial fats and oils.** The research on fish oils is mixed. Eating fish or taking fish oils has been shown to have an anti-inflammatory effect on psoriasis for some people. Fatty acids contribute to healthy skin, hair, and nails, and fish oils promote production of anti-inflammatory prostaglandins. It is also possible that fish oils increase the activity of vitamin D and sunlight. Eat cold-water fish—salmon, halibut, mackerel, sardines, tuna, and herring— two to four times per week or take EPA/DHA capsules along with a balance of omega-6 fatty acids such as evening primrose oil, borage oil, or black currant seed oil.
- **Enjoy some sunlight and get your vitamin D.** Sunlight stimulates our bodies to manufacture vitamin D, which has been shown to be an effective treatment for psoriasis. Ask your doctor to test your vitamin D levels. If low, supplement.

Cod liver oil is a good source of vitamin D because it also contains fish oil and vitamin A, both of benefit in psoriasis. In general, slow tanning improves psoriasis, with sunshine and sunlamps prescribed as part of standard therapy. Get your vitamin D levels tested. Normal levels are between 32 and 100 ng/ml. Many integrative clinicians consider levels of 60 to 100 ng/ml to be optimal for people with autoimmune illnesses. Dosage depends on levels. For maintenance, take 2,000 IU of D_3 daily. If deficient, then take 5,000 to 10,000 IU of D_3 daily for 8 to 12 weeks, and then retest.

A recent study done in Israel at the Dead Sea, long renowned for its treatment of psoriasis, showed that natural sunlight stimulated significant improvement in disease activity. One group was given just sunlight therapy, and the other received additional therapy in mud packs and sulfur baths. Both groups showed significant improvement in skin symptoms and with psoriatic arthritis, where present. Sunlight and ultraviolet light therapy are regular therapies for psoriasis.

- **Take zinc supplements and/or eat zinc-rich foods.** Many studies have determined that people with psoriasis have lower levels of zinc than people in control groups. However, studies using oral zinc supplementation haven't always shown a clear improvement in psoriasis, though such studies have been of short duration—only 6 to 10 weeks. Even though they didn't show improvement in the skin, they did show improvement in immune function and dramatic improvement in joint symptoms. It's possible that either zinc needs to be used along with other nutrients, or the time frame of these studies was too brief to see improvement. Take 50 mg zinc daily.

- **Try chondroitin sulfate.** Several studies have reported improvement in psoriasis in people taking chondroitin sulfate. Take 800 mg daily. Continue at least two months to see if this is effective for you.

- **Try milk thistle (silymarin).** Extracts of the herb milk thistle have been used since the 15th century for ailments of the liver and gallbladder. Milk thistle, also known as silymarin, contains anti-inflammatory flavonoid complexes that promote the flow of bile and help tone the spleen, gallbladder, and liver. An excellent liver detoxifier, milk thistle has also been shown to have a positive effect on psoriasis. Take three to six capsules of 175 mg standardized 80 percent milk thistle extract daily with water before meals.

- **Try Honduran sarsaparilla.** Sarsaparilla, a flavoring in root beers and confections, has proven to be effective in treating psoriasis, especially the more chronic, large-plaque-forming type. Sarsaparilla binds bacterial endotoxins. Take 2 to 4 teaspoons liquid extract daily, or 250 to 500 mg solid extract daily.

- **Try lecithin and phosphatidylcholine.** Lecithin was used in a 10-year study from 1940 to 1950. People consumed 4 to 8 tablespoons of lecithin daily, along with small amounts of vitamins A, B_1, B_2, B_5, B_6, and D, thyroid and liver preparations, and creams. Out of 155 patients, 118 people responded positively. Lecithin-rich foods include soybeans, wheat germ, nuts, seeds, whole grains, eggs, and oils from soy, nuts, and seeds. Lecithin granules can be purchased in health-food stores and added to foods as a cooking ingredient. Lecithin can also be purchased in capsule form, as can the active ingredient in lecithin, phosphatidylcholine. Take 4 to 8 tablespoons of lecithin daily or one to four capsules of phosphatidylcholine daily.

- **Try high-dose folic acid.** There is much research on folate deficiency caused by the drug methotrexate, which is a folate antagonist medication often used for psoriasis. This seems ironic, because folic acid is one of the primary nutrients needed for proper skin formation. Jonathan Wright, M.D., recommends extremely high-dose folic acid therapy for psoriasis—50 to 100 mg daily. Alan Gaby, M.D., reports on a study of seven people with long-standing psoriasis. They were given 20 mg of folic acid four times daily. Improvements were seen in three to six months of beginning this regimen. Dr. Gaby warns that this is not a good plan for people who have taken methotrexate because it may cause adverse reactions. Be aware that if folic acid is taken by someone with a vitamin B_{12} deficiency, nerve damage can go undetected. If you are going to use high levels of folic acid, have your doctor test your vitamin B_{12} status with serum B_{12}, or more accurately methylmalonic acid testing. I also wonder if the same results could be obtained by using a more absorbable form of folic acid, such as methyltetrahydrofolate at lower doses.

- **Take selenium.** Many studies have shown that people with psoriasis are deficient in selenium. Selenium is part of a molecule called *glutathione peroxidase*, which protects against oxidative damage (free radicals). Giving supplemental selenium to people with psoriasis showed an increase in glutathione peroxidase levels and improvement in immune function, though not an improvement in skin condition. However, these were studies of short duration with selenium as the only supplement. This underscores the concepts of patience when using natural therapies and of using more than one nutrient or approach at a time. Take 200 mcg daily, which you can get in a good multivitamin. Selenium can be toxic, so more is not necessarily better. Brazil nuts are an excellent source of selenium. Eat one to two daily to get 200 mcg.

■ **Try Saccharomyces boulardii.** Saccharomyces boulardii is a cousin to baker's yeast. It has been shown to raise levels of secretory IgA, which are low in psoriatic arthritis and psoriasis. Take three to six capsules daily.

Topical Treatments to Reduce Skin Inflammation and Symptoms

■ **Use aloe vera cream.** A placebo-controlled study of 60 people with psoriasis found that a 0.5 percent aloe vera cream cured 86 percent of the subjects. Each person used the aloe vera cream three times each day for a period of one year, and the researchers concluded that aloe vera cream is a safe and effective cure for psoriasis.

■ **Try other topical creams.** Many topical creams, oils, and ointments help psoriasis. Capsaicin, a cayenne pepper cream, helped 66 to 70 percent of the people who used it in a recent trial. The main side effect was that of a burning feeling associated with chili peppers, which quickly subsided. Vitamins A and E have also been used topically with success; one physician alternates them, one each day. Creams containing zinc are also effective, as are salves containing sarsaparilla. Goldenseal ointment or oral supplements can also be helpful.

■ **Practice stress-management skills.** Flare-ups of psoriasis often occur after a stressful event. Because stress has to do with our own internalization of an event, even a mildly stressful situation can trigger psoriasis. Learning stress-modification techniques can change your attitude about stressful situations, allowing you to let them roll by more easily. In a recent study, 4 out of 11 people showed significant improvement in psoriatic symptoms with meditation and guided imagery. Hypnotherapy, biofeedback, and walks in nature are other effective tools. Regular aerobic exercise is a powerful stress reducer.

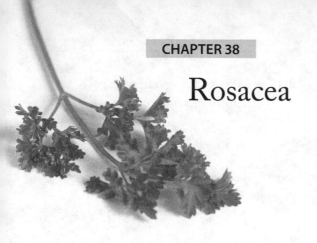

CHAPTER 38

Rosacea

Rosacea is a chronic inflamed facial condition. It is characterized by redness on the cheeks, nose, chin, and forehead with small bumps or pimples on the face. More rarely it can occur on the scalp, neck, chest, or ears. Over time the redness can become more persistent. You can often also see small blood vessels on the face.

People with rosacea often have watery, bloodshot, or irritated eyes. The condition affects 16 million Americans and is becoming more prevalent. It flares up and goes into remission. Rosacea is a tough illness socially. It affects people's self-esteem, career, and social life.

According to the National Rosacea Society, the most common triggers include sunshine, emotional stress, hot or cold weather, wind, heavy exercise, alcohol consumption, hot baths, spicy foods, indoor heat, and some skin care products.

Research on rosacea and digestion is sparse, yet what is available points to a large component that is digestive in nature. I have seen remarkable improvements in my clients on a gluten-free diet and also with use of betaine HCl to increase stomach acids. Research by Andrea Parodi and colleagues discovered small intestinal bacterial overgrowth (SIBO) in 46 percent of participants (52 out of 113). After treatment with Rifaximin, lesions cleared in 71 percent (20 out of 28) and greatly improved in 21 percent (6 out of 28).

SIBO is associated with lower levels of hydrochloric acid. A few old studies (1920 and 1948) measured hydrochloric acid sufficiency and found rates of insufficiency to be higher in people with rosacea.

There have also been several studies linking Candida species with rosacea.

One researcher reported finding low levels of lipase (fat-splitting enzymes) in people with rosacea. He reported improvements by giving pancreatic enzyme supplements.

Functional Laboratory Testing

- Breath test for small intestinal bacterial overgrowth
- Candida antibodies in serum, or candida in stool analysis
- Organic acid testing
- Stool testing for pancreatic function
- HCl testing
- Food sensitivity testing
- Celiac testing
- Vitamin D levels
- Red blood cell zinc levels
- Vitamin A levels

Healing Options

- **Get tested for SIBO.** Since about 90 percent of people with SIBO and rosacea improved after treatment for the SIBO, this is the first place to begin. If discovered, eat a low-carbohydrate diet for several months.
- **Rule out candida.** Take the self-test for candida in Chapter 11. Get tested through organic acid testing, stool, or serum antibodies. If discovered, eat a low-carbohydrate diet and treat the candida with medications and/or natural therapies such as oil of oregano, grapefruit seed extract, garlic, or pau d'arco.
- **Take digestive enzymes.** One researcher reported finding low levels of lipase (fat-splitting enzymes) in people with rosacea. He reported improvements by giving pancreatic enzyme supplements. I would probably use lipase-loaded enzymes. Take one with meals.
- **Try an elimination diet.** I have found that this works extremely well for people with rosacea. Gluten and dairy seem to be the biggest culprits, but any food could be inflammatory. See Chapter 15.
- **See if HCl levels are normal.** Take the HCl self-test in Chapter 11.
- **Take probiotics and eat probiotic-rich food.** While there is no research on this, if dysbiosis and gluten sensitivity are main underlying causes of rosacea, it makes sense to protect the gut with probiotics and probiotic-rich foods.
- **Eat brewer's yeast or nutritional yeast.** A study of 96 people with rosacea reported that about 1½ teaspoons daily of brewer's yeast offered great improvement in their rosacea. This was not duplicated by taking synthetic B-complex vitamins.

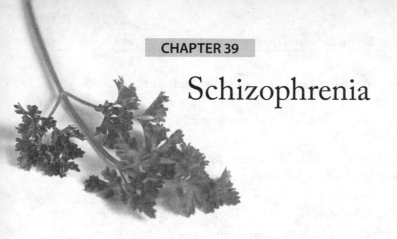

CHAPTER 39

Schizophrenia

Schizophrenia is a chronic, disabling brain disease. People with schizophrenia experience altered realities, including hallucinations, hearing voices, delusions, and confused or paranoid thoughts. Speech and behavior of people with schizophrenia can be very disorganized, which can be disturbing or confusing to those around them. During acute periods, people with schizophrenia experience a loss of energy, sense of humor, and interest in living. It affects one million Americans each year, and 1 percent of us will have it during our lifetime. It's one of the top 10 worldwide causes of disability. It can be progressive or episodic. Schizophrenia has an autoimmune component, which may be a result of the disease itself. A large number of studies find correlation between prenatal and postnatal infections, including flu, herpes, polio, German measles, toxoplasmosis, and respiratory infections, and increased incidence of schizophrenia.

Medication is useful for many people with schizophrenia, but some are not greatly helped by it. Fortunately there are other therapies.

This is definitely an illness where a complete approach must be taken to get the best results. An entire field of nutritional medicine, called orthomolecular medicine (named by Linus Pauling), is based on treatment of schizophrenia and other mental illnesses, although its original definition was broader. Specific testing of amino acids, food sensitivities, fatty acids, heavy metals, and gut health will reveal information relevant to each person. Often, studies of schizophrenia using nutritional models have been disappointing because all patients are lumped into one group.

When groups are broken into subtypes or patients are treated individually, improvements are seen.

Deficiencies in vitamin C, niacin, and folic acid have been found in people with schizophrenia.

Abram Hoffer, M.D., and Humphry Osmond, M.D., were pioneers in the field. Their protocols are based around use of niacin at 3,000 mg daily (vitamin B_3), vitamin C at 3,000 mg daily, and loving care. Niacin therapy works best when used early after the diagnosis. Be patient: it can take months before it begins to work. Niacin causes a skin flush brought on by the release of prostaglandins in the skin; in people who don't flush, it probably indicates a fatty acid deficiency. A niacin challenge offers a simple way to test for this group of people. Loving care expedites the healing process.

Carl Pfeiffer, M.D., Ph.D., found that some people with schizophrenia had faulty metabolism of specific B-complex vitamins. He once stated, "For every drug that yields a beneficial result, there is a nutrient that can produce the same effect."

Fatty acid metabolism is faulty in people with schizophrenia, and schizophrenics have shown altered fatty acid panels. Levels of arachidonic acid and the omega-3 fatty acids EPA and DHA are often low. Schizophrenics are found to have high levels of interleukin-2, an inflammatory substance known to have the potential to cause symptoms similar to schizophrenia. Fish oils can help reduce levels of interleukin-2 and cytokines. Doing a fatty acid test would make sense.

People with schizophrenia have an increased need for antioxidant nutrients. Other antioxidants have also been found to be deficient. Poor free radical protection can damage fat-dependent membranes, the nervous system, and the brain. Testing for specific antioxidants would be advised.

GLUTEN AND SCHIZOPHRENIA

The incidence of gluten intolerance in people with schizophrenia is higher than average. It's speculated that where the two meet is having a leaky gut and being undernourished. Review studies indicate that between 2.6 and 4.2 percent of people with schizophrenia also have celiac disease. It has been estimated that 10 percent of people with schizophrenia will improve on a gluten-free trial. The earliest reports were published by Lauretta Bender, M.D., in 1953, who noticed an increase of celiac disease in children diagnosed with schizophrenia when 4 out of 37 boys admitted that year for schizophrenia also had celiac disease.

F. C. Dohan noted less schizophrenia during World War II in five countries when wheat was scarce, while in the United States both wheat consumption and schizophrenia increased. Dohan also used anthropological data from the South Pacific islands to show that as wheat, barley, beer, and rice consumption increased, so did schizophrenia. He subsequently compared two groups of schizophrenic males. Forty-seven were assigned a grain-free diet; 55 ate a high-grain diet. Sixty-two percent of those on the gluten-free diet were released to a non-locked ward within seven days, compared to 36 percent on a high-gluten diet. Wheat sensitivity can stimulate the production of chemicals in the brain that resemble opiates and cause hallucinations and behavior disturbances.

M. M. Singh and S. R. Kay studied 14 people with schizophrenia who were in a locked research ward. They followed a gluten-free diet for six weeks and were rated on 33 psychopathology measures and 6 social measures of social avoidance and participation. Treatment was blinded from the people who did the outcome measurements. There was significant improvement on 30 of 39 measures.

It appears that for the most part, people with schizophrenia and gluten intolerance have different genetics than people with celiac disease. In 2010, Diana Samaroo and colleagues found that people with schizophrenia did not have elevated tissue transglutaminase antibodies or HLA-DQ2 or HLA-DQ8 genotypes (95 percent of people with celiac have these genotypes), and most did not have high levels of deaminated gliaden. Nonetheless, they found high levels of antigliaden antibodies, indicating gluten sensitivity.

Although gluten intolerance and celiac disease are not present in all people with schizophrenia, it is important to screen for it.

CASEIN AND FOOD SENSITIVITIES

Checking for additional food allergies and sensitivities can be useful. Elevated IgA antibodies to the dairy proteins beta-lactoglobulin and casein have been reported. Casein can have opioid-like effects in the brains of people with schizophrenia and autism. There are four specific types of casein in milk, and 13 genetic variations of beta-casein. It is believed that the A1 variant leads to the type of bioactive peptide beta-casomorphin 7 (BCM-7). High levels of BCM-7 have been found in the urine of people with schizophrenia and autism. This peptide crosses the intestinal mucosa, gets absorbed into the blood, and passes through the blood-brain barrier, causing an opioid-like response.

Other classic food offenders in schizophrenia include dairy products, food additives, and chocolate, although nearly any food can cause problems.

COULD A LOW-CARBOHYDRATE DIET HELP?

In 2009 Bryan D. Kraft and Eric C. Westman reported on a schizophrenic woman whose auditory hallucinations resolved on a ketogenic diet. A ketogenic diet is a very low-carbohydrate diet, such as the Atkins Diet. The woman's hallucinations resolved by day 19 of the diet and remained so over the next 12 months, even though she had a couple of lapses during the winter holidays. Dohan and colleagues previously have noted an association between schizophrenia and consumption of grains. Others have noted an association specifically with gluten-containing grains. Still others have noted an increased incidence of psychotic episodes immediately after eating a carbohydrate load.

SCHIZOPHRENIA AND THE GUT

People with schizophrenia have an increased risk of developing stomach and duodenal ulcers. Others have found that when there is an ulcer, H. pylori–associated gastritis, or motor disorders of the upper GI, schizophrenic episodes are less severe.

Functional Laboratory Testing
- Celiac testing
- Food allergy testing—IgE and IgG, plus IgM and IgA if possible
- Nutrient testing
- Essential fatty acid testing
- Urinary amino acid testing
- Genetic testing for methylenetetrahydrofolate reductase gene (MTHFR)
- Homocysteine testing

Healing Options
Schizophrenia is a complex illness. Digestive issues do not play a role in all people with schizophrenia, but for the subset of those whom it does affect, resolving these issues can be life changing.

- **Rule out celiac disease and food sensitivities.** Do blood testing for food allergies and sensitivities. Try an elimination diet.
- **Look for nutritional deficiencies.** Checking for specific nutrients and supplementing will give the best results because each person's needs will be different. Beginning with a good multivitamin and mineral supplement can help but probably won't fill in the gaps if there are severe deficiencies in specific nutrients.
- **Take niacin.** Abram Hoffer, M.D., long used niacin therapy for schizophrenia. It is believed that there is faulty niacin metabolism in this condition, because people with schizophrenia often do not experience the intense flushing that usually occurs with niacin ingestion. Take up to 3,000 mg daily.
- **Increase intake of 5-hydroxytryptophan (5-HTP).** In 14 patients tested, dietary restriction of tryptophan worsened their symptoms. Tryptophan can easily be converted to niacin, which may be one reason why it is of benefit. Tryptophan is also a precursor to serotonin, which affects mood, behavior, sleep, and carbohydrate cravings. At a recent conference Bill Walsh, Ph.D., medical director at Great Plains Laboratory, expressed concern about possible negative effects of tryptophan and recommended using only 5-HTP. To err on the side of caution, I am recommending 5-HTP. Take 300 to 600 mg 5-HTP.
- **Increase consumption of good fats.** Schizophrenics often have low omega-3 fatty acid levels, low arachidonic acid levels, and low levels of polyunsaturated fatty acids. Benefit would be found by increasing good fats in the diet from sources such as nuts, seeds, whole grains, unprocessed vegetable oils, and cold-water fish, including salmon, halibut, tuna, mackerel, sardines, or herring. Twenty hospitalized patients were given 10 grams of fish oil daily. There were significant improvements in psychological symptoms, behavior, and tardive dyskinesia (uncontrollable movements) after six weeks. Another study used a smaller dose: 180 mg EPA, 120 mg DHA, plus 400 IU vitamin E and 500 mg vitamin C twice daily. There was improvement in lab testing and also in schizophrenic symptoms.
- **Try serine.** Research indicates that high-dose glycine is beneficial for schizophrenia. Concern has been posted as to the possible long-term neurological effects of high-glycine supplementation, however. The mechanism of the response was believed to be the effect on the receptor sites for NMDA, a neurotransmitter. NMDA function is low in people with schizophrenia. Newer research on serine, by Toru Nishikawa, shows that the positive effects of enhancing NMDA function can be achieved by taking serine, without the risks of high-dose glycine.

Dosage in one study was 0.8 grams of serine per kilogram of body weight daily. It would be advisable to do a urine amino acid test before using this type of therapy. Work with a physician.

- **Check your MTHFR gene and homocysteine levels.** Homocysteine levels are often high in people who have schizophrenia. There are many studies looking at genetic variations in the MTHFR gene in people with schizophrenia. These studies have mixed results. Nonetheless, if you do have a genetic variation of this gene, you are less able to utilize folic acid from food and supplements. People with this genetic variation (MTHFR gene 677 C>T) benefit from supplements that have preformed folic acid, called methyltetrahydrofolate. People who have this genetic variation and schizophrenia are more likely to develop metabolic syndrome.

- **Take magnesium.** Magnesium deficiency can produce depression, agitation, confusion, and disorientation. In one study, 20 schizophrenic patients were evaluated for serum magnesium levels. Twenty-five percent were found to be magnesium deficient. Serum magnesium is not a sensitive test of magnesium deficiency, so if red blood cell magnesium had been analyzed, the results would probably have been much higher. Half of the magnesium-deficient patients were exhibiting psychotic behavior, including hallucinations. In drug-treated schizophrenics, magnesium levels have been found to be consistently low. Supplementing with magnesium does not always show improvement in symptoms. Magnesium injections or use of choline citrate may be necessary at first to "prime the pump." Because so many enzymes are dependent on magnesium, a deficiency could affect other nutrients, including vitamins B_1, B_6, E, and C and minerals such as zinc, copper, and selenium.

CHAPTER 40

Scleroderma
(Systemic Sclerosis)

Scleroderma is an autoimmune connective-tissue disease characterized by a thickening and loss of elasticity in the skin, joints, digestive tract (especially in the esophagus), lungs, and thyroid; and scarring in the heart and kidneys. The most common initial complaint is loss of circulation in toes or fingers (Raynaud's syndrome), characterized by swelling and a thickening of skin. About 300,000 Americans have scleroderma. Like all autoimmune conditions, scleroderma is linked to genetics and your environment. Scleroderma has been linked to bacterial and viral infections as possible triggers that set up the molecular mimicry that causes cell damage. So far parvovirus B19, cytomegalovirus, Epstein-Barr virus, and retroviruses have been implicated.

There are two forms of the disease: localized, affecting one or two locations, and systemic (also called diffuse), which is found throughout the body. The diffuse form can rapidly progress and can be quite serious. Generalized symptoms include fatigue, muscle pain, and arthritis.

People with the more limited form of scleroderma have less involvement, which is mostly confined to the skin on the fingers and face. Changes occur more slowly in this type of scleroderma but in a typical way that has been defined as CREST, which represents the initials of the symptoms. You may have only a few of these signs.

Calcinosis: These are tiny calcium deposits in the skin. They look like hard, whitish areas and are most common on elbows, knees, and fingers. This is not as common as the other indicators.

Raynaud's phenomenon: In Raynaud's there are spasms of tiny arteries and your fingers, toes, nose, ears, and tongue can lose circulation. This is typically triggered by cold, heat, or dampness.

Esophageal issues: The lower two-thirds of the esophagus are often affected by poor muscle function. This can lead to gastroesophageal reflux (GERD), which can lead to scarring and narrowing of the esophagus.

Sclerodactyly: This is the thickening that occurs on fingers and toes. It can look shiny and can limit your flexibility and ability to use fingers and toes.

Telangiectasias: These are tiny red areas that most often occur on your face and hands, inside your mouth, and inside of your lips. If you press on them, they turn white.

TREATMENT

Medical treatment of scleroderma consists of dealing with symptoms and medical issues as they arise. Proton-pump inhibitors are used for GERD. Small intestinal bacterial overgrowth (SIBO) is treated with antibiotics. If your lungs or kidneys are affected, those are treated as well. If blood pressure is high, that is also treated.

Integrative treatment consists of looking for underlying triggers and modulating inflammation, use of elimination diets and celiac testing, stress management, looking for and treating infections, looking for allergies and sensitivities to food and environmental chemicals, and anything else that may be of benefit in alleviating symptoms and slowing down the course of the disease.

In one study, use of vitamin B_6 and a Chinese medication called Xuefu Zhuyu Decoction were used in 33 people with localized scleroderma. Reductions in inflammation of interleukin-6 (IL-6) and TNF-alpha were similar in both groups. It is believed that the B_6 and herbal combination activated blood circulation.

DIGESTION AND SCLERODERMA

GI issues are present in 50 to 90 percent of people with scleroderma. There can be issues in any one of the DIGIN areas, so look at all of them carefully. The most common manifestations of scleroderma are in the esophagus with reflux and difficulty swallowing. If left untreated this can lead to Barrett's esophagus. There can also be constipation or diarrhea, SIBO, and food sensitivities. SIBO occurs 17 to 58 percent of the time in people who have scleroderma. When treated, symptoms improve.

Delayed gastric emptying is found in 10 to 75 percent of people with systemic scleroderma. This correlates well with symptoms of early satiety, bloating, and vomiting.

H. pylori can be an issue in people who have scleroderma and GERD. Kanako Yamaguchi and colleagues tested 64 patients with scleroderma who had not been treated for GI imbalances. Thirty-seven (57.8 percent) tested positive for H. pylori. Significantly more people without GERD had high H. pylori levels.

CELIAC, GLUTEN, AND SCLERODERMA

There is a high overlap of celiac disease in people with scleroderma. Eduardo Rosato and colleagues report that of 50 people studied, 5 had elevated tissue transglutaminase levels. When biopsied, four of the five had celiac disease, for an incidence of 8 percent. Remember that celiac disease is diagnosed only when there is serious erosion of the villi and microvilli. This study did not look at simple gluten intolerance.

DAMPENING INFLAMMATION

Free radical damage underlies the pathology of scleroderma. There are elevated levels of Th-2 cytokines (IL-6) in the early stages of scleroderma that lead to the thickening of tissues. Antioxidants are beneficial in people with scleroderma. Raynaud's causes a surge of free radicals that need to be quenched. Studies have shown that blood levels of vitamin C, vitamin E, selenium, and carotenoids are all lower in people with scleroderma, despite normal levels in their diets. G. Fiori and colleagues report that vitamin E used topically increases healing and reduces pain. It's also speculated that taurine can be used as an antioxidant. Supplementation with antioxidant nutrients and testing for antioxidant status to see if levels are adequate is advisable. Specific use of N-acetyl cysteine increases glutathione levels and is also advised. Use of several antioxidant supplements may be necessary for optimal results.

Homocysteine may be elevated in people with scleroderma. The higher the homocysteine level, the more progressive the disease. Screening for homocysteine can be extremely useful. Use of vitamin B_6, B_{12}, folic acid, and betaine (TMG) may be helpful in normalizing levels.

Low serum zinc levels have been found with frequency in people with scleroderma. In a recent study 17 people with localized scleroderma were given 60 to 90 mg of zinc gluconate daily. Fifty-three percent had benefits. Five people had partial remissions, and four people had complete remissions.

SCLERODERMA AND THE ENVIRONMENT

There is no single known cause of scleroderma. It is caused by a combination of genetics and environmental factors. Evidence suggests that prolonged exposure to silica, silicone, and chemical solvents significantly increases the risk of developing scleroderma.

In some individuals, solvents trigger the illness. An evaluation was made of 178 people with scleroderma, in comparison to 200 controls. People with scleroderma were more likely to have higher concentrations of and levels of exposure to solvents, especially trichloroethylene.

Silicosis has been well studied in scleroderma. People with silicosis from industrial exposure are 24 times more likely to be diagnosed with scleroderma. They are also two to eight times more likely to develop rheumatoid arthritis or systemic lupus erythematosus. Risk is greater in men. In a small study, 44 women and 6 men went through extensive testing and examination to see if there was a relationship between their work and autoimmune disease. They had been working for an average of six years in a factory that produced scouring powder with a high silica content. Thirty-two, or 64 percent, showed symptoms of a systemic illness, six with Sjögren's syndrome, five with scleroderma, three with systemic lupus, five with a combination syndrome, and thirteen who didn't fit into any definite pattern of disease. Seventy-two percent had elevated ANA (antinuclear antibodies), an indicator of autoimmune connective tissue diseases. The conclusion was that workers who are continually exposed to silica have a high probability of developing an autoimmune problem.

The research on breast implants is mixed. Silicone breast implants may also play a role in some women with scleroderma, yet no relationship between autoimmune antibodies was found (for rheumatoid arthritis, ANA, and Scl-70 for scleroderma). Twenty-six women with either lupus or scleroderma had breast implants removed. Three had complete remission of at least two years. Saline implants have a silicone casing that may also cause problems. If you have breast implants, testing for silicone and chemical antibodies would help you determine if you might benefit from their removal.

Natural therapies can work along with medical therapies for scleroderma. Infections must be treated and beneficial flora given. Nutrients that help with collagen maintenance and repair are essential to help prevent loss of elasticity in skin and organs. Consider supplementing with vitamin C, quercetin, zinc, glucosamine, and chondroitin. Foods and supplements that help reduce production of arachidonic acid will reduce inflammation and pain. Good-quality oils, fish, nuts, and seeds work in this way. It's also important to increase circulation and oxygen supply to the tissues. Finally, a nutrient-dense food plan must be developed that works to offset the problems of malnutrition, which are common.

Functional Laboratory Testing

- Breath test for small intestinal bacterial overgrowth
- Vitamin D levels
- Comprehensive digestive stool analysis
- Testing for food and environmental sensitivities
- DHEA and cortisol testing
- Liver function profile
- Testing for silicone antibodies (for women with breast implants)
- Nutrient testing, including homocysteine
- H. pylori testing
- Essential fatty acid testing

Healing Options

Scleroderma isn't one illness; it's many, and finding your own triggers and solutions will be a personal journey. Here are ideas that will help you on the journey. Very little research on using nondrug approaches has been done; you will be a pioneer.

- **Look for and treat infections.** H. pylori, esophageal and oral candidiasis, and other infections are associated with scleroderma. I could find only rare references to SIBO in association with scleroderma; however, my instincts tell me to at least explore the possibility. You may be able to keep the infections at bay with use of colloidal silver, berberine from goldenseal or Oregon grapes, grapefruit seed extract, oregano oil, garlic capsules, or combination herbs. Each of these substances has wide antimicrobial properties, low toxicity, and a low incidence of negative side effects. Your doctor may prescribe antibiotics or antifungal medications.
- **Test for hydrochloric acid sufficiency.** See Chapters 3 and 11.
- **Try an elimination-provocation diet and make dietary changes.** Explore the relationship between your scleroderma and food and environmental sensitivities. While I cannot find any research on this, I have seen this approach work for several of my own clients who have scleroderma.
- **Check for food sensitivities and celiac.** Gluten sensitivity and food sensitivities are common in people with scleroderma. Try the elimination diet. (See Chapter 15.)

- **Check for high homocysteine levels.** Methylation issues can be demonstrated by checking homocysteine levels. High homocysteine levels are common in people with scleroderma. There are also labs offering methylation panels that delve deeper.
- **Check hormone levels.** In a case study with two women, estriol treatment provided considerable beneficial effects.
- **Check vitamin D.** Low levels of 25-OH D have been found in many studies of people with scleroderma. More than 80 percent were found to be vitamin D insufficient and 23 to 32 percent vitamin D deficient. As with other autoimmune diseases, bringing levels up to at least 50 ng/ml and possibly toward the upper normal range of between 80 and 100 ng/ml may be optimal. For maintenance take 2,000 IU vitamin D_3 daily; to bring levels up take between 5,000 to 10,000 IU vitamin D_3 daily for 8 to 12 weeks and retest.
- **Test for essential fatty acids.** Supplement accordingly. People with scleroderma have oxidation of fats due to a lack of antioxidants.
- **Take zinc.** You can test for red blood cell zinc levels, or do taste testing for zinc sufficiency with liquid zinc sulfate. People are often zinc deficient. Take 50 mg zinc daily. Try this for two to three months. Work with a clinician on this because you can take too much zinc and possibly deplete copper as a result.
- **Increase antioxidants.** The best food sources include fruits, vegetables, legumes, nuts, and seeds. Fresh vegetable and green juice is a concentrated source. Using green powders such as spirulina, blue-green algae, wheatgrass juice extract, or mixtures of powdered "reds" or "greens" can also give quite an antioxidant kick. Think about taking several grams or more daily of mineral ascorbates (vitamin C). Consider adding 200 to 1,000 IU of vitamin E. Vitamin E can also be used topically on skin to soothe and soften it. Consider selenium at 200 mcg daily. Taurine has antioxidant properties; take 1,000 to 2,000 mg daily. Try N-acetyl cysteine or whey protein to boost glutathione levels; take 500 to 1,000 mg N-acetyl cysteine daily. Consider taking antioxidant supplements. You can often check to see if you are doing enough by how much symptom relief you are getting and also by checking your first morning urinary pH. (See Chapter 17.)
- **Detoxify.** A liver function panel can determine whether your phase one and phase two liver detoxification pathways are working normally. Because the risk of scleroderma increases with solvent exposure, a liver detoxification program may be of significant benefit. In the few people I've worked with who have scleroderma, this has proven to be an effective starting point.
- **Try DHEA.** DHEA is an adrenal hormone that has been found to be beneficial for people with scleroderma, especially in perimenopausal women. Because

DHEA is a hormone, I recommend that you first have a free DHEA/cortisol saliva test to determine if you actually need supplementation and to monitor your dosage levels. Dosages will vary, depending on your personal needs.

- **Take a multivitamin with minerals.** Poor diet, loss of movement in the digestive tract, loss of elasticity of the organs, infections, and medications all contribute to the malabsorption of nutrients. Selenium and vitamin C deficiencies are common in people with scleroderma. At least 20 nutrients are essential for formation of bone and cartilage, so it's important to find a supplement that supports these needs. Look for a supplement that contains 10,000 IU vitamin A, 800 to 1,000 mg calcium, 400 to 500 mg magnesium, 400 IU vitamin E, at least 250 mg vitamin C, 50 mg vitamin B_6, 15 to 50 mg zinc, 5 to 10 mg manganese, 12 mg copper, and 200 mcg selenium in addition to other nutrients. Follow the dosage on the bottle to get nutrients in appropriate amounts.
- **Take vitamin C.** Vitamin C is vital for formation of cartilage and collagen, which is a fibrous protein that forms strong connective tissue necessary for bone strength. Vitamin C also plays an important role in immune response, helping protect us from disease-producing microbes. It also inhibits formation of inflammatory prostaglandins, helping to reduce pain, inflammation, and swelling. If you have candidiasis or bacterial overgrowth, vitamin C can boost your body's ability to defend itself. Vitamin C is also an antioxidant, needed to counter free radical formation noted in sclerotic conditions. Take 1 to 3 grams daily in an ascorbate or Ester-C. For best results, do the vitamin C flush. (See Chapter 18.)
- **Try gamma-linolenic acid (GLA).** One gram of evening primrose oil was given to four women with scleroderma three times daily for one year. They experienced a reduction in pain, with improved skin texture and healing of sores; red patches on skin due to broken capillaries were much improved. The researchers suggest that 6 grams daily may be of greater benefit. Take 3 to 6 grams of evening primrose oil, borage oil, or flaxseed oil daily.
- **Follow suggestions for GERD if it is present.** See Chapter 20.
- **Try nattokinase.** I have not seen research on this, but it makes sense to me. Protein-digesting enzymes taken on an empty stomach can help to break down fibrous tissues throughout the body. Nattokinase works to help break down blood clots, so I would probably begin with that. You could eat natto, a traditional Japanese food with an unusual flavor, at 2 to 15 ounces daily. Or you can purchase nattokinase in capsules. Products differ, so use as directed.

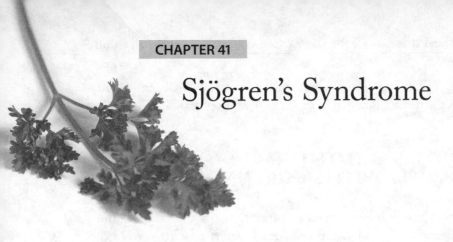

CHAPTER 41

Sjögren's Syndrome

Sjögren's syndrome is an autoimmune disease in which moisture-producing glands are destroyed by white blood cells. Typically the first signs of Sjögren's syndrome are dry eyes and dry mouth. However, virtually all organs can be affected. More than 4 million people have Sjögren's in the United States. Ninety percent are women. Half of people with Sjögren's syndrome will have a second autoimmune disease, and it is often connected with rheumatoid arthritis, lupus, or scleroderma. Primary Sjögren's syndrome is when it occurs without other autoimmune illnesses; secondary Sjögren's is when you also have a second autoimmune disease. Like all autoimmune diseases, it can take on many forms and can flare up and improve.

Current medical treatments are aimed at symptom relief. People are told to chew gum, use artificial tears, and use bile stimulants to increase saliva production. Steroid and other immunosuppressive medications are also used. I suggest that you look further. Several people with Sjögren's syndrome whom I have worked with have benefited from dietary changes, supplements, and exploration of the DIGIN model.

DIGESTIVE CONNECTION AND SJÖGREN'S

There is a high incidence of digestive distress in people with Sjögren's. They are more likely to have irritable bowel syndrome and delayed gastric emptying. If you have Sjögren's, you are more likely to develop oral candidiasis. H. pylori infection has been associated with Sjögren's syndrome, but studies have not consistently confirmed that the incidence is really higher than in the general population.

FOOD SENSITIVITIES AND OTHER ALLERGIES IN PEOPLE WITH SJÖGREN'S

People with Sjögren's have a high prevalence of allergies to drugs (46 percent) and more skin contact allergies. Maria Liden and colleagues report that 20 percent of people with Sjögren's who also have the DQ1 gene type have mucosal inflammation when challenged with rectal gluten even though they don't have celiac disease. Dr. Liden labels them as gluten sensitive with a possible risk of developing celiac disease. Inflammation was measured by increases in nitric oxide and mucosal granules from neutrophils.

The same group gave rectal challenges of dried milk powder to 21 people (2 males, 19 females) with Sjögren's syndrome and 18 healthy controls. Eight of the 21 people with Sjögren's had a reaction two standard deviations above the mean of the controls, although IgG and IgA antibodies to casein, beta-lactoglobulin, and alpha-lactalbumin were similar in patients and controls. All people were also tested with a rectal challenge to soybean; none had any adverse reaction. Those with Sjögren's were also tested for the genetics for celiac. No association was seen between reaction to cow's milk and their genotypes. In fact, the two people who had the most inflammation had no reaction to gluten and were negative for the DQ2 and DQ8 genes associated with celiac. The researchers report that 2 out of 21 reacted to gluten only (one was subsequently diagnosed with celiac disease); 5 out of 21 were reactive to cow's milk; and 3 out of 21 reacted to both gluten and cow's milk. These patients also reported other allergies: 13 of 21 reported allergies to avocado, apple, peanut, strawberry, shellfish, pollen, dust, animals, or mold. GI symptoms were reported by 16 of 21 (76 percent), and 10 of 21 (48 percent) attributed their GI issues to food reactions from dairy products and wheat. Thirteen out of 21 (62 percent) met the criteria for irritable bowel syndrome.

Functional Laboratory Testing
- Celiac testing
- Breath test for small intestinal bacterial overgrowth
- Comprehensive digestive stool analysis
- Organic acid test

- Food sensitivity and allergy testing
- Fatty acid testing
- DHEA and cortisol testing
- Vitamins D, E, K, and A levels

Healing Options

- **Discover dysbiosis.** Do testing for small intestinal bacterial overgrowth, stool testing, and/or organic acid testing to discover whether these issues play a role in your illness.
- **Try an elimination diet.** I have seen an elimination diet work wonders in women with scleroderma. Also rule out celiac disease. See Chapter 15.
- **Increase good-quality omega-6 fats in your diet.** In a couple of studies, evening primrose oil was used at levels between 1,000 mg and 6,000 mg daily. Changes were seen in pain reduction, healing of ulcers, improved skin texture, and fewer attacks of Raynaud's. High omega-6 fats can also be found in nuts and seeds, borage oil, and black currant seed oil.
- **Check for HCl.** In six women who were tested for gastric acid sufficiency, four were deficient. Take the HCl self-test or Heidelberg capsule test or ask a gastroenterologist to test you for this.
- **Practice relaxation and stress management.** Stress plays a role in this illness, so relax as much as possible and do things that give you pleasure. See Chapter 16 for more on this topic.
- **Optimize fat-soluble vitamins.** Fat-soluble vitamins have anti-inflammatory effects. Get yours tested. In one study, people with more severe Sjögren's had lowered levels of vitamin A.

AFTERWORD

We've covered a lot of ground in the past 400 or so pages. We've explored how the digestive system works, the DIGIN method for assessing underlying triggers and components of digestive and systemic disease and imbalances, lifestyle and nutritional recommendations, and finally chapters on dozens of specific digestive and systemic disease. Hopefully, you have a deeper understanding of how the digestive system works and what to do when it's out of balance.

There's so much more that I wanted to include in the book. You'll find all of the extras at http://www.digestivewellnessbook.com. You'll find all of the references that I used to research *Digestive Wellness*. You'll also find resources for nutritional supplements and functional laboratories. Also, take a look at the expanded elimination diet, a candida diet, a four-day rotation diet, and more.

Thanks for coming with me on the journey.

INDEX

Page numbers in italics refer to figures or tables.

ABOUT THE AUTHOR

Liz Lipski, Ph.D., CCN, CHN, holds a doctorate in clinical nutrition and is board certified in both clinical nutrition and holistic nutrition. Liz is the director of Doctoral Studies and Educational Director at Hawthorn University, is on the faculty at Saybrook University, and is on the faculty at Institute for Functional Medicine (IFM) and the Autism Research Institute. She sits on the advisory board for "Food as Medicine" and is an alumni of the Nutrition Advisory Board at IFM. She is also the founder of Access to Health Experts, an educational membership website for consumers and health professionals. Liz is the author of *Leaky Gut Syndrome* and *Digestive Wellness for Children*. She speaks all over the country at professional meetings and is frequently interviewed for media of all types. She's the mom of Kyle and Arthur, stepmom of Aron and Cora, and grandmother of Jasper. She lives in the Atlanta area with her husband, Chris.

Liz has a small private practice and is available for consultations in person and via phone.

You can discover more about her and her work at the following websites:

http://www.innovativehealing.com
http://www.digestivewellnessbook.com
http://www.accesstohealthexperts.com
http://www.hawthornuniversity.org